■ Brain Death

Also by Eelco F.M. Wijdicks

The Comatose Patient
Neurologic Complications of Critical Illness, Third Edition
The Practice of Emergency and Critical Care Neurology

Brain Death

SECOND EDITION

Eelco F.M. Wijdicks, MD, PhD, FACP

Professor of Neurology, College of Medicine
Chair, Division of Critical Care Neurology
Consultant, Neurosciences Intensive Care Unit
St. Marys Hospital, Mayo Clinic
Rochester, Minnesota

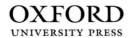

OXFORD
UNIVERSITY PRESS

Oxford University Press, Inc., publishes works that further Oxford University's objective of excellence in research, scholarship, and education.

Oxford   New York
Auckland   Cape Town   Dar es Salaam   Hong Kong   Karachi   Kuala Lumpur
Madrid   Melbourne   Mexico City   Nairobi   New Delhi   Shanghai   Taipei   Toronto

With offices in
Argentina   Austria   Brazil   Chile   Czech Republic   France   Greece   Guatemala   Hungary   Italy
Japan   Poland   Portugal   Singapore   South Korea   Switzerland   Thailand   Turkey   Ukraine
Vietnam

Published by Oxford University Press, Inc.
198 Madison Avenue, New York, New York 10016

www.oup.com

Oxford is a registered trademark of Oxford University Press

Library of Congress Cataloging-in-Publication Data
Brain death/Eelco F.M. Wijdicks.—2nd ed.
    p.; cm.
    Includes bibliographical references and index.
ISBN 978-0-19-979336-5 (hardcover)
1. Brain death. I. Wijdicks, Eelco F. M., 1954-
[DNLM: 1. Brain Death. W 820]
QP87.B73 2011
616.07'8—dc22   2010038781

9 8 7 6 5 4 3 2 1

Printed in the United States of America on acid-free paper

This book is about a neurologic condition that medically and legally defines death. The clinical criteria for brain death have been well defined, and many hospitals, certainly those with a Level 1 Trauma Center designation, have a protocol in place. In a sense, therefore, its diagnosis is an incontrovertible fact, and virtually all practicing physicians would agree. Much has been written about this clinical state, and advances have been made in clinical research. Therefore, one of the principal aims of this book is to compress an amazing amount of scholarship, opinions, and clinical research into one small volume. Another aim is to present a practical book that can be used at the bedside. This completely rewritten book is a work with primary source research and includes material published in recent years. Mayo Clinic has detailed data on over 300 brain death determinations, and I performed many of them personally. I have retained sections and chapters I wrote in the prior edition of this book but greatly expanded and updated them.

There are several new features in this book, including a discussion of the development of criteria for brain death using new research about the Harvard Ad Hoc Committee. The book also expands on the current criteria used in countries throughout the world and highlights the often inexplicable differences among them. There is a comprehensive discussion of the new 2010 American Academy of Neurology guidelines on determining brain death.

I began with the proposition that brain death means not only a nonsapient state but death, and this book describes it without ambiguity. Brain death has undeniable fascination, and some scholars find its diagnosis inaccurate. Any definition of death progresses through controversy and this book brings to the fore a few of the polarities involved. Without necessarily being a critic of critics, I have devoted one chapter to these arguments and, after having read all that has been said, I tried to approach the topic commonsensically in order to cut through a vast array of philosophical positions.

The complexities of the clinical diagnosis and evaluation of potential pitfalls in brain death remain substantial. Because this is such an important topic, I believe the reader benefits from a discussion of common practice problems. To help the reader in finding the topics, I have added in Chapter 6 a number of familiar concerns when dealing with the neurologic examination and management of organ donors. This chapter answers over 50 questions and I believe the most pertinent ones.

This book will do more than help readers to review the knowledge on brain death. Each chapter stands on its own. The book can be read one chapter at a time, not necessarily sequentially, and can be picked up when a problem arises. Its main purpose is to provide a clinically useful text for practitioners who care for patients with acute catastrophic neurologic disorders evolving to brain death. This is a determinedly objective work and touches on many aspects of critical care neurology, but also bioethics, law, philosophy, society, beliefs and traditions, personal values, and, most profoundly, the art of medicine. I hope it will appeal to neurologists, neurointensivists, neurosurgeons, neurocritical care fellows, neuro-science and intensive care nursing staff, allied health staff in the ICU, anesthesi-ologists, trauma surgeons, transplantation surgeons, and organ procurement organizations.

■ ACKNOWLEDGMENTS

Sources for this book came from many angles. I learned much over the years by spending considerable time in our Neurosciences Intensive Care Unit and I appreciate the care of the nursing staff; they always have to carry this heavy load. I thank the numerous physicians and health care workers who called and e-mailed me with prodding questions on the diagnosis of brain death and its potential pitfalls. Many of these questions led to a good deal of thinking and they are the basis for the problems deconstructed in this book.

I offer my sincere thanks to the many librarians who helped me find the historical sources, in particular Jack Eckert of the Center for History of Medicine at the Francis A. Countway Library of Medicine.

I appreciate all the medical illustrations provided by the distinguished David Factor, and I thank Paul Honermann for his help in formatting the figures. The cover representing a disintegrated brain is artfully designed by Jim Rownd. The secretarial help has been outstanding, and special thanks to Tammy Drees and Donna Larkin for doing all the work needed to complete the book. I thank the copy editors and proofreaders (Kenna Atherton, Alissa Baumgartner, Ann Ihrke, and John Hedlund) of the Mayo Clinic Section of Scientific Publications. I am grateful to our organ transplantation agency LifeSource, which is intimately involved in the care of organ donors and their families. Sara Schlichting provided crucial information about procurement and protocols.

I am again very impressed by the professionalism of everyone associated with Oxford University Press (in particular my editor, Craig Panner) and the publisher's continued commitment to produce my books. It was a great joy during the production process to work with Aparna Shankar from Glyph International and production editor Karen Kwak.

On a personal level, I own a great debt of gratitude to my family, my greatest good fortune. My wife, Barbara, and my children, Coen and Marilou, have lived with my book projects for so many years that they always ask what the next one will be.

In modern times, brain death cannot be seen without considering the possibility of organ or tissue donation. I therefore dedicate this book to all families who faced the worst loss but gained by giving life to others.

CONTENTS

1   History of Brain Death   3

2   Neurology of Brain Death   27

3   Beliefs and Brain Death   69

4   Critics and Brain Death   81

5   Procurement after Brain Death   97

6   Clinical Problems in Brain Death   149

   Clinical Problem 1: The Qualification of the Examiner   150
   Clinical Problem 2: Clinical Mimics   155
   Clinical Problem 3: Acid-Base Disturbances   158
   Clinical Problem 4: Electrolyte Abnormalities   160
   Clinical Problem 5: Acute Intoxications   162
   Clinical Problem 6: Reliability of Ancillary Tests   165
   Clinical Problem 7: Ancillary Tests and Confounders   168
   Clinical Problem 8: Primary Brainstem Lesion   171
   Clinical Problem 9: Uncertainty About Interpreting Spinal Reflexes   174
   Clinical Problem 10: Ventilator Autocycling   177
   Clinical Problem 11: Chronic CO_2 Retention and the Apnea Test   179
   Clinical Problem 12: Terminating the Apnea Test   181
   Clinical Problem 13: Breathing During the Apnea Test   184
   *Clinical Problem 14: Cardiopulmonary Resuscitation and
        Brain Death*   187
   *Clinical Problem 15: Extracorporeal Membrane Oxygenation
        (ECMO) and Brain Death*   190
   Clinical Problem 16: Anencephaly and Brain Death   193
   Clinical Problem 17: Shaken Baby Syndrome and Brain Death   196
   Clinical Problem 18: Maternal Brain Death   200
   Clinical Problem 19: Legal Challenges in Brain Death   204
   Clinical Problem 20: Family Opposition to Accepting Brain Death   209
   Clinical Problem 21: Sperm and Oocyte Retrieval in Brain Death   211
   *Clinical Problem 22: Organ Donation and the Hemodynamically
        Unstable Donor*   214
   Clinical Problem 23: Organ Donation in Prisoners   218
   Clinical Problem 24: Organ Donation, Consent, and Costs   220
   Clinical Problem 25: Organ Donation and Directing the Gift   222

   Index   225

■ Brain Death

1   History of Brain Death

It is startling to be reminded that it took many thousands of years to link the brain to the mind. The cardiocentric view prevailed in antiquity, and the unimportance of the brain can be inferred from the practice of the Egyptian embalmers, who commonly removed the brain by trephining the orbit. The brain was discarded, unlike viscera, which were buried with the dead. The Egyptians did not know what the brain was for; as far as they were concerned, intellectual activity took place in the heart.

The physicians who followed Hippocrates can be credited with connecting the brain to the mind. It is difficult to say where the thought started, but Herophilus of Chalcedon (circa 300 BC), after performing human dissections, emphasized that the brain transmitted motor impulses from the soul to the extremities through nerves. There was fierce opposition by Aristotle, who maintained the central position of the heart. The embryo developing within an egg had a beating heart as the first sign of life; thus, Aristotle argued its physiologic primacy. He theorized that the naturally cold brain served as a refrigerator to cool the blood's heat and to adjust the organism as a whole. Galen (circa 160 AD) discovered that perception and cognition were affected by brain injury and delineated the cranial nerves. It was only in the 1600s that Thomas Willis further differentiated the cerebral functions and championed neuroanatomy, culminating in his work *Cerebri Anatome*.

We came to understand that the brain in humans has originated from a more primitive brainstem structure with proportionate increases in the volume of the neocortex when species evolve. We learned that consciousness, personality, insights, perception, motion, emotion, memory, learning, language, and things we do every day all originate in the brain.

Until the mid-twentieth century, severe brain injury led to respiratory arrest due to the inability to keep an open upper airway and insufficient respiratory drive. Circulatory arrest soon followed after collapse of the blood pressure in an apneic, cyanotic patient. After the introduction of the mechanical ventilator and, in particular, endotracheal intubation, comatose patients could be supported. This unprecedented intervention in patients with a massive brain injury resulted in the emergence of a new neurologic condition. This neurologic state was characterized by coma, irreversibly absent brainstem reflexes and apnea, uncontrolled diuresis, and loss of vascular tone. With the additional absence of electroencephalographic (EEG) tracings and profound brain necrosis at autopsy, this state became known as brain death. With this additional definition of death, however, clinical criteria had to be developed, but there was a good understanding among neurologists what this state meant. Henry Beecher, chairman of the Harvard Ad Hoc Committee to Examine the Definition of Brain Death said that "we should, first, abandon the ancient sign of death—the cessation of the heartbeat."[1] This chapter chronicles the development of these neurologic criteria.

■ DEFINING NEUROLOGIC CRITERIA FOR DEATH

In the United States, the initial attempt to determine death based on neurologic criteria is often attributed to the 1968 Harvard Criteria,[1] but the first steps toward using loss of cerebral function to define death actually began a decade earlier.

In 1956, Lofstedt and von Reis[24] reported six mechanically ventilated patients with absent reflexes, apnea, hypotension, hypothermia, and polyuria. Cerebral blood flow, determined by angiography, was absent. However, death was declared following cardiac arrest, which occurred in 2 to 26 days. Cerebral necrosis was present at autopsy in all cases. In 1959, Wertheimer, Jouvet, and Descotes were among the first to propose criteria for these new clinical states ("À propos du diagnostic de la mort système nerveux…"). This article largely focused, like many before it, on the significance of the isoelectric EEG, but it also documented shutting off the ventilator to stimulate the respiratory centers with increasing respiratory acidosis. Absent medulla oblongata function was further confirmed with no change in pulse rate with carotid compression, ocular pressure, and intravenous injection of atropine and amphetamine. Both of these articles, although introducing new findings, lacked the logic to distinguish brain death from other neurologic conditions.[20,42] Several months later in 1959, Mollaret and Goulon[28] published an article entitled "Le coma dépassé" and more comprehensively defined death based on neurologic criteria. It was an extension of earlier anecdotal observations of comatose patients with isoelectric EEG recordings, absent intracranial flow, or total or near-complete brain necrosis at autopsy.

This article is considered a signature piece in the development of clinical criteria of death by neurologic standards[28] (Figure 1-1). The authors presented 23 cases from the Claude Bernard Hospital in Paris with a new type of coma they called *coma dépassé*—coma that went well beyond (*dépassé*) the deepest comas so far described. It is best translated as "irretrievable coma" (M. Goulon, personal communication), but currently French physicians translate it as "brain death." Although both authors (Figure 1-2) used the term in their hospital service for several years before publication, they were dissatisfied with it. In fact, they encouraged readers to propose a better term.[28]

Mollaret and Goulon correctly asked the most critical ethical questions: Do we have the right to stop resuscitation using criteria that attempt to define the boundary of life and death? Does life support have to be maintained as long as the heart beats and perfuses vital organs? How about the religious position? Professor Goulon felt that *coma dépassé* was a disturbing condition for an observer, and it led him to question "where the patient's soul dwelled" (M. Goulon, personal communication).

In addition to their foresight regarding future ethical quandaries, Mollaret and Goulon presented a well-documented description of what is now called *brain death*. In retrospect, their article's details of the neurologic examination are striking. *Coma dépassé* was said to be characterized by immobility of the eyeballs in a neutral position, mydriasis, absent light reflex, absent blinking with stimuli,

REVUE NEUROLOGIQUE

MEMOIRES ORIGINAUX

LE COMA DEPASSE
(MEMOIRE PRÉLIMINAIRE)

PAR MM.

P. MOLLARET et M. GOULON

Après quatre années de réflexion, nous croyons venu le moment d'ajouter un chapitre nouveau au domaine traditionnel des comas.

Précisons de suite que ce problème du coma dépassé a été mis, l'année dernière, au programme de la prochaine Journée de Réanimation de l'Hôpital Claude-Bernard du 7 octobre 1959, en vue d'une mise au point intégrale.

La présente communication, qui n'a ainsi qu'une valeur préliminaire, peut être offerte, peut-être, en hommage à la XXIIIᵉ Réunion Neurologique Internationale, qui a accepté de tenir une de ses séances dans le Centre de Réanimation où fut élaboré ce travail. Précisons également que le coma dépassé a déjà conquis droit de cité dans l'important volume qui vient de paraître de H. Fischgold et P. Mathis (*Obnubilations, comas et stupeurs*, Masson édit., Paris, 1959, p. 5 et pp. 51-52) ; nous remercions ces auteurs d'être venus se faire présenter les premiers malades et d'avoir donné place à quelques-uns de nos documents.

Figure 1-1 Original cover page of the article "Le Coma Dépassé."

absence of swallowing reflexes, drooping of the jaw, absence of motor responses to any stimuli, muscle hypotonia, tendon areflexia, equivocal plantar reflexes, absence of spontaneous respiration after discontinuation of ventilation, immediate cardiovascular collapse as soon as vasopressors are stopped, and a disturbance of thermoregulation with core temperature, that depends on the environmental temperature.

The EEG is flat, without any noticeable reactivity, and it remains so until cardiac arrest occurs. The authors here warn the reader, very appropriately, that a flat EEG by itself does not permit a diagnosis of *coma dépassé*. They cite personal observations in which a flattening of the EEG alone can be followed by resumption of normal electrical cerebral activity, but details about the cause in such cases were not provided.

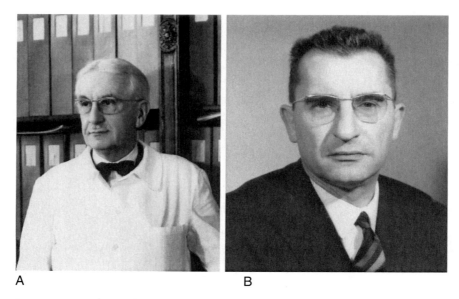

Figure 1-2 Neurologists (A) Pierre Mollaret (1896–1987) and (B) Maurice Goulon (1919–2008).

Mollaret and Goulon noted cases in which mechanical ventilation was uncomplicated in the first days, only to deteriorate later, and they documented oxygen desaturation, acute hypercapnia, and combined respiratory and metabolic acidosis. Polyuria was present in most cases, and intramuscular injection of *d'hormone posthypophysaire* resulted in reduced diuresis and concentration of urine. Hyperglycemia and glycosuria were observed, but there was a normal response to insulin. The heart rate slowed to 40 to 60 beats per minute and was not changed by pressure on the eyeballs, the carotid artery, or by intravenous injection of atropine. This condition ended ultimately with cardiac arrest.[15,28]

The article by Mollaret and Goulon is a landmark for a number of reasons. For one thing, it distinguished *coma dépassé* from other types of comatose states. Before this term was introduced, French neurologists, notably Déjèrine, classified coma as *coma leger* ("light coma"), *coma profond* ("deep coma"), *coma carus* ("deepest coma," with reflexes abolished but with the patient still breathing), and *coma vigil* ("vegetative state").[21] Mollaret and Goulon's new term, *coma dépassé* would be another category. Moreover, this article provided a comprehensive clinical and EEG description together with the observations of diabetes insipidus, vascular collapse, and neurogenic pulmonary edema, all major derangements facing modern neurointensivists and neurosurgeons. The paper was published in *Revue Neurologique* but was unnoticed outside Europe and perhaps even outside France.

Back in the US, unsettling ethical questions were surfacing. The appearance of persistently comatose patients with no brainstem reflexes on ventilators begged the question of futility. If care was futile, why not define it better? Moreover, the question of what to do after withdrawal of support was on the minds of some physicians (in particular, transplant surgeons). These two developments (defining neurologic criteria of death and transplantation) were bound to cross.[25]

During these years, organ transplantation was in its infancy. Joseph Murray, a transplant surgeon, a future member of the Harvard Ad Hoc Committee, and a future Nobel laureate, recalls in his biography one of the great dilemmas: "When anticipating the availability of an organ from a critically ill patient, how could a doctor decide between trying to save one patient while another waited in the next room desperately hoping for a donor?"[30] It is useful to remember that there was considerable controversy about retrieving organs from patients whose cardiac function had not yet ceased; to illustrate this, the following event is noteworthy. In 1966, the proceedings of a CIBA symposium on transplantation were published. Murray's paper described what he saw as the options for the future of organ transplantation.[29] This was followed by a dialogue among several transplant surgeons that included discussion of potential sources of organ donors (relatives, cadavers, heart-beating donors without brain function, and even prisoners). Despite the fact that organs from heart-beating donors who had lost all brain function were considered the best option for the recipients, there was formidable resistance to this approach. Some felt that there was not sufficient evidence to justify a legal redefinition of death. Most telling of all in this discussion, Guy Alexandre (a Belgian transplant surgeon) suggested that two separate teams be involved, one working to resuscitate the patient and the other dealing with transplantation. In addition, he proposed adoption of the criteria that had already been applied by his group in nine patients with severe cerebral injuries to procure organs.[29]

These criteria were basically extracted from Mollaret and Goulon's paper,[28] which was known to Alexandre (who was versed in French) but not to other members of the symposium. The criteria were as follows: "(a) complete bilateral mydriasis, (b) complete absence of reflexes in response to pain, (c) complete absence of respiration for 5 min, (d) falling blood pressure necessitating increasing doses of vasopressors, and (e) a flat EEG for several hours."[29]

These criteria—incomplete by today's standards—were by no means accepted, and the responses reflected not only uneasiness but also strong opposition. Thomas Starzl, a pioneer in liver transplantation, stated, "I doubt if any of the members of our transplantation team could accept a person as being dead as long as there was a heartbeat." Another transplant surgeon, Roy Calne, noted: "Although Alexandre's criteria are medically persuasive according to traditional definitions of death, he is in fact removing kidneys from live donors. I feel that if a patient, has a heartbeat, he cannot be regarded as a cadaver." Calne predicted that this would become a very sensitive issue: "Any modification of the means of diagnosing death to facilitate transplantation will cause the whole procedure to fall into disrepute with the rest of the profession." Only Murray expressed enthusiasm: "Those criteria are excellent." "This is the kind of formulation that we will need before we can approach the legal profession."[29] During this symposium, Jean-Pierre Revillard—a transplant immunologist—proposed, in what seemed an overture to expansion of the criteria in future European legislation, (1) a consultation with three physicians, one of whom should be the hospital chief of service, and (2) a written report of the evaluation to be prepared, with a copy for each signatory, the hospital and the authorities. The CIBA conference—a window into the sentiments at the time—ended without a consensus statement or final recommendations. Similarly, in the early 1960s, meetings were held in Europe (involving ethical and legal work groups in Paris, Sweden, and Ghent) but none of them produced a well thought out document.

In the US during the conception of earlier guidelines, neurologists appeared conspicuously absent, but this would soon change. Robert Schwab can be credited with providing a more detailed description of an isoelectric EEG in brain death and merging the EEG into diagnostic criteria, as well as with coining the term *brain death*. The following criteria would allow the physician to indicate that the patient was dead: (1) absence of spontaneous respiration, (2) no tendon reflexes of any type, (3) no pupillary reflexes, (4) absence of an oculocardiac reflex (eyeball pressure slowing the heart rate), and (5) 30 minutes of isoelectric EEG.[35]

These early observations in 1963 were a prelude to a more comprehensive definition of brain death. This focused effort would appear in 1968. In Boston, the Harvard Medical School's Ad Hoc Committee to Examine the Definition of Brain Death set out to "define irreversible coma as a new criterion for death."[1] The committee consisted of Raymond Adams (neurology), A. Clifford Barger (physiology), William Curran (law), Derek Denny-Brown (neurology), Dana Farnsworth (public health), Jordi Folch-Pi (biochemistry), Everett Mendelson (history), John Merrill (transplant neurology), Ralph Potter (social ethics), Robert Schwab (neurology) and William Sweet (neurosurgery). The Ad Hoc Committee was chaired by Henry Beecher, an anesthesiologist and a distinguished ethics scholar, who was the main motivator of this committee. (Figures 1-3 and 1-4). The criteria of brain death were based on the collective experience of the committee members.[45]

In a letter, Murray summarized the major themes after reading Beecher's manuscript on the issue. This correspondence between Beecher and Murray identified two parallel lines of thought.[45] Organ donation could follow if a person died after the brain was irreversibly destroyed.

The subject has been thoroughly worked over in the past several years, and by now areas for action are crystallized into two categories. First is the dying patient, and the second, distinct and unrelated, is the need for organ for transplantation.

The first problem requires merely a definition of death. Brain death is the essential requirement, and the faculty of the Harvard Medical School is in a suitable position to make a definite statement about this medical definition of death. This will require the opinions of the neurologists, neurosurgeons, anesthetists, general surgeons and physicians who deal with terminal patients. When to declare death is a problem to be solved whether or not organ transplantation follows. The second question regarding organs for donation is really simple. Once the patient is dead, the legal mechanism then applies. All that is now required is proper permission from either the patient or the next of kin.

The next question posed by your manuscript, namely, "Can society afford to lose organs that are now being buried?" is the most important one of all. Patients are stacked up in every hospital in Boston and all over the world waiting for suitable donor kidneys. At the same time patients are being brought in dead to emergency wards and potentially useful

HARVARD MEDICAL SCHOOL
BOSTON, MASSACHUSETTS

OFFICE OF THE DEAN

January 4, 1968

Dr. Joseph Murray
Peter Bent Brigham Hospital
721 Huntington Avenue
Boston, Massachusetts 02115

Dear John:

At a recent meeting of the Standing Committee on Human Studies,
Dr. Henry K. Beecher reviewed some basic material on the ethical
problems created by the hopelessly unconscious man. Dr. Beecher's
presentation re-emphasized to me the necessity of giving further
consideration to the definition of brain death. As you are well
aware, many of the ethical problems associated with transplantation and other developing areas of medicine hinge on appropriate
definition.

With its pioneering interest in organ transplantation, I believe
the faculty of the Harvard Medical School is better equipped to
elucidate this area than any other single group. To this end
I ask you to accept appointment to an ad hoc committee. Assuming
your acceptance of this added responsibility for the School, the
committee membership will be as follows:

Dr. Raymond D. Adams
Dr. A. Clifford Barger
Dr. William Curran
Dr. Derek Denny-Brown
Dr. Dana L. Farnsworth
Dr. Jordi Folch-pi
Professor Everett I. Mendelsohn
Dr. John P. Merrill
Dr. Joseph Murray
Dr. William Sweet
Dr. Henry Beecher, chairman

Sincerely yours,

Robert H. Ebert, M. D..
Dean

Figure 1-3 Letter finalizing the membership of the Harvard Ad Hoc Committee.

*kidneys are being discarded. This discrepancy between supply and demand is soluble
without any further medical knowledge; it requires merely an educational program aimed
at the medical profession, the legal profession, and the general public.*

The committee worked quickly on six drafts, and the manuscript improved
after circulating among the members. Murray did annotate the drafts, but he
largely accepted the writings of Adams and Schwab. Murray did not agree with
the term *irreversible coma*, but his edits to replace it with *death* did not make
the final draft. Transplantation was not really mentioned, but correspondence

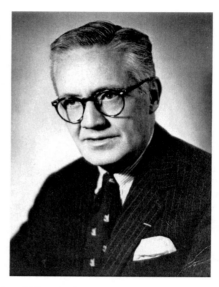

Figure 1-4 Henry Beecher (1904–1976).

suggests that there was appropriate sensitivity by the committee not to link this work to transplantation.

A notable change from the first draft was Schwab's preference to use his triad. This triad consisted of the following: (1) A patient in this state has fixed and dilated pupils; there are no elicitable reflexes and no spontaneous muscle movements; (2) there is no spontaneous respiration of any type; (3) there is an isoelectric EEG. Notable edits in drafts by Adams were the following: (1) no need to document "visual evidence of irretrievable brain damage," (2) more details on brainstem reflexes, and (3) specific mention of central nervous system (CNS)–depressing drugs and hypothermia as confounders.

Curran contributed the legal section of the manuscript and in his correspondence listed anticipatory problems. These included concern about the examination "to be repeated 24–48 hours later and even 75 hours later. I presume this would give great difficulty for vital organ transplant. . . . there is too wide a span here for legal guidance" and additional legal safeguards for the doctor in charge. "I see no justification in the memorandum that the following of these three steps would establish legal safeguards in all 50 states. There is no indication of legal research here at all, in one state let alone 50."

Beecher decided to send the penultimate draft to Adams one more time for a last review, which resulted in a major addition. Adams added a complete new paragraph entitled "Unreceptivity and Unresponsiveness" (which in the original paper became "unresponsivity"), and Adams remembered that the two terms seemed to encompass the total of the clinical state (Wijdicks, personal communication).

TABLE 1-1 *Harvard Criteria (1968)*

- Unreceptivity and unresponsivity
- No movements or breathing
- No reflexes
- Flat electroencephalogram
  - ➤ All of the above tests shall be repeated at least 24 hours with no change.
  - ➤ Exclusion of hypothermia (below 90°F or 32.2°C) or central nervous system depressants.

The Harvard Criteria (Table 1-1) were published in the *Journal of the American Medical Association* on August 5, 1968 (Figure 1-5). The document, a collection of brief statements, included a definition of brain death, a legal commentary, and an address by Pope Pius XII. Overwhelmed with other news, the media relegated the Harvard Criteria to the category of minor interest. Some major newspapers, such

A Definition of Irreversible Coma

Report of the Ad Hoc Committee of the Harvard Medical School to Examine the Definition of Brain Death

Our primary purpose is to define irreversible coma as a new criterion for death. There are two reasons why there is need for a definition: (1) Improvements in resuscitative and supportive measures have led to increased efforts to save those who are desperately injured. Sometimes these efforts have only partial success so that the result is an individual whose heart continues to beat but whose brain is irreversibly damaged. The burden is great on patients who suffer permanent loss of intellect, on their families, on the hospitals, and on those in need of hospital beds already occupied by these comatose patients. (2) Obsolete criteria for the definition of death can lead to controversy in obtaining organs for transplantation.

Irreversible coma has many causes, but *we are concerned here only with those comatose individuals who have no discernible central nervous system activity.* If the characteristics can be defined in satisfactory terms, translatable into action—and we believe this is possible—then several problems will either disappear or will become more readily soluble.

More than medical problems are present. There are moral, ethical, religious, and legal issues. Adequate definition here will prepare the way for better insight into all of these matters as well as for better law than is currently applicable.

The Ad Hoc Committee includes Henry K. Beecher, MD, *chairman;* Raymond D. Adams, MD; A. Clifford Barger, MD; William J. Curran, LLM, SMHyg; Derek Denny-Brown, MD; Dana L. Farnsworth, MD; Jordi Folch-Pi, MD; Everett I. Mendelsohn, PhD; John P. Merrill, MD; Joseph Murray, MD; Ralph Potter, ThD; Robert Schwab, MD; and William Sweet, MD.
Reprint requests to Massachusetts General Hospital, Boston 02114 (Dr. Henry K. Beecher).

Characteristics of Irreversible Coma

An organ, brain or other, that no longer functions and has no possibility of functioning again is for all practical purposes dead. Our first problem is to determine the characteristics of a *permanently* nonfunctioning brain.

A patient in this state appears to be in deep coma. The condition can be satisfactorily diagnosed by points 1, 2, and 3 to follow. The electroencephalogram (point 4) provides confirmatory data, and when available it should be utilized. In situations where for one reason or another electroencephalographic monitoring is not available, the absence of cerebral function has to be determined by purely clinical signs, to be described, or by absence of circulation as judged by standstill of blood in the retinal vessels, or by absence of cardiac activity.

1. *Unreceptivity and Unresponsivity.*—There is a total unawareness to externally applied stimuli and inner need and complete unresponsiveness—our definition of irreversible coma. Even the most intensely painful stimuli evoke no vocal or other response, not even a groan, withdrawal of a limb, or quickening of respiration.

2. *No Movements or Breathing.*—Observations covering a period of at least one hour by physicians is adequate to satisfy the criteria of no spontaneous muscular movements or spontaneous respiration or response to stimuli such as pain, touch, sound, or light. After the patient is on a mechanical respirator, the total absence of spontaneous breathing may be established by turning off the respirator for three minutes and observing whether there is any effort on the part of the subject to breathe

Figure 1-5 Publication of the Harvard Criteria in the *Journal of the American Medical Association.*

as the *New York Times,* did report their publication on the front page (Figure 1-6) and gave the committee high marks. The Harvard Criteria did not foster a public debate.

Almost immediately after this publication, the need for EEG in this situation was questioned. In 1969, Adams and Jequier emphasized that brain death was a clinical diagnosis and should not rely on EEG. "The physician who would permit such a crucial decision to be made by a machine, ingenious as it might be, leaves himself (and his patient) in a highly vulnerable position."[2]

Harvard Panel Asks Definition of Death Be Based on Brain

By ROBERT REINHOLD

A special faculty committee at Harvard University has recommended that the definition of death be based on "brain death," even though the heart may continue to beat. The committee offered a set of guidelines for physicians to determine when such death occurs.

The 13-man panel was drawn from the university's faculties of medicine, public health, law, divinity and arts and sciences.

The panel said its action was prompted by the possibility that "obsolete criteria" for death might lead to controversy in organ transplants and in modern resuscitative methods, which can maintain heartbeat in comatose patients with irreversible brain damage.

In a report, to be published today in the Journal of the American Medical Association under the title "A Definition of Irreversible Coma," the committee urges physicians to accept new standards for determining the moment of death as a prelude to a change in the legal definition.

Figure 1-6 Front page article in the *New York Times.*

In 1969, Beecher wrote in an editorial in the *New England Journal of Medicine* that the definition of irreversible coma proposed by the Ad Hoc Committee was well accepted by the medical community but not in legal circles. He also pointed out that "the committee was unanimous in its belief that an EEG was not essential to a diagnosis of irreversible coma, but it could provide valuable supporting data."[8]

In a development that turned out to be crucial for the way brain death was diagnosed, Mohandas and Chou published the Minnesota Code of Brain Death Criteria, also briefly known as the Minnesota Criteria.[27] Major changes from the Harvard Criteria included a definition of the period of apnea (4 minutes of disconnection), exclusion of metabolic derangements, and a shorter observation time of 12 hours; however, none of these criteria had validating data. Mohandas and Chou should be credited with introducing into the literature the concept that damage of the brainstem was a critical component of severe brain damage. They stated, "What are we attempting to define and establish, beyond reasonable doubt, is the state of irreversible damage to the brainstem. It is the point of no return." In addition, they stressed the irrelevance of the EEG: "We also had instances in which there was electrical activity of the brain recorded; but pathologically, the brainstem was completely autolyzed in one case and extensively hemorrhagic in the other two cases." "If the clinical-neurophysiological criteria of brain death are met, the value of an EEG examination is extremely questionable."[27] Interestingly, the Minnesota Criteria, with their deemphasizing of electrodiagnostic tests, became the basis of the United Kingdom criteria and were in line with the British pragmatic approach to neurologic conditions.

After the Harvard criteria were published, work began in the United Kingdom in the late 1970s. The Joint Committee of the Royal Colleges of Physicians consisted of a multidisciplinary working group and published three guidelines in 1976 (Figure 1-7), 1979, and 1995.[12,13] The members of the working group included Sir Douglas Black (chairman) and Sir Leslie Turnberg (president of the Royal College of Physicians), together with other physicians, most notably Christopher Pallis. The title "The Diagnosis of Brain Death"[12] in 1976 changed in 1995 to "Criteria for the Diagnosis of Brain Stem Death."[13] The document resulted from 2 years of discussion among anesthesiologists, neurologists, neurophysiologists, and neurosurgeons in the United Kingdom. The United Kingdom's position was that if the brainstem is dead, the brain is dead, and if the brain is dead, the person is dead. Detailed and meticulous as it was, the Conference of the Royal Colleges did require that the cause of the condition be fully established and a search made for factors that could potentially mimic loss of brainstem function. The absence of CNS-depressing drugs, neuromuscular blocking agents, respiratory depressants, and metabolic or endocrine disturbances was emphasized. A flexible period of observation was recommended, such that prolonged observation was needed in cases of hypoxic or ischemic injury, whereas a few hours might be needed following severe head injury or intracerebral hemorrhage. Finally, the technique for apnea testing was better described to include preoxygenation, continued oxygen administration during apnea, administration of 5% CO_2 to raise arterial CO_2 to at least 50 mm Hg, and expert investigation in patients with advanced chronic

Clinical Topics

Diagnosis of brain death

Statement issued by the honorary secretary of the Conference of Medical Royal Colleges and their Faculties in the United Kingdom on 11 October 1976

British Medical Journal, 1976, **2**, 1187-1188

With the development of intensive care techniques and their wide availability in the United Kingdom it has become common-place for hospitals to have deeply comatose and unresponsive patients with severe brain damage who are maintained on artificial respiration by means of mechanical ventilators.

This state has been recognised for many years and it has been the concern of the medical profession to establish diagnostic criteria of such rigour that on their fulfilment the mechanical ventilator can be switched off, in the secure knowledge that there is no possible chance of recovery.

There has been much philosophical argument about the diagnosis of death, which has throughout history been accepted as having occurred when the vital functions of respiration and circulation have ceased. With the technical ability to maintain these functions artificially, however, the dilemma of when to switch off the ventilator has been the subject of much public interest. It is agreed that permanent functional death of the brain stem constitutes brain death and that once this has occurred further artificial support is fruitless and should be withdrawn. It is good medical practice to recognise when brain death has occurred and to act accordingly, sparing relatives from the

their effects persist, and they are commonly used as anti-convulsants or to assist synchronisation with mechanical ventilators. It is therefore recommended that the drug history should be carefully reviewed and adequate intervals allowed for the persistence of drug effects to be excluded. This is of particular importance in patients whose primary cause of coma lies in the toxic effects of drugs followed by anoxic cerebral damage.

(*b*) Primary hypothermia as a cause of coma should have been excluded.

(*c*) Metabolic and endocrine disturbances that can cause or contribute to coma should have been excluded. Metabolic and endocrine factors contributing to the persistence of coma must be carefully assessed. There should be no profound abnormality of the serum electrolytes, acid base balance, or blood glucose concentrations.

(2) *The patient is being maintained on a ventilator because spontaneous respiration had previously become inadequate or had ceased altogether.*

Relaxants (neuromuscular blocking agents) and other drugs should have been excluded as a cause of respiratory inadequacy or failure. Immobility, unresponsiveness, and lack of spontaneous respiration may be due to the use of neuromuscular blocking drugs, and the persistence of their effects should be excluded

Figure 1-7 Publication of the Conference of the Royal College of Physicians (1976).

respiratory insufficiency (Table 1-2). The 1995 document also specifically mentioned that (1) certain endocrinologic abnormalities may be a consequence of brain death rather than a confounder or potential mimicker, stated that (2) neurophysiologic or imaging investigations have no place in the criteria and should have no role in the diagnostic requirements, and (3) warned of overlapping neurologic syndromes associated with critical illness.[13] A working group of the British Pediatric Association published guidelines much later, in 1991, and concluded that the brain death criteria in children over the age of 2 months should be the same as those in adults.[10]

Notwithstanding the clarity and comprehensiveness of the document, the public trust in the Royal College of Physicians criteria was undermined by a BBC

TABLE 1-2 *United Kingdom Criteria (1976)*

- Establish etiology
- Exclude mimicking conditions
- Absent motor response
- Absent brainstem reflexes in comatose patients
- Apnea testing using arterial PCO_2 target of 50 mm Hg
- Prolonged observation in anoxic-ischemic injury

program produced by *Panorama TV* viewed by 8 million people under the title "Transplants—Are the Donors Really Dead?"(October 13, 1980).[19] Three far-reaching arguments were put forward and echoed some of the earlier concerns raised in the United States after dissemination of the Harvard Criteria: (1) brain death criteria were not properly discussed and vetted before their publication, (2) the criteria were developed because of the need to find organs, and, more disturbing, (3) the criteria were not reliable. American physicians interviewed about the criteria in the United Kingdom claimed that, due to emphasis on the brainstem alone, their patients not infrequently recovered. The television broadcast fueled controversy and newspaper coverage ("Donors tearing up cards"; "TV shock of 'live' donors"). A subsequent program made by physicians nominated by the Royal College of Physicians left little room for misinterpretation and went a long way toward restoring the public's trust. Prompted by the refusal of the BBC to apologize for the mistakes in the *Panorama TV* feature, Pallis was commissioned by the editor of the *British Medical Journal,* Stephan Lock, to write a series of articles collected in a classic work known as the *ABC of Brain Stem Death*[31] (Figure 1-8). The UK criteria have remained unchanged since.

The only prospective attempt to develop evidence-based guidelines for the declaration of death based on neurologic criteria in the world was made by the National Institutes of Health (NIH)–sponsored multicenter U.S. Collaborative Study of Cerebral Death in 1977.[7] The project sought to identify prospectively neurologic factors that would predict cardiac arrest within 3 months despite continued cardiopulmonary support.

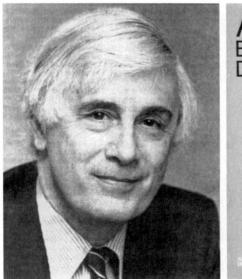 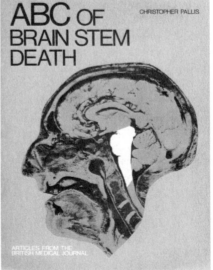

Figure 1-8 Left, Christopher Pallis (1923–2005) kindly provided by his wife Jeanne Pallis. *Right*, ABC of Brain Stem Death.

To be enrolled in the study, a patient had to demonstrate cerebral unresponsivity and apnea. Of the 503 patients who met these criteria, 87% had a cardiac arrest within 3 months. Only 19 of the 503 patients met the Harvard Criteria, and all 19 succumbed to cardiac arrest. The Harvard Criteria were considered 100% specific but very insensitive. Therefore, a third set of criteria was applied: cerebral unresponsiveness, apnea, and one isoelectric EEG. Of the 189 patients who met these criteria, 187 had a cardiac arrest; the 2 who survived had drug intoxication.

In the collaborative study, there was a high–but far from perfect—completion rate with pupil, corneal, oculocephalic, auditory blink reflexes assessed in 97–99% of the patients but substantially less documentation of pharyngeal, swallow and cough reflexes (83–85%). In addition there was—by current standards—a poor definition of apnea. Apnea was determined after no overriding of the ventilator or disconnection for 3 minutes (the investigators felt that "it was considered hazardous to an already damaged brain to undergo such tests for 3 minutes or more). The implicit message of these results is that there is a general lack of focus by the examiner on the medulla oblongata function and that apnea testing might have been insufficient in some patients.

The final recommended NIH criteria required one examination at least 6 hours after the onset of coma and apnea (unlike the 24 hours required by the Harvard Criteria). The examination had to demonstrate cerebral unresponsivity, dilated pupils, absent brainstem reflexes, apnea, and an isoelectric EEG. Apnea was defined as the need for controlled ventilation for at least 15 minutes, that is, the patient made no effort to override the ventilator but was not disconnected from it. Although it was recognized that not all brain-dead patients had dilated pupils, the requirement was included to avoid incorrect diagnosis in cases of drug intoxication. It was noted that spinal cord reflexes were poor indicators of loss of brain function and were present in approximately a third of the patients who died. Additional confirmatory tests to demonstrate absence of cerebral blood flow were recommended when an early diagnosis was desired, particularly when brainstem reflexes were unable to be tested or when sedatives had been administered.

More definitively, less than 5 years later, the President's Commission for the Study of Ethical Problems in Medicine and Biomedical and Behavioral Research published guidelines in 1981 (Figure 1-9) that represented a distillation of practice at that time.[16,32] The commission, chaired by attorney Morris Abram, wrote, "We have concluded that, in light of the ever increasing powers of biomedical science and practice, a statute is needed to provide a clear and socially-acceptable basis for making determinations of death."[32] The President's Commission heard philosophical, political, and religious testimony and set a day apart to hear testimony from five expert witnesses in vascular surgery (Keith Veith), neurology (Ronald Cranford, Gaetano Molinari, and Julius Korein), and neurosurgery (Earl Walker). They attempted to develop criteria that (1) eliminated error in classifying a living person as dead, (2) allowed as few errors as possible in classifying a dead person as alive, (3) allowed a determination to be made without unreasonable delay, and (4) were explicit, adaptable, and accessible to verification. Brain death was defined as the "irreversible cessation of all [clinically ascertainable] function of the entire brain including

Defining Death

Medical, Legal and
Ethical Issues in the
Determination of Death

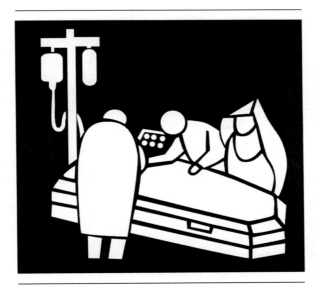

President's Commission for the Study of
Ethical Problems in Medicine and
Biomedical and Behavioral Research

Figure 1-9 Cover page of the report by the President's Commission for the Study of Ethical Problems in Medicine and Biomedical and Behavioral Research.

the brainstem." This was to be demonstrated by unreceptivity, unresponsivity, absent brainstem reflexes, and apnea. Irreversibility was assured by (1) establishing the cause of the coma, (2) excluding the possibility of recovery of any brain function (exclusion of reversible conditions), and (3) a period of observation. Apnea testing was described in detail to include preoxygenation, passive flow of oxygen during apnea, and hypercapnea of at least 60 mm Hg confirmed by arterial blood gas sampling. The report specifically indicated that true decerebrate or decorticate posturing or seizures were inconsistent with the diagnosis of death. This report was the first to include shock as a confounder. The period of observation was considered a matter of clinical judgment, but the President's Commission did define time periods. These periods were: 6 hours in complicated cases with a confirmatory EEG or test of cerebral blood flow, 12 hours with a well-established

TABLE 1-3 *President's Commission Criteria (1981)*

- Unreceptive and unresponsive coma
- Absent pupillary, corneal, oculocephalic, oculovestibular, oropharyngeal reflexes
- Apnea with arterial PCO_2 greater than 60 mm Hg
- Absence of posturing or seizures
- Irreversibility demonstrated by establishing cause and excluding reversible conditions (sedation, hypothermia, shock, and neuromuscular blockade)
- Period of observation determined by clinical judgment
- Use of cerebral blood flow tests when brainstem reflexes are not testable, sufficient cause cannot be established, or to shorten period of observation

The signatories were: Jesse Barber, MD; Don Becker, MD; Richard Behrman, MD, JD; Donald Bennett, MD; Richard Beresford, MD, JD; Reginald Bickford, MD; William Black, Jr, MD; Benjamin Boshes, MD, PhD; Philip Braunstein, MD; John Burroughs, MD, JD; Russell Butler, MD; John Caronna, MD; Shelley Chou, MD, PhD; Kemp Clark, MD; Ronald Cranford, MD; Michael Earnest, MD; Albert Ehle, MD; Jack Fein, MD; Sal Fiscina, MD, JD; Terrance Furlow, MD, JD; Eli Goldensohn, MD; Jack Grabow, MD; Phillip M. Green, MD; Ake Grenvik, MD; Charles Henry, PhD; John Hughes, MD, PhD, DM; Howard Kaufman, MD; Robert King, MD; Julius Korein, MD; Thomas Langfitt, MD; Cesare Lombroso, MD; Kevin M. McIntyre, MD, JD; Richard L. Masland, MD; Don Harper Mills, MD, JD; Gaetano Molinari, MD; Byron Pevehouse, MD; Lawrence H. Pitts, MD; A. Bernard Pleet, MD; Fred Plum, MD; Jerome Posner, MD; David Powner, MD; Richard Rovit, MD; Peter Safar, MD; Henry Schwartz, MD; Edward Schlesinger, MD; Roy Selby, MD; James Snyder, MD; Bruce F. Sorenson, MD; Cary Suter, MD; Barry Tharp, MD; Fernando Torres, MD; A. Earl Walker, MD; Arthur Ward, MD; Jack Whisnant, MD; Robert Wilkus, MD; and Harry Zimmerman, MD.

irreversible cause of coma without a confirmatory test, and 24 hours for anoxic brain damage. Finally, the observation period could be reduced if tests showed an isoelectric EEG or absent cerebral blood flow for 10 minutes in an adult without drug intoxication, hypothermia, or shock. The President's Commission recognized that isoelectric EEG could be caused by drugs ingested in toxic quantities (Table 1-3).

The President's Commission specifically reviewed the "British viewpoint" and felt that it was "closer to a prognostic approach" but preferred a "diagnostic approach" in seeking evidence that all functions of the brain had ceased irreversibly. These guidelines remained the gold standard for more than a decade. The report led to the Uniform Determination of Death Act (UDDA; Chapter 2). "An individual who has sustained either (1) irreversible cessation of circulatory and respiratory functions, or (2) irreversible cessation of all functions of the entire brain, including the brain stem, is dead. A determination of death must be made in accordance with accepted medical standards."

The President's Commission was mostly concerned with avoiding equating persistent vegetative state with death and hence its emphasis on the brainstem in the formulated statements. The President's Commission concluded that "it is not necessary—indeed it would be a mistake—to enshrine any particular medical criteria, or any requirements for procedure or review, as part of the statute."[32]

Over the years, further refinements followed and mostly involved better definition of the apnea test. Apneic diffusion oxygenation to test apnea in brain death was first reported by Milhaud et al. in 1974 using the technique of oxygenation by Hirsch and Vohance described in 1905.[26] Forty patients were tested for only 15 minutes to limit the development of severe hypercapnic acidosis. Marked acidosis was recognized as potentially causing cardiac arrhythmias and myocardial depression. A target arterial PCO_2 was not suggested but in a later study, an arterial PCO_2 threshold of 60 mm Hg was recommended by Shafer and Caronna, remarkably on the basis of testing only three patients. These patients started to breathe at levels varying from 45 to 56 mm Hg (five trials total).[36] This arterial PCO_2 threshold became accepted but was rightly challenged by Ropper et al., who found much lower breathing thresholds in four patients varying from 30 to 39 mm Hg (seven trials).[34] This arterial PCO_2 threshold will be debated until a collective study involving a large group of patients is published. Theoretically, too low an arterial PCO_2 (e.g., <30 mm Hg) would mean insufficient stimulation of the impaired respiratory centers; too high an arterial PCO_2 (e.g., >100 mm Hg) would depress possible brain function through CO_2 narcosis. The apneic oxygen diffusion technique remains the most reliable technique and is used in most intensive care units (Chapter 2).

In early 1993, the Quality Standards Subcommittee of the American Academy of Neurology (AAN) investigated ways to develop practice parameters using an evidence-based approach to the literature. The areas of need were defined as follows: (1) unequivocal definition of clinical testing of brain function, (2) description of conditions that may mimic brain death, (3) clinical observations that are compatible with brain death but raise doubts for the attending physician, (4) a clear description of the apnea testing procedure, and (5) critical review of the value of confirmatory laboratory tests. A comprehensive review became the basis for a practice parameter.[43] These guidelines were approved by the AAN Executive Board in 1995[5] (Figure 1-10).

Practice parameters for determining brain death in adults
(Summary statement)

Report of the Quality Standards Subcommittee of the American Academy of Neurology

Overview. Brain death is defined as the irreversible loss of function of the brain, including the brainstem. Brain death from primary neurologic disease usually is caused by severe head injury or aneurysmal subarachnoid hemorrhage. In medical and surgical intensive care units, however, hypoxic-ischemic brain insults and fulminant hepatic failure may result in irreversible loss of brain function. In large referral hospitals, neurologists make the diagnosis of brain death 25 to 30 times a year.

Justification. Brain death was selected as a topic for practice parameters because of the need for standardization of the neurologic examination criteria for the diagnosis of brain death. Currently, there are differences in clinical practice in performing the apnea test and controversies over appropriate confirmatory laboratory tests. This document outlines the clinical criteria for brain death and the procedures of testing in patients older than 18 years.

acute CNS catastrophe that is compatible with the clinical diagnosis of brain death
2. Exclusion of complicating medical conditions that may confound clinical assessment (no severe electrolyte, acid-base, or endocrine disturbance)
3. No drug intoxication or poisoning
4. Core temperature ≥32 °C (90 °F)
B. The three cardinal findings in brain death are coma or unresponsiveness, absence of brainstem reflexes, and apnea.
1. Coma or unresponsiveness—no cerebral motor response to pain in all extremities (nail-bed pressure and supraorbital pressure)
2. Absence of brainstem reflexes
   a. Pupils
      (i) No response to bright light
      (ii) Size: midposition (4 mm) to dilated (9 mm)
   b. Ocular movement

Figure 1-10 American Academy of Neurology guidelines (1995).

The new 2010 AAN brain death guidelines separated evidence-based data from opinion-based data. The guidelines noted that (1) no recoveries in adults have been reported since the adoption of the AAN 1995 guidelines, (2) the apnea test is safe using the apneic oxygenation method, (3) confirmatory tests are less reliable and useful than has been suggested and should be used sparingly, and (4) adequate documentation may be facilitated with a checklist.[47]

The acceptance of brain death in children was advanced by a publication of an ad hoc committee of Boston Children's Hospital and a special task force of neurologists and pediatricians.[3] The recommendations included age brackets with different recommendations for the time of observation and electrophysio-logic tests. The time of observation and the use of EEG were taken from the adult Harvard Criteria. These guidelines became readily accepted. Important data in newborns by Ashwal and Schneider followed these guidelines and suggested extension to preterm and term infants.[6] The pediatric brain death guidelines have been recently reassessed by a multidisciplinary group appointed by the Society of Critical Care Medicine and American Academy of Pediatrics. The guidelines will be published in 2011. The criteria are discussed in Chapter 2.

■ CURRENT INTERNATIONAL GUIDELINES

Neurologic criteria for the declaration of death have been developed in many countries throughout the world.[44] In Europe, many countries have statutes that allow for the declaration of death based on neurologic criteria. Several Asian countries (Indonesia, Malaysia, the Philippines, Singapore, and Taiwan) have laws allowing organ transplantation. Others (e.g., the People's Republic of China) have no laws or laws only for kidney transplantation. Differences among countries are notable; the most striking differences are shown in Figure 1-11.[44,46] Confirmatory tests are not mandatory in many countries, probably because they are not readily available.

The Latin American Network and the Council of Donation and Transplant includes 21 countries, and all Latin American countries except Nicaragua have legally accepted brain death as death of the person.[14] Two or three physicians are needed to declare brain death. The procedures are similar to those in other countries, but in more than a third, an atropine test (Chapter 2) is mandated. Confirmatory tests are needed in only 40% of the 21 countries.[14,44]

In 2000, the Canadian Neurological Care Group published guidelines for the diagnosis of brain death that closely mirror the AAN guidelines,[11] and a 2005 forum convened by the Donation Committee of the Canadian Council for Donation and Transplantation organized by anesthesiologist Sam Shemie has clarified diagnosis and management in Canada.[37]

In Europe there is fairly uniform agreement regarding the criteria for the clinical evaluation of brain death, although there is considerable variation in the use of ancillary tests. In 11 of 25 countries, guidelines require a confirmatory test for the diagnosis, and in the remaining 14 countries this test "facilitates" the diagnosis.[18] Half of the surveyed countries require that more than one physician be involved in the clinical determination of brain death. In Ireland,

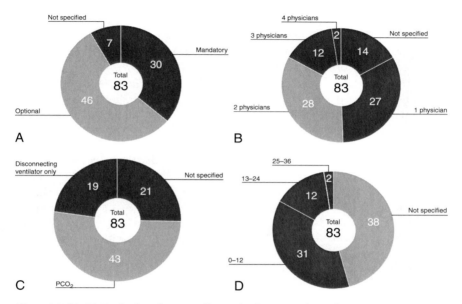

Figure 1-11 (A–D) Lack of uniformity of brain death criteria throughout the world.
(A) Confirmatory tests; (B) Number of examiners; (C) Method of apnea test;
(D) Time of observation between 2 tests.

two sets of tests must be carried out, performed by a consultant and a physician with more than 5 years' experience with patient care at the acute hospital level. Several countries have longer observation periods when anoxia is the cause of brain death. For example, in Hungary, "secondary brain damage" extends the observation time to 72 hours.

Another level of complexity has been introduced by Germany. The German criteria stipulate EEG, evoked potentials, or absent blood flow with infratentorial lesions and 72 hours of observation, and in situations with "secondary brain damage (hypoxia or cardiopulmonary resuscitation resulting in anoxic-ischemic encephalopathy)."[33]

In a surprise move, Poland recently changed to more comprehensive guidelines and now includes mandatory confirmatory tests (preferably cerebral blood flow studies) in patients with infratentorial processes and in children younger than 2 years.[9]

Virtually all African countries are without legal provisions for organ transplantation, and brain death criteria are difficult to obtain. Tunisia and South Africa have developed guidelines,[45] but most East and West African countries do not have them. Official guidelines for brain death determination have not been drafted in most countries of the Middle East. Guidelines for brain death were approved by the Pan-Islamic Council on jurisprudence in Jordan in 1986 and in Saudi Arabia in 1988.[44] The procedure in Iran is unique. After the diagnosis of brain death is made, the minister of health appoints five physicians (an internist, a neurologist, a neurosurgeon, an anesthesiologist, and a specialist in forensic medicine). In addition, 12, 24, and 36 hours of observation (and presumably repeat examinations) are mandatory.[44] In Israel, the director general of the Ministry of Health published criteria for brain death in 1991 that were revised in 1996. A team of two physicians are required to accompany the treating physician.

The concept of death based on neurologic criteria has not been uniformly accepted in Asia, and major differences in regulations exist. In Turkey, an organ harvesting law has been passed; it requires a cardiologist, a neurosurgeon, a neurologist, and an anesthesiologist to examine the patient, followed by confirmatory testing that often requires a combination of tests.[17] In India, the Rajya Sabha passed the Transplantation of Human Organs Bill in 1993.[39] Brain death determination follows the British criteria of brainstem death but involves a panel consisting of (1) the doctor in charge of the patient, (2) the doctor in charge of the hospital where the patient was treated, (3) an independent specialist (unspecified), and (4) a neurologist or neurosurgeon. The burden of proof rests with the specialist in the neurosciences, with the other member of the panel confirming the diagnosis.

China has no legal criteria for the determination of brain death, and there are indications of the reluctance of medical staff to disconnect the ventilator. Nonetheless, hundreds of medical institutions are involved in organ transplantation. There remains an unease with the public and abuse and lack of transparency are perceived concerns. Family members may fear being accused of murder. These factors remain major obstacles.

In Japan, brain death determination has been the subject of considerable controversy and the path taken seems muddled. In 1968, heart surgeon Toshiro Wada was charged with murder after removing a heart from a patient who was allegedly not brain dead and transplanting it into a recipient who was allegedly not sick enough to receive a graft.[22,23] This transplant not only fostered suspicion of tampering, but the procedure by an American-trained Japanese heart surgeon (1 year after Barnard's pioneering transplant) was considered "un-Japanese." Sadly, the recipient died 83 days after the transplant was performed. The judge dismissed the murder case, but it was 30 years before another heart transplant was performed. This second case also received massive media attention, with photographers chasing the car carrying the donor's organ.[38] In 1985, the Ministry of Health and Welfare set up a Brain Death Advisory Council that established new brain death criteria but did not define brain death as human death. Three years later, the Japanese Medical Association voted to accept brain death as the end of human life, but several medical specialty societies refused to accept this position. Additionally, the Ministry of Justice, the National Police Agency, and the Public Prosecutors Office all continue to resist recognition of brain death as the end of human life. In 1997, in order to facilitate organ transplantation, Japan legalized the declaration of death using neurologic criteria only when the patient was to be an organ donor, creating an unfortunate double standard. Additional controversy arose in 1999 when the Japanese Health and Welfare Ministry aborted a transplantation when it was discovered that the potential donor had a ruptured tympanic membrane.[22,23,41] Subsequently, the guidelines were amended to not allow brain death testing in patients with ruptured tympanic membranes (even though it in fact enhances the test) or trauma to the eyeballs.

The Japanese criteria have the following additional unique features: (1) a computed tomography (CT) scan should detect irreparable lesions; (2) when cardiac arrest has occurred, its cause should be known; (3) the ciliospinal reflex should be tested; (4) the apnea test should be performed after loss of seven brainstem reflexes and only after isoelectric EEG; (5) brain death determination is allowed only if intact tympanic membranes exist; and (6) children less than 6 years old should be excluded. Currently, the discussion in Japan is focusing on the type of confirmatory test in brain death. A combination of tests may be recommended after facial or eye trauma in an attempt to reduce the chance of a misdiagnosis of brain death. The Japanese organ law was revised in 2009 and removed the double standard on brain death (the diagnosis of brain death is allowed only if the patient had given previous written consent to be an organ donor). This change stipulated that brain death was equal to legal death. However, according to Aita, a national survey showed that only 40% of the Japanese population supported brain death; 39% did not.[4] (For a further cultural perspective, see Chapter 3.)

The Australian and New Zealand Intensive Care Society's statement and guidelines on brain death were published in July 1993 and are being revised. They state that brain death for donation purposes should be determined by two medical practitioners. The first formal examination is performed after at least 4 hours have elapsed; the second examination occurs 2 hours after the first examination except following primary hypoxic brain injury; in the latter situation, the first examination should not be performed until 12 hours have elapsed.[40]

■ CONCLUSION

History must consider the development of brain death in many ways and from many angles: the rapid development of intensive care allowing life support, the interest of the transplant specialty, and continuous refinement of criteria with endless nuances. The development of neurologic criteria of death or brain death once seemed both straightforward and unambiguous. Today, many committees in different countries are buoyed by a desire to introduce safeguards, and this has led to more elaborate criteria. The embarrassing variability of operational guidelines serves little purpose and probably only fuels criticism.

The diagnosis of brain death is complex in its clinical testing, in the determination of confounding conditions, and in the interpretation of ancillary tests. A uniform guideline accepted by most countries of the world should be a priority of major medical organizations.

■ REFERENCES

1. A definition of irreversible coma. Report of the Ad Hoc Committee of the Harvard Medical School to Examine the Definition of Brain Death. *JAMA* 1968;205:337–340.
2. Adams RD, Jequier M. The brain death syndrome: hypoxemic panencephalopathy. *Schweiz Med Wochenschr* 1969;99:65–73.

3. Ad Hoc Committee on Brain Death. The Children's Hospital, Boston. Determination of brain death. *J Pediatr* 1987;110:15–19.
4. Aita K. Japan approves brain death to increase donors: will it work? *Lancet* 2009;374: 1403–1404.
5. American Academy of Neurology Practice Parameters for Determining Brain Death in Adults (summary statement). *Neurology* 1995;45:1012–1014.
6. Ashwal S, Schneider S. Brain death in the newborn. *Pediatrics* 1985;84:429–437.
7. An appraisal of the criteria of cerebral death, a summary statement of a collaborative study. *JAMA* 1977;237:982–986.
8. Beecher HK. After the "definition of irreversible coma." *N Engl J Med* 1969;281: 1070–1071.
9. Bohatyrewicz R, Bohatyrewicz A, Zukowski M, et al. Reversal to whole-brain death criteria after 15-year experience with brain stem death criteria in Poland. *Transplant Proc* 2009;41:2959–2960.
10. British Pediatric Association. Diagnosis of brainstem death in infants and children. Report of a working party. London: British Pediatric Association; 1991.
11. Canadian Neurological Care Group. Guidelines for the diagnosis of brain death. *Can J Neurol Sci* 2000;26:64–66.
12. Conference of Medical Royal Colleges and Faculties of the United Kingdom. Diagnosis of brain death. *BMJ* 1976;2:1187–1188.
13. Criteria for the diagnosis of brain stem death: review by a working group convened by the Royal College of Physicians and endorsed by the Conference of Medical Royal Colleges and Their Faculties in the United Kingdom. *J R Coll Phys Lond* 1995;29: 381–382.
14. Escudera D, Matesanz R, Soratti CA, et al. Brain death in Ibero-America. *Med Intensiva* 2009;33:415–423.
15. Goulon M, Nouailhat F, Babinet P. Irreversible coma [French]. *Ann Med Interne (Paris)* 1971;122:479–486.
16. Guidelines for the determination of death: report of the medical consultants on the diagnosis of death to the President's Commission for the Study of Ethical Problems in Medicine and Biomedical and Behavioral Research. *JAMA* 1981;246:2184–2186.
17. Haberral M, Moray G, Karakayali H, et al. Ethical and legal aspects and the history of organ transplantation in Turkey. *Transplant Proc* 1996;28:382–383.
18. Haupt WF, Rudolf J. European brain death codes: a comparison of national guidelines. *J Neurol* 1999;246:432–437.
19. Jennett B. Brain death. *Br J Anaesth* 1981;53:1111–1119.
20. Jouvet M. Coma and other disorders of consciousness. In: Vinken PJ, Bruyn GW, eds. *Handbook of Clinical Neurology*. Vol. 3: *Disorders of Higher Nervous Activity*. Amsterdam: North-Holland; 1969:62–79.
21. Koehler PJ, Wijdicks EFM. Historical study of coma: looking back through medical and neurological texts. *Brain* 2008;131:877–889.
22. Lock M. Contesting the natural in Japan: moral dilemmas and technologies of dying. *Culture, Med Psychiatry* 1995;19:1–38.
23. Lock M. The problem of brain death: Japanese disputes about bodies and modernity. In: Younger SJ, Arnold RM, Schapiro R, eds. *The Definition of Death: Contemporary Controversies*. Baltimore: Johns Hopkins University Press; 1999:239–256.
24. Lofstedt S, von Reis G. Intracranial lesions with abolished passage of x-ray contrast throughout the internal carotid arteries. *PACE* 1956;8:99–202.
25. Machado C, Korein J, Ferrer Y, et al. The concept of brain death did not evolve to benefit organ transplants. *J Med Ethics* 2007;33:197–200.
26. Milhaud A, Ossart M, Gayet H, et al. L'epreuve de débrancher en oxygéne. *Test de Mort Cérébrale, Special III* 1974;15:73–79.
27. Mohandas A, Chou SN. Brain death—a clinical and pathologic study. *J Neurosurg* 1971;35:211–218.

28. Mollaret P, Goulon M. Le coma dépassé (memoire préliminaire). *Rev Neurol* 1959; 101:3–15.
29. Murray JE. Organ transplantation: the practical possibilities. In: Wolstenholme GEW, O'Conner M, eds. *Ciba Foundation Symposium: Ethics in Medical Progress.* Boston: Little, Brown: 1966:54–77.
30. Murray JE. *Surgery of the Soul: Reflections on a Curious Career.* Boston: Science History, 2001.
31. Pallis C. *The ABC of Brainstem Death.* London: British Medical Journal Publishing Group; 1983.
32. President's Commission for the Study of Ethical Problems in Medicine and Biomedical and Behavioral Research 1981. Defining death: a report on the medical, legal and ethical issues in the determination of death Washington, D.C.: Government Printing Office, 1981.
33. Richtlinien zur Feststellung des Hirntodes. *Deutsches Arzteblatt* 1997;95:A1861–A1868.
34. Ropper AH, Kennedy SK, Russel L. Apnea testing in the diagnosis of brain death. *J Neurosurg* 1981;55:942–946.
35. Schwab RS, Potts F, Mathis P. EEG as an aid in determining death in the presence of cardiac activity. *Electroenceph Clin Neurophysiol* 1963;15:147.
36. Shafer JA, Caronna J. Duration of apnea needed to confirm brain death. *Neurology* 1978;28:661–666.
37. Shemie SD, Doig C, Dickens B, et al. Severe brain injury to neurological determination of death: Canadian forum recommendations. *CMAJ* 2006;14:174:S1–13.
38. Takeshita H. Coma and brain death. In: Cucchiara RF, Black S, Michenfelder JD, eds. *Clinical Neuronanesthesia.* 2nd ed. New York: Churchill Livingstone; 1998:643–665.
39. The Transplantation of Human Organs Bill, 1993. Bill No. LIX-C of (1992), Republic of India.
40. Transplantation and Anatomy Ordinance 1978. Australian Capital Territory.
41. Watts J. Brain-death guidelines revised in Japan. *Lancet* 1999;354:1011.
42. Wertheimer P, Jouvet M, Descotes J. A propos du diagnostic de la mort du système nerveux dans les comas avec arrêt respiratoire traités par respiration artificielle. *Presse Med* 1959;67:87–88.
43. Wijdicks EFM. Determining brain death in adults. *Neurology* 1995;45:1003–1011.
44. Wijdicks EFM. Brain death worldwide: accepted fact but no global consensus in diagnostic criteria. *Neurology* 2002;58:20–25.
45. Wijdicks EFM. The neurologist and Harvard criteria for brain death. *Neurology* 2003;61:970–976.
46. Wijdicks EFM. The clinical criteria of brain death throughout the world: why has it come to this?. *Can J Anaesth* 2006;53:540–543.
47. Wijdicks EFM, Varelas PN, Gronseth GS, et al. Evidence based guideline update: determining brain death in adults. Report of the Quality Standards Subcommittee of the American Academy of Neurology. *Neurology* 2010;74:1911–1918.

2 Neurology of Brain Death

It starts with an acute catastrophic injury to the brain. Brain death, if it occurs, evolves often rapidly and many patients have irreversibly lost brain function within the first days of admission.[216] Common mechanisms of severe injury leading to brain death are shift and compression of the brainstem caused by an acute large mass or a more direct diffuse injury to the cortex, diencephalic structures, and brainstem.

The clinical diagnosis of brain death, however, remains uncommon in a neurosciences intensive care unit (NICU). On average, in NICUs or trauma ICUs in the United States, brain death is diagnosed in two or three patients a month.[49,176,216] In pediatric units, brain death accounts for slightly more than 1% of all pediatric critical care unit admissions.[154] In one European study, brain death could be established in less than 10% of all deaths in general ICUs.[191] Most comatose patients—despite having severe damage to the brainstem—will retain some brainstem reflexes and a breathing drive.

Because only a fraction of patients lose all brain function it is pertinent to identify patients that are imminently brain dead. This designation was created by transplant organizations in order to identify patients who could become donors early. This obviously does not absolve the clinician from the duty to treat the patient aggressively. The decision to pursue aggressive medical or neurosurgical management and the decision to consider organ donation are totally independent of each other and always have been. Some criteria for imminent brain death apply to ventilator supported patients with absence of at least three brain stem reflexes. A more recent study suggested the use of the Full Outline of UnResponsiveness (FOUR) score coma scale, in particular a sum FOUR score of 0 (no eye opening to pain; no motor response to pain; absent pupil, corneal, and cough reflexes; and no triggering of the ventilator). Using the FOUR score not only increased recognition, but also the donor conversion rate[45,46] (Chapter 5). Aside from these neurologic indicators, precipitous loss of blood pressure, new-onset hypothermia, or polyuria are further characteristic clinical indicators that the brain has been irreversibly damaged.

This chapter concentrates on the many tests needed to evaluate the patient accurately. The overriding principle is that the diagnosis of brain death is a stepwise, systematic clinical process. The main purpose of establishing the clinical diagnosis of brain death is to bring closure. It is a legally and medically accepted way of determining the person's death. The next step is to activate the process of asking consent of the next of kin to donate organs and tissue. Problems surfacing with this determination are further discussed in Chapter 6.

▪ THE PATHOLOGY OF BRAIN DEATH

The clinical findings on examination has been linked to findings at autopsy. Loss of brain function—assessed clinically—may have a neuropathologic correlate, but the degree of abnormalities—albeit profound—may be variable. One would expect diffuse brain swelling, significant shift of the brainstem, intrinsic damage to the brainstem, and other brain tissue shift (uncal and tonsillar herniation). Least common is diffuse anoxic-ischemic encephalopathy after cardiac arrest or exsanguination. Prolonged cardiopulmonary resuscitation—often after multiple defibrillation attempts and use of vasoactive drugs—may eventually result in resumption of circulation, but it could leave a comatose patient with no apparent brainstem reflexes. Similar scenarios may occur in patients with self-poisoning resulting in anoxic-ischemic injury. When patients declared brain dead after cardiopulmonary resuscitation come to autopsy, extensive diffuse neuronal ischemic damage is found in most brain samples.[215,140,146]

The major pathophysiologic mechanism is shown in Figure 2-1. The mechanism of terminal destruction is displacement of the thalamus-brain stem complex,

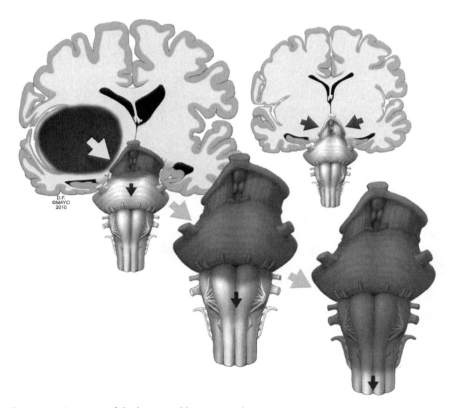

Figure 2-1 Drawing of the brain and brainstem showing rostrocaudal progression leading to brain death. *See* Figure 2-1 in the color insert.

either downward, sideways, or a combination of both, leading to progressive loss of function. Displacement of the brainstem may be a result of diffuse brain edema or it may be caused by a single mass compressing this structure (Figure 2-1). Damage of the pons alters the breathing drive, and breathing stops altogether when the medulla oblongata becomes involved. Simultaneously, with involvement of the brainstem, the control of vasomotor tone by the rostral ventrolateral neurons of the medulla oblongata is lost, resulting in hypotension.

At the same time, intracranial pressure (ICP) rises substantially and seriously reduces or causes stagnation of cerebral perfusion, leading eventually to virtual intracranial standstill. This leads to additional brain injury culminating in complete loss of brain function. One would expect this to occur with cerebral perfusion pressures (CPPs) in the 10–20 mm Hg range (for example, mean arterial blood pressure [MAP] of 70 mm Hg and ICP of 60 mm Hg; CPP = MAP-ICP). Brain perfusion is nonexistant with these critical CPPs, resulting in reverberating (*pendel flüss*) and ineffective blood flow.[125] The intracerebral vascular collapse is permanent, leading to further cerebral necrosis. Once cerebral blood flow stops in an apneic patient with no brainstem reflexes and no confounders, cerebral blood flow and brainstem function do not return. The exact time course is not known and would require serial blood flow studies and neurologic examinations. Overall, a certain degree of brainstem injury resulting in loss of all brainstem reflexes is the defining event. Injury mostly progresses from the thalami to the lower medulla, although not necessarily in a gradual fashion. The medulla oblongata has the longest survival time, and that important finding places emphasis on damage to the lower centers to determine brain death.[74]

The degree of neuropathological findings varies substantially (Figure 2-2). The typical finding of a "respirator brain"—total necrosis with a musky brain and disintegration when the cerebrum is removed from the skull—is uncommon and in the past was always a consequence of prolonged support in a poorly perfused or nonperfused brain.[114,128] The most recognizable finding is a herniated, swollen brain with autolysis of herniated cerebellar tonsils. In extreme cases, pieces of necrotic tonsils may break off and displace in the intrathecal space. If not carefully sought, these fragments may be missed.[97] Widespread ischemic neuronal changes are found throughout the brain in addition to the primary lesions that led to the patient's rapid demise.[204] The microscopic abnormalities surprisingly may spare vulnerable areas such as the hippocampus. The Purkinje cell layer may also be normal, except in patients with severe anoxic-ischemic injury. Microscopic examination of the cerebellum mostly reveals the effects of congestion, with a washout pattern of the granular layer but preservation of the molecular layer. Areas of severe ischemic injury may be next to areas with mild abnormalities. In one study, sporadically appearing ischemic neuronal loss may occur in one-third of the brain lobes, in one-third of the thalami, and in more than one-half of the samples of the brain stem.[215]

The pituitary gland is of special interest in brain death because it can be normal in more than 50% of cases. When it is examined carefully, patchy softenings can be found. When the pituitary gland is normal it is likely that early preservation of

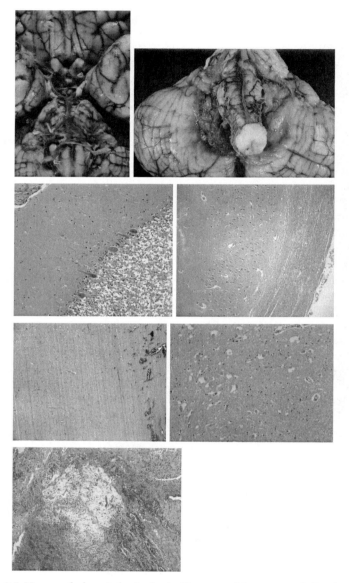

Figure 2-2 Neuropathology in brain death. *Upper row*: Macroscopy: diffuse brain swelling, tonsillar herniation, and third nerve grooving; necrotic tip of the cerebellar tonsil. *Second row*: Microscopy: preserved Purkinje cells, hippocampus. *Third row*: Preserved occipital area next to hemorrhage, but severe neuronal injury to the brainstem. *Fourth row*: necrotic areas in the pituitary gland. (*Continues*)

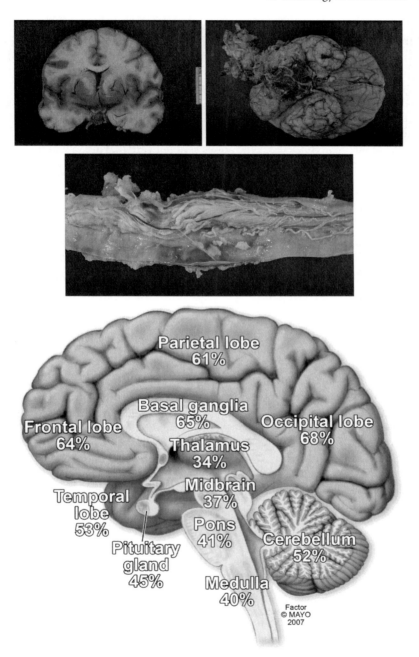

Figure 2-2 (Continued) Musky brain known as classic "respirator brain" seen in modern times only with prolonged support showing fragmentation and cerebellar remnants in spinal cord. Illustration shows distribution of severe neuronal injury to the brain.
From Wijdicks and Pfeifer.[215] Used with permission from *Neurology*.
See Figure 2-2 in the color insert.

these hormones is a consequence of extracranial blood supply to the pituitary gland and possibly even to some areas of the hypothalamus (Chapter 6). However, if injury is present, ischemia to the supraventricular and paraventricular hypothalamic nuclei results in immediate loss of vasopressin and large amounts of dilute urine. When measured, antidiuretic hormone levels are undetectable in three-fourths of all brain-dead patients.

The spinal cord usually appears normal except for upper cervical segments where tonsillar compression has resulted in ischemia. The spinomedullary junction (C1-C2 segments) is an arterial end zone (between vertebral blood and spinal artery perfusion) and, when compromised, leads to necrosis, edema, and petechial hemorrhages.[142]

Autopsies are rarely performed in the modern era of transplantation. (This may be a consequence of the difficulty of asking families to consent to two requests (organ donation and autopsy). Earlier descriptions of "total brain necrosis" or "liquid fatty soup" may have appeared in the heyday of intensive care and organ donation, but it has become clear that clinical brain death does not require complete destruction to become apparent and to remain irreversible. The degree of necrosis is likely a consequence of the amount of time a no-flow state has been present. Thus, one would expect to see extensive, widespread necrotic destruction in patients with a no flow-extreme ICP state who are maintained for several days and mosaic-like ischemic destruction in patients who come to autopsy soon. To give an indication of such a correlation, in the Collaborative Study[204,205] a "respirator brain" was more common after 24 hours and occurred in only 7 of 34 (21%) brains examined less than 24 hours after brain death. In order to determine the exact correlation between the degree of necrosis and the amount of time patients without cerebral blood flow are supported in the ICU, a large series of patients with cerebral blood flow studies and detailed neuropathology studies would be required. This variability in neuropathologic findings may have possible consequences in forensic and legal cases. There are no sufficient distinctive neuropathologic characteristics in brain death when brains come to autopsy and are examined thoroughly. Mild ischemic changes (less than 5%) may be seen in some patients (in 2 of 41 autopsies)[215] diagnosed with brain death and some neuropathologists may see a near normal brain and may find it curious to have to write that in the report.

Clinical Examination in Adults

Assessment of brain death in a comatose patient should proceed with the following principles in mind: exclude major confounders, establish the cause of coma, ascertain the futility of any intervention, test the absence of a motor response, accurately document brainstem reflexes at all levels of the brainstem, and determine conclusively the lack of a respiratory drive. Clinical examination should proceed only if certain prerequisites are met. A checklist has been developed (Table 2-1). This section closely follows this step-by-step assessment of determining brain death in a comatose patient.[159,214,216]

TABLE 2-1 *25 Assessments to Declare a Patient Brain Dead*

Prerequisites (ALL MUST BE CHECKED)	
1. Coma, irreversible and cause known	☐
2. Neuroimaging explains coma	☐
3. Sedative drug effect absent	☐
(if indicated, order a toxicology screen)	
4. No residual effect of paralytic drug	☐
(if indicated, use peripheral nerve stimulator)	
5. Absence of severe acid-base, electrolyte, endocrine abnormality	☐
6. Normal or near-normal temperature	☐
(Core temperature ≥36°C)	
7. Systolic blood pressure >100 mm Hg	☐
8. No spontaneous respirations	☐

Examination (ALL MUST BE CHECKED)	
9. Pupils non-reactive to bright light	☐
10. Corneal reflexes absent	☐
11. Eyes immobile, oculocephalic reflexes absent *(tested only if C-spine integrity ensured)*	☐
12. Oculovestibular reflexes absent	☐
13. No facial movement to noxious stimuli	☐
at supraorbital nerve or TMJ. Absent snout or rooting reflexes *(neonates)*	
14. Gag reflex absent	☐
15. Cough reflexes absent to tracheal suctioning	☐
16. No motor response to noxious stimuli in all 4 limbs	☐
(spinally-mediated reflexes are permissible and triple flexion is most common)	

Apnea Testing (ALL MUST BE CHECKED)	
17. Patient is hemodynamically stable, systolic blood pressure ≥ 100 mm Hg	☐
18. Ventilator adjusted to normocapnia ($Paco_2$ 35–45 mm Hg)	☐
19. Patient pre-oxygenated with 100% Fio_2 for 10 minutes (Pao_2 ≥ 200 mm Hg)	☐
20. Patient maintains oxygenation with a PEEP of 5 cm H_2O	☐
21. Disconnect ventilator	☐
22. Provide oxygen via an insufflation catheter to the level of the carina at 6 liters/min or attach T-piece with CPAP valve @ 10 cm H_2O	☐
23. Spontaneous respirations absent	☐
24. ABG drawn at 8–10 minutes, patient reconnected to ventilator	☐
25. $Paco_2$ ≥60 mm Hg, or 20 mm Hg rise from normal baseline value	☐
or	
Apnea test aborted and ancillary test (EEG or blood flow study) confirmatory	☐

Abbreviations: ABG, arterial blood gas; CPAP, continuous positive airway pressure; PEEP, positive end-expiratory pressure; TMJ temporomandibular joint.

Source: Adapted from Wijdicks et al. with permission of *Neurology*.[217]

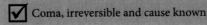 Coma, irreversible and cause known

The cause of coma can usually be established by the history, examination, neuroimaging, and laboratory tests. A certain period of time should have passed since the onset of brain injury to exclude the possibility of recovery (in practice, usually many hours), and the neurologic examination should not be rushed. No physician should determine brain death hours after a patient has entered the emergency room or after transfer from another facility. In these situations, the history is often scanty, use of sedative or analgesic drugs is unknown or unverifiable, and more likely the complete clinical picture (and prognosis) may not be clear at all. Irreversibility is determined by two factors. First, the patient should have been treated aggressively, such as administration of osmotic agents, surgical evacuation of a mass causing displacement of the brainstem (particularly in the cerebellum), ventriculostomy placement, or other measures to reduce ICP.[1] Second, irreversibility is linked to the findings on examination. When the patient meets these criteria—assuming no confounders—the clinical findings are implicitly irreversible. No intervention—medical or surgical—is able to reverse these findings when they present in combination. Mimics, if any, are very uncommon; they are discussed further in Chapter 6. Most commonly, resembling conditions involves profound accidental hypothermia or major drug intoxication and several cases of severe Guillain-Barré syndrome but none are truly identical to the clinical findings seen in brain death.[71,109,151,156,166,194]

✓ Neuroimaging explains coma

In the vast majority of patients, computed tomography (CT) scanning shows a new mass with a profound shift, multiple hemispheric lesions with brain edema, or brain edema alone. Obviously, a CT scan abnormality compatible with brain death does not obviate a search for confounders. Drug or alcohol ingestion may have resulted in a fatal brain injury (e.g., subdural hematoma). Conversely, albeit uncommon, a normal CT scan can be seen early after cardiac or respiratory arrest and in patients with fulminant meningitis or encephalitis. In circumstances of overwhelming infection, examination of cerebrospinal fluid (CSF) should reveal diagnostic findings, such as pleocytosis, an elevated erythrocyte count, or a positive Gram stain. Some viruses, parasites, and bacteria can be detected by polymerase chain reaction (PCR), although not in due time.

Interpretation of the CT scan in a patient suspected of being brain dead requires knowledge of the patterns that are compatible with brain death. For example, in cases of traumatic brain injury, multiple contusions or a subdural or epidural hematoma should be present, displacing the septum pellucidum from its midline position. Effacement of the basal cistern and sulci is a common finding in patients with diffuse, profound cerebral edema (Figure 2-3). When major discrepancies exist between the clinical examination and the CT scan, a repeat CT study is warranted and often will document expansion of the mass, more shift, or edema. If the CT scan remains incongruent with loss of brain function, other confounders should be excluded, particularly drugs or poisons.

✓ Sedative drug effect absent

The presence of a central nervous system-depressing drug effect may be excluded by history, drug screen, and with calculation of clearance using five times

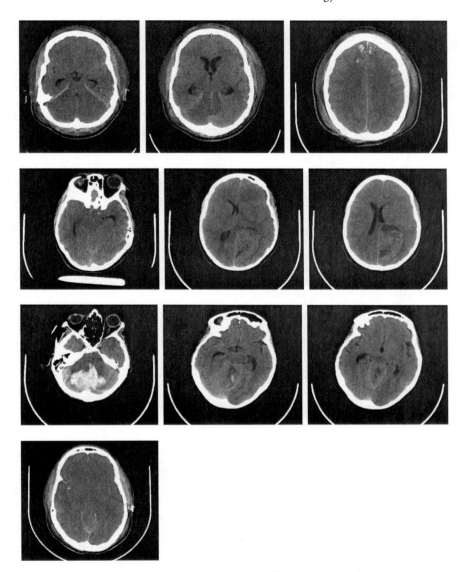

Figure 2-3 Examples of common CT scans abnormalities in brain death. *First row*: traumatic brain injury with anoxic-ischemic injury. *Second row*: tumor with mass effect, obliteration of cisterns, and acute hydrocephalus. *Third row*: massive cerebellar hemorrhage with hydrocephalus. *Fourth row*: diffuse loss of gray matter–white matter differentiation in anoxic-ischemic injury.

the drug's half-life (assuming normal hepatic, renal function, normothermia and no prior therapeutic hypothermia). If possible, drug plasma levels should be measured (Table 2-2). Commonly used drugs include short-acting benzodiazepines and opioids, but the half-life can be prolonged in patients who have

TABLE 2-2 *Half-Life (t½) of Central Nervous System-Depressant Drugs*

Amitriptyline	24 hours
Atracurium	½ hour
Clonazepam	20 hours
Codeine	3 hours
Diazepam	40 hours
Fentanyl	6 hours
Ketamine	2.5 hours
Lorazepam	15 hours
Midazolam	6 hours
Morphine	3 hours
Pancuronium	2 hours
Phenobarbital	100 hours
Primidone	20 hours
Rocuronium	1 hour
Thiopental	20 hours
Vecuronium	2 hours

received therapeutic hypothermia. Doubling the five times half-life rule may be too conservative, and caution is advised, and in a stable just-rewarmed patient, several days of observation may be needed before proceeding with a full examination. In some of these patients with prior use of sedatives and analgesics neurologic examination for brain death should not proceed at all. It is equally important to emphasize that patients with anoxic-ischemic encephalopathy after cardiopulmonary resuscitation often do not meet the criteria of brain death. Thus, when asked to evaluate these patients after therapeutic hypothermia, every physician should anticipate that the patient may not meet these criteria (Chapter 6). The legal alcohol limit for driving (blood alcohol content 0.08%) is a practical threshold with a reliable examination below this level.

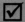 No residual effect of paralytic drug

Muscle relaxants are used with intubation and the effect is shortlived. Its use in surgical and medical ICU's is currently much less frequent due to its serious side effects. When the drug is withdrawn after an infusion, elimination varies. Plasma levels cannot be routinely measured. Absent neuromuscular blocking effect can be confirmed by the presence of four twitches with maximal ulnar nerve stimulation. However more simply, presence of tendon reflexes excludes an important effect of the neuromuscular blockers.[112]

☑ Absence of severe acid-base, electrolyte, and endocrine abnormality

No severe electrolyte or endocrine abnormality should be evident. A major acid-base disturbance may indicate an ingested compound not found on a drug screen. Metabolic acidosis may be seen with acetaminophen, alcohols, salicylates, isoniazid, cyanide, cocaine, strychnine, papaverine, and toluene. Respiratory acidosis is seen with opiates, ethanol, barbiturates, and other anesthetics.

The acidosis seen in some patients may be due to uncoupled oxidative phosphorylation (salicylates), seizures (isoniazid, cocaine), or anaerobic glycolysis (cyanide). Metabolic or respiratory alkalosis is seldom a manifestation of poisoning. Antidotes (naloxone or flumazenil) may need to be administered, but they may not eliminate all the confounding effects. (For further discussion, see Chapter 6.)

☑ Normal or near-normal core temperature ≥ 36°C

The diagnosis of brain death cannot proceed in a markedly hypothermic patient. Brainstem reflexes are generally resistant to hypothermia unless core temperatures decrease below 27°C. All brainstem reflexes may be lost in a profoundly hypothermic patient (<20°C), such as after environmental exposure. The patient with mild hypothermia is usually quite simple to correct, but a warming blanket or direct contact pads may be needed to raise the core bladder temperature to ≥36°C. In addition, to avoid delaying an increase in partial arterial pressure of carbon dioxide ($PaCO_2$)—a result of metabolism—a normal or core temperature is preferred during the apnea test.

☑ Systolic blood pressure >100 mm Hg

A normal blood pressure—systolic blood pressure (SBP) >100 mm Hg—should be achieved, using vasoconstrictive agents such as phenylephrine or vasopressin. Hypotension from loss of peripheral vascular tone or hypovolemia (diabetes insipidus) is common. The neurologic examination is usually reliable with an SBP >100 mm Hg. Clinical examination should not proceed when there is evidence of shock.

☑ No spontaneous respirations

The ventilator should indicate no respirations triggered by the patient. This observation is generally unreliable and a formal apnea test is needed. Conversely, if triggering is present, it may not indicate that the patient is breathing. A brief switch to pressure sensitivity and decreasing sensitivity may be needed to exclude ventilator autocycling (see Chapter 6).

☑ Pupils nonreactive to bright light

The response to bright light should be absent in both eyes. Round, oval, or irregularly shaped pupils are compatible with brain death. Most pupils in brain death are in the midposition (4 to 6 mm) (Figure 2-4).[186] More dilated pupils are compatible with brain death because intact sympathetic cervical spine pathways connected to the radially arranged fibers of the dilator muscle may remain intact.

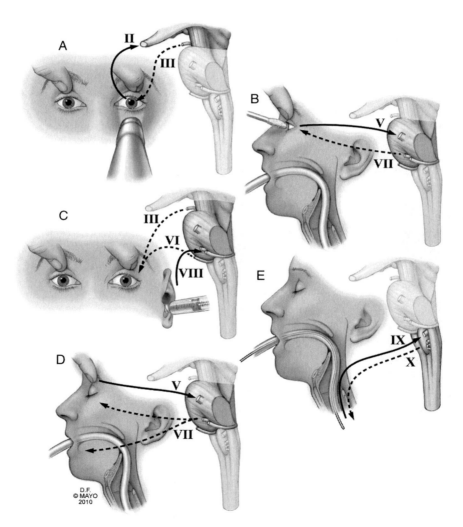

Figure 2-4 (A) Pupil size and light response. (B) Corneal reflexes. (C) Oculovestibular reflexes. (D) No facial movement to pressure on supraorbital nerve. (E) Cough and gag reflex. Roman numerals refer to cranial nerves. *See* Figure 2-4 in the color insert.

Many drugs can influence pupil size, but the light response remains intact. In conventional doses, atropine given intravenously has no marked influence on the pupillary response.[75] Short-term neuromuscular blocking drugs do not noticeably influence pupil size, but a recent report involving escalating doses of atracurium and vecuronium documented reversible mydriasis and, ultimately, nonreactive light responses.[81,181] Topical ocular instillation of drugs and trauma to the cornea or bulbus oculi may cause abnormalities in pupil size and can produce nonreactive pupils. Preexisting anatomic abnormalities of the iris or effects of previous surgery should be excluded.

☑ Corneal reflexes absent

Absent corneal reflexes should be confirmed with squirting water on the cornea or touch with a cotton swab (Figure 2-4B). Blinking requires intact brain stem reflex pathways and is not compatible with brain death. Facial myokymias may be due to muscle contraction from denervation or deafferentation of the facial nucleus and thus are compatible with brain death. Severe facial and ocular trauma may limit or preclude interpretation of these brainstem reflexes.

☑ Eyes immobile, oculocephalic reflexes absent

The eyes are immobile, although they may assume a slightly divergent or skewed position. Mostly they are frozen in the eye socket and thus spontaneous movements (including nystagmus beats) do indicate intact brain stem function. Eye deviation also implies stimulation of either the frontal or pontine eye field. The oculocephalic reflex, elicited by fast turning of the head from the middle position to 90 degrees on both sides, may not be sensitive enough to document the absence of ocular movements.

☑ Oculovestibular reflexes absent

Ocular movements are also absent after caloric testing with ice water (Figure 2-4C). Caloric testing should preferably be done with the head elevated to 30 degrees followed by irrigation of the tympanum on each side. With 30 degrees of elevation, the horizontal canal becomes vertical. Irrigation of the tympanum can best be accomplished by inserting a small suction catheter into the external auditory canal and connecting it to a 50 mL syringe filled with ice water. A cold stimulus results in sedimentation of the endolymph and stimulation of the hair cells. The normal response in a comatose patient is a slow deviation of the eyes directed toward the cold stimulus. The response is absent in brain death. Absent eye movement after caloric testing may be very difficult to appreciate; placement of pen marks on the lower eyelid at the level of the pupil may be helpful. One should allow up to 1 minute of observation after injection, and the time between stimulation on each side should be at least 5 minutes to reduce a possible overriding effect from the opposite irrigated ear.

Clotted blood or cerumen in the ear may diminish the caloric response, and repeat testing is required. It is prudent to inspect the tympanum directly and to document free access with cold water injection. Prior exposure to toxic levels of certain drugs can diminish or completely abolish the caloric response.[189] Typical examples are aminoglycosides, tricyclic antidepressants, anticholinergics, antiepileptic drugs, and chemotherapeutic agents, among others. Such confounders are rarely considered relevant in practice. More commonly, eyelid edema and chemosis of the conjunctiva due to direct trauma may limit movement of the globes. Basal fracture of the petrous bone abolishes the caloric response only unilaterally and may be identified by the presence of an ecchymotic mastoid process (Battle's sign).

☑ No facial movement to noxious stimuli

Absent grimacing to pain can be documented by applying deep pressure with a blunt object on the nail beds, pressure on the supraorbital nerve, or deep pressure on both condyles at the level of the temporomandibular joint (Figure 2-4D). The jaw reflex may be performed. Rooting and sucking reflexes should be absent in neonates.

☑ Cough and gag reflex absent

In orally intubated patients, the gag response may be difficult to interpret and is probably unreliable. Lack of a cough response to bronchial suctioning should be demonstrated by passing a catheter through the endotracheal tube and providing suctioning pressure for several seconds (Figure 2-4E). Although not required as a test, 2 mg atropine will not produce tachycardia. No change in heart rate after suctioning or atropine administration is further confirmation of destruction of the central parasympathetic pathways.

☑ No motor response to noxious stimuli in all 4 limbs

The depth of coma can be assessed by examining motor responses with the use of standard stimuli such as pressure on the supraorbital nerve, nail bed pressure, and temporomandibular joint compression (Figure 2-5). Other stimuli, such as sternal rubbing, rubbing the knuckles against the ribs in the axilla, twisting the forearm or nipples, and applying pin pricks on several body locations, may be equally effective but have not been accepted as the norm.

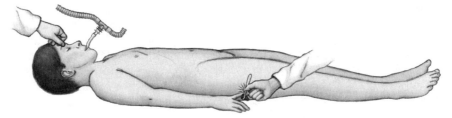

Figure 2-5 Motor responses to stimuli is absent (nailbed and supraorbital nerve compression). *See* Figure 2-5 in the color insert.

Noxious stimuli should produce no motor response other than spinally mediated reflexes (Figure 2-5) Motor responses may be absent due to a severed cervical cord, which may be suggested on a plain x-ray.[207] The clinical differentiation of spinal responses from retained motor responses associated with brain activity requires expertise (Chapter 6).

Motor responses may occur spontaneously, after stimulation, and during apnea testing, particularly when hypoxemia or hypotension appears. These spinal responses include brief, slow movements in the upper limbs, flexion in the fingers, fine finger tremors,[10] or arm lifting, and they do not become integrated into coordinated decerebrate or decorticate responses.[33,42,134,171,178] They extinguish with repeated stimulation. Ocular "micro tremors" and eyelid opening have been incidentally noted.[26,177,178] Slow head turning to one side has been observed but again is extremely rare.[38]

Vermicular twitching resembling fascilations have been noted on pectoralis, arm and abdominal muscles and are likely generated from ischemic anterior horns cells in the spinal cord.[21] Plantar reflexes are usually absent, although some toe flexion may occur, often in combination with a triple flexion response.[91,110,137,222] The Babinski sign is mostly absent.[43]

■ THE APNEA TEST

Apneic oxygenation-diffusion is the most commonly used technique to demonstrate lack of ventilatory drive.[5,23,63,104] This diagnostic tool involves placement of a source of 100% oxygen in the trachea, which, through convection, results in a flow of oxygen into the lungs.[53] Preoxygenation eliminates the nitrogen stores in the respiratory tract and facilitates oxygen transport. On the basis of animal experiments and clinical observations, a target $PaCO_2$ of 60 mm Hg has been proposed as the level at which the respiratory centers are maximally stimulated. However, it has been assumed that the respiratory centers are reset higher due to malfunction from brainstem injury.[95,160] The target, therefore, may be much lower, because in the few reported patients who started to breathe after disconnection of the ventilator, many $PaCO_2$ levels were in the 30–40 mm Hg range (Chapter 6). Breathing can be easily detected by noticing chest expansion, clavicle elevation, and abdominal excursions, but it may be a single brief gasp that may or may not return during the short testing period.

The increase in PaCO$_2$ is biphasic, with a steep increase in the first minutes due to equilibration of arterial carbon dioxide with mixed central venous carbon dioxide. During the apnea test, oxygen flow ensures uptake of oxygen in pulmonary capillaries, but carbon dioxide exhalation does not take place and therefore there is a rapid rise of PaCO$_2$ due to metabolic production of carbon dioxide.[58,65,90] An increase in PaCO$_2$ results in a decrease in CSF pH, which is sensed by the respiratory centers in the medulla oblongata and, when they function, results in a respiratory drive.[30,133] This rapid increase in PaCO$_2$ to 60 mm Hg or 20 mm Hg above normal baseline maximally stimulates these centers, also because CSF is unable to buffer acidosis with bicarbonate owing to its slower diffusion than carbon dioxide.

Many neurointensivists and neurosurgeons prefer disconnection of the ventilator and use of oxygen flow through an endotracheally placed catheter.[168,173] The method is free from hindrances and simple. In addition to monitoring of oxygen saturation, pulse, and blood pressure, visual inspection of thoracic and abdominal movement is required. This is the only way to ensure adequate testing for apnea and to reduce artifact reading of breathing on the ventilator display.[214]

An approach that can be inconvenient is switching the ventilator to a CPAP mode and monitoring for apnea. Most modern ICU ventilators have a maximum apnea time of 60 seconds. The ventilator would go into a backup volume or pressure controlled mode of ventilation and this cannot be turned off. Moreover, interpretation of flow and pressure wave forms on the ventilator display remains difficult and distinquishing artificial CPAP breathing from true breathing requires a particular expertise.

Another group has suggested a possibly attractive method of carbon dioxide augmentation to reduce observation time, but an overshoot to potentially dangerous hypercarbia is a concern.[122,123] Monitoring carbon dioxide by using a transcutaneous device may reduce carbon dioxide target overshoot, but discrepancies between transcutaneous and arterial carbon dioxide may be substantial.[124,199] This method however can be considered in patients on extracorporeal membrane oxygenation (Chapter 6).

Alternatively, manipulating PaCO$_2$ upward by using hypoventilation with end-tidal carbon dioxide monitoring devices has been suggested. It can be cumbersome, not only because of the inability to predict PaCO$_2$ but also because the method may lead to gradual CSF buffering and thus failure to produce acute acidosis in the CSF compartment.

Testing for apnea in a patient with otherwise absent brainstem reflexes is standard, and a positive test (no breathing with target PaCO$_2$) confirms brain death. The procedure, however, has generated some debate. The arguments against the apnea test are as follows. First, in the event of preserved respiration, the outcome is similar. True, no report has been published of an adult patient who, with otherwise absent brainstem reflexes but spontaneous breathing, "recovers" to a persistent vegetative state or better. However, physicians have a responsibility to declare a patient brain dead if this is very likely (for legal issues, Chapter 6). Moreover, the apnea test determines whether the organ donor—assuming consent—will follow a donation after cardiac death (DCD) or a donation after brain death (DBD) protocol. The two procurement protocols are very different (Chapter 5).

Second, the procedure may induce hypotension and hypoxemia, which potentially may render organs unsuitable for transplantation. There are no data in the transplant literature to support this contention. The apnea test may be very difficult to perform—because of failure to assure adequate oxygenation—in patients with marginal lung function due to contusion or pulmonary edema. Some have argued, and incorrectly so, that hypoxemia or acidosis will result in the death of some viable neurons and thus cause brain death (Chapter 4).[39]

 Conditions for the apnea test are acceptable

The apnea test is generally safe with careful precautions. First, hypothermia should be avoided. In hypothermia, carbon dioxide production may be delayed because of decreased metabolism. Moreover, in hypothermia, the oxyhemoglobin dissociation curve shifts to the left, resulting in decreased oxygen release. Second, persistent hypotension should be corrected, which often requires a bolus of 5% albumin or an increase in administration of intravenous dopamine. It is prudent to have 100 μg phenylephrine available in the event blood pressure declines, but it is rarely needed. A blood pressure of 90 to 100 mm Hg is probably acceptable before an apnea test. Before disconnection from the ventilator, the positive endexpiratory pressure (PEEP) requirement should be reduced to 5 cm water. If this does not lead to oxygen desaturation, maintenance of oxygenation during oxygen insufflation can be expected.

At the start of the apnea test, a $PaCO_2$ within the normal range (35 to 45 mm Hg) is preferred. One can expect the $PaCO_2$ to increase 3 to 6 mm Hg per minute.[57] If one adheres to these strict conditions, the apnea test is generally safe (Figure 2-6).

 Insert the oxygen insufflation catheter, providing oxygen at a rate of 6 L/min after disconnecting the ventilator

An oxygen insufflation catheter has an advantage over a suction catheter. With an oxygen insufflation catheter (Figure 2-7), the position can be more exactly determined. (Usually it is placed 1 cm beyond the tip of the endotracheal tube.) This will avoid traumatic injury as a result of placement and possibly even a pneumothorax. In the first minutes after insertion, oxygenation should be watched closely before proceeding.

 No breathing with the apnea test

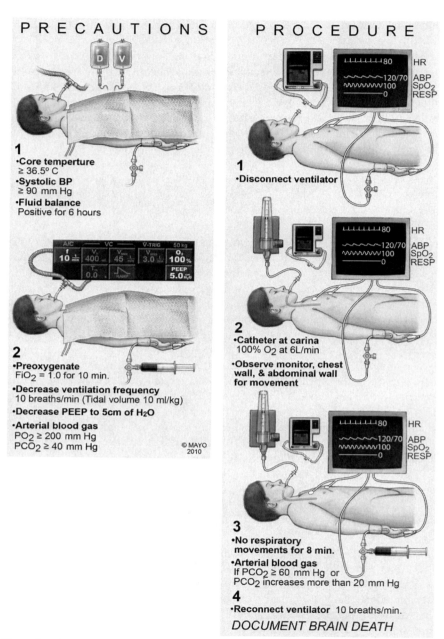

PRECAUTIONS

1
•Core temperture
≥ 36.5° C
•Systolic BP
≥ 90 mm Hg
•Fluid balance
Positive for 6 hours

AC   VC   V-TRIG   50 kg
f 10 $\frac{1}{min}$ V_t 400 V_{max} 45 $\frac{L}{min}$ V_{sens} 3.0 O_2 100%
T_h 0.0   RAMP   PEEP 5.0 $\frac{cm}{H_2O}$

2
•Preoxygenate
FiO_2 = 1.0 for 10 min.
•Decrease ventilation frequency
10 breaths/min (Tidal volume 10 ml/kg)
•Decrease PEEP to 5cm of H_2O
•Arterial blood gas
PO_2 ≥ 200 mm Hg
PCO_2 ≥ 40 mm Hg

© MAYO 2010

PROCEDURE

80   HR
120/70   ABP
100   SpO_2
0   RESP

1
•Disconnect ventilator

80   HR
120/70   ABP
100   SpO_2
0   RESP

2
•Catheter at carina
100% O_2 at 6L/min
•Observe monitor, chest
wall, & abdominal wall
for movement

80   HR
120/70   ABP
100   SpO_2
0   RESP

3
•No respiratory
movements for 8 min.
•Arterial blood gas
If PCO_2 ≥ 60 mm Hg or
PCO_2 increases more than 20 mm Hg

4
•Reconnect ventilator 10 breaths/min.

DOCUMENT BRAIN DEATH

Figure 2-6 Apnea test procedure. *See* Figure 2-6 in the color insert.

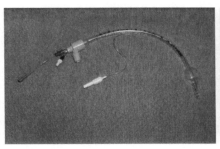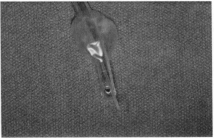

Figure 2-7 Oxygen insufflation catheter. Note the tip of the catheter just out of the endotracheal tube. The port jet ventilator adaptor has an insufflation catheter that is measured from the distal tip approximately 1 cm beyond the end of the endotracheal tube and is estimated to be just above the carina. This will prevent injury and a sandblasting effect. *See* Figure 2-7 in the color insert.

When the $PaCO_2$ is in the normal range, 8 minutes of disconnection should be sufficient to reach the target level of 60 mm Hg or to produce an increase of 20 mm Hg.[133] Apnea is determined by visual inspection only. Visual inspection of the rib cage and abdomen typically may show minimal movement synchronous with the heartbeat; less frequently, there is some intercostal retraction in the upper thorax. If breathing occurs and is constant, the patient should be reconnected to the ventilator to measure the tidal volume.

In our experience with the oxygen-diffusion technique, the apnea test was safe; it was aborted in only 3% of 212 tests. The expected changes of arterial pH, PCO_2, and PO_2 are shown in Figure 2-8. The mean arterial pH decreased from 7.38 to 7.18, the mean arterial PCO_2 increased from 40 to 70 mm Hg, and the PO_2 decreased from 265 to 236 mm Hg.[216]

Hypotension is the most common complication of the apnea test, and the patient should be reconnected to the ventilator when SBP drops precipitously to 70 mm Hg.[79,103,210,219] Failure to preoxygenate remains an important cause of hypotension during apnea testing.[79] However the induced acidosis may reduce myocardial contractility, usually when pH reaches 7.2. Moderate hypercapnia associated with respiratory acidosis does not induce ventricular dysfunction as measured by transesophageal echocardiography.[149] Hypotension without hypoxemia during the apnea test often indicates that the $PaCO_2$ has significantly exceeded 60 mm Hg. Cardiac arrest resulting from the procedure is extremely rare and we have noted only 1 instance in over 350 procedures. Cardiac arrhythmias generally occur in patients in whom hypoxemia is not corrected with oxygen supplementation during the apnea test. Patients who have had cardiac arrhythmias during the evolution of the neurologic catastrophe may not have them during the apnea test, and their presence should not preclude apnea testing. When hypoxemia occurs despite adequate preoxygenation and oxygen supply, some have suggested to retry the procedure with a T-piece, CPAP valve of 10 cm water, and 100% oxygen at a rate of 12 L/minute (Chapter 6).[129]

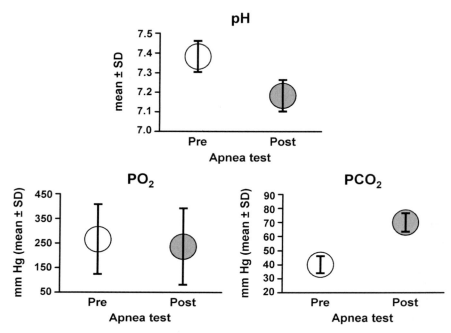

Figure 2-8 Changes in arterial pH, PCO_2, or PO_2 during the apnea test. Circles are group means; error bars represent SD. All differences were statistically significant ($p < 0.05$). From Wijdicks et al.[216] with permission of *Neurology*.

■ ANCILLARY TESTS IN ADULTS WITH BRAIN DEATH

In the earlier days of refining criteria for the clinical state of brain death, there was a desire to show additional absent electrical function or absent blood flow to the brain, which by implication would mean neuronal death. As early as 1942, animal experiments showed that acutely increased ICP results in disappearance of electroencephalogram (EEG) when the ICP exceeds the blood pressure.[69] Later studies documented the failure to opacify the intracranial vessels with contrast medium in patients who had increased ICP.[86,130] A correlation with the clinical examination was not apparent in the medical literature until the clinical diagnosis of brain death was better defined by the French neurologists Mollaret and Goulon[80] and by the Ad Hoc Committee of the Harvard Medical School.[2] Thereafter, investigators used cerebral angiography to make the diagnosis of "angiographic brain death."

However, before angiographic studies became a way of documenting absent intracranial flow, the EEG was considered the most important laboratory test.[4,67]

In the United States, the EEG became part of the clinical examination of these patients after publication of the Harvard Criteria (Chapter 1). Several EEG studies were used to support its use in the determination of brain death and details were published later.[187,188] The American Neurological Association in 1977 stated

TABLE 2-3 *Emerging Ancillary Tests in Brain Death*

Study Year and Authors	Ancillary Test
1959 Löfstedt and von Reis[130]	Cerebral angiogram
1959 Fischgold and Mathis[67]	EEG
1969 Goodman et al.[78]	Nuclear brain scan
1974 Yoneda et al.[220]	TCD
1976 Starr[192]	BAEP
1978 Rappaport et al.[163]	CT angiogram
1978 Rangel[162]	CT angiogram
1981 Goldie et al.[77]	SSEP
1992 Jones and Barnes[107]	MRI

Abbreviations: BAEP, brainstem auditory evoked potential; CT, computed tomogram; EEG, electroencephalogram; MRI, magnetic resonance imaging; SSEP, somatosensory evoked potential; TCD, transcranial Doppler.

Source: From Wijdicks.[213] Used with permission of *Neurology*.

that the EEG was "a valuable confirmatory indicator of brain death and its use is strongly recommended."

The report of the medical consultants on the diagnosis of death to the President's Commission for the Study of the Ethical Problems in Medicine and Biomedical and Behavioral Research expanded on the usefulness of the EEG and the cerebral blood flow test.[88] It added that electrocerebral silence or cessation of cerebral blood flow could reduce the time of observation.

During the years since that report appeared, additional ancillary tests have been introduced in the medical literature. It may be a contradiction of our time not to rely entirely on technologic devices to confirm brain death, but these tests have only been used to confirm the clinical examination or have been used when there are some uncertainties about the reliability of certain aspects of the examination, and in situations when the apnea test could not be performed (Table 2-3).

The tests can be divided into those that evaluate neuronal function and those that assess blood flow. Electrophysiologic tests along with an EEG with specific settings include early component evoked potentials, auditory evoked potentials, and somatosensory evoked potentials. Tests of brain blood flow include a four-vessel cerebral angiogram, a transcranial Doppler (TCD) ultrasonographic scan,

TABLE 2-4 *Current Recommendations to Determine an Isoelectric EEG in Brain Death*

- A minimum of eight scalp electrodes
- Interelectrode impedances between 100 and 10,000 Ω
- Interelectrode distance of at least 10 cm
- Sensitivity increase up to 2 V and time constant of 0.3 to 0.4 second
- High frequency filter > 30 Hz
- Low frequency filter <1 Hz
- Recording of 30 minutes
- Testing of EEG reactivity to noxious stimuli and flashlight

Abbreviation: EEG, electroencephalogram.

Source: American Electroencephalographic Society.

TABLE 2-5 *Criteria for Interpretation of Cerebral Perfusion Scintigraphy in Brain Death*

- Flow images show lack of flow to the middle cerebral artery, the anterior cerebral artery, and the posterior cerebral artery.
- Lack of tracer activity in the superior sagittal sinus during venous phase of flow study.
- Tracer flow is present from the carotid arteries to the skull vertex.
- Blood flow superior to the circle of Willis circulation is completely absent.
- Delayed images show no tracer uptake in the brain.
- CSF shunts and ICP monitoring system can cause hyperemia and increased scalp flow, causing a false-negative study.
- Color tables may underrepresent low activity, causing a false-positive study (gray scale is preferred).

Abbreviations: CSF, cerebrospinal fluid; ICP, intracranial pressure.

Source: Adapted from Donohoe et al.[50]

a magnetic resonance angiogram, a CT angiogram, and a nuclear brain scan. Each of these tests has difficulties, and none have been rigorously validated.

Recent tests include the bispectral index scale (a mathematical algorithm of the EEG),[60,200] venous oxygen saturation in the jugular bulb,[48] and brain tissue oxygenation.[153] More studies are expected, with the new technology aiming to show direct (electrical activity) or indirect (no blood flow) loss of neuronal functioning.

Cerebral angiography,[7,84,179] EEG,[85] transcranial ultrasonography,[157] and cerebral perfusion scintigraphy (nuclear scan) can be useful ancillary tests.[221] Validation of most of these tests is lacking, and in the United States, only consensus papers on EEG and nuclear scanning have been published (Tables 2-4 to 2-6).

Unfortunately, situations arise in which an ancillary test is performed before the formal clinical evaluation for possible brain death. In certain circumstances, an ancillary test may show the presence of blood flow or EEG activity despite the absence of all brain function. This occurs in patients in whom ancillary tests were performed very early in the determination of brain death, particularly in those in whom the mechanism was something other than increased ICP.[32] It is appropriate not to rely on technical confirmatory tests when their findings are at odds with those of a clinical neurologic examination (Chapter 6).

The most commonly used ancillary tests are shown in Figure 2-9. Flow studies are aimed at documenting no intracranial flow.[34,102,155] A cerebral angiogram using

TABLE 2-6 *Criteria to Determine Absent Cerebral Blood Flow by TCD in Brain Death*

- Confirmation of cerebral circulatory arrest with extra- and intracranial Doppler sonography, bilaterally on two examinations 30 minutes apart.
- Systolic spikes or oscillating flow in any cerebral artery (anterior and posterior).
- Diagnosis established by intracranial examination must be confirmed by the extracranial bilateral recording of the common carotid, internal carotid, and vertebral arteries.
- Disappearance of intracranial flow signals together with typical extracranial signs can be accepted as proof of circulatory arrest when no intracranial signal is found.
- Exclusion of patients with ventricular drains or large craniotomy.

Abbreviation: TCD, transcranial Doppler.

Source: Adapted from Ducrocq et al.[55]

the Seldinger technique through the femoral artery should document nonfilling of intracranial arteries. Increased ICP leads to increased cerebral vascular resistance, extreme slowing of flow, and circulatory arrest. Perivascular glial swelling and subintimal bleb formation from ischemia cause collapse of the smaller vessels, leading to increased cerebrovasular resistance. Another mechanism of absent intracranial flow is destruction of the intracerebral vascular tree in conjunction with necrosis of the brain.

The following anatomy needs to be understood. The common carotid artery commonly bifurcates at C3-C4 into the internal and external portions. The carotid bifurcation to the skull base is called the cervical segment until it enters the carotid canal. The petrous segment ascends 1 cm, then becomes horizontal until it enters the intracranial space at the foramen lacerum. The carotid artery then continues as the cavernous segment. The vertebral artery pierces the dura after traversing the atlanto-occipital membrane; this transition can sometimes be seen as a smooth band on a normal film. The carotid circulation will demonstrate circulatory arrest first, but the vertebral circulation can still show filling. This can be due to a supratentorial mass that has not transferred pressure to the posterior fossa, resulting in cerebellar tonsillar herniation.[96]

Contrast is injected under high pressure into both the anterior and posterior circulations. With current standardized injection force, it is unlikely that flow can

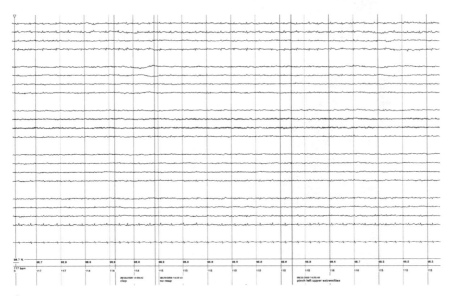

A

Figure 2-9 Examples of electrophysiologic tests and flow studies. (A) Isoelectric EEG but EKG artifact. (*Continues*)

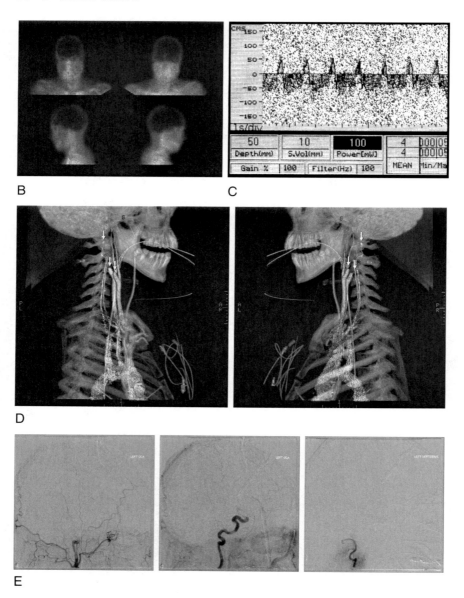

Figure 2-9 (Continued) (B) Nuclear scan showing absent intracranial uptake. (C) Transcranial Doppler ultrasound showing reverberating flow. (D) CTA showing absent intracranial flow in both vertebral and carotid circulation (arrows). (E) Cerebral angiogram showing flow mostly in the extracranial circulation, barely filling the syphon and no intracranial posterior circulation.

be artificially created by increasing the injection pressure. Normally, the intracranial arteries fill first (low-resistance system), followed by the external arteries (high-resistance system). This order is reversed with brain death.[102,155] Arch aortography with lateral and anteroposterior views will show the contrast column in the carotids, usually arresting abruptly at the level of the skull base in the petrous region of the internal carotid arteries. It should not fill beyond the siphon.[118] The external carotid circulation remains patent and fills rapidly and early, as opposed to slow filling of the remaining portion of the carotid circulation. The vertebral system will opacify from the aortic arch injection and a selective vertebral artery injection is not needed. The dye column in the vertebral artery arrests at the atlan-to-occipital junction, and the contrast level may reach C1 to C2 in 50% of patients. Delayed visualization of the superior sagittal sinus results from perfusion through meningeal vessels from the external carotid artery supply or from emissary veins. Some protocols consider at least two injections of contrast medium given at an interval of 20–30 minutes to establish persistently absent flow to the brain and, by implication, total brain necrosis. Criteria for confirmation of brain death using cerebral angiography have not been developed by neuroradiologic societies.[25,28]

The CT angiogram is widely used in the United States, Europe, and Canada. Its validity has been insufficiently tested.[11,41,56,59,161,162,163] Studies have often found residual opacified cerebral arteries. There are few comparative studies with the cerebral angiogram, the nuclear scan, and EEG, although a specificity of 100% has been found.[24,70] The study appears to be helpful if flow is not detected or even if it stops before entry into the dura, but filling of callosal and basilar arteries may occur in 6% to 50% of studies. False-positive CT angiography results have been reported.[82]

TCD is a validated ancillary test, with sensitivity varying from 91% to 99% and with a specificity of 100%.[44,51,54,121,144,157,158,159,165,172,196,220,223] A Doppler device probe is used with insonating of both middle cerebral arteries through the temporal bone above the zygomatic arch. Absent flow intracranially may be due to transmission difficulties and may occur in 10–20% of patients. In brain death, the typical TCD signals, produced by the contractive forces of the arteries, are oscillating flow, defined by signals with forward and reverse flow components in one cardiac cycle.[64,89,94,114,119] Most of the time, small (less than 50 cm/second) peaks in early systole, indicating very high vascular resistance, are recorded. The pulsatility index is very high. All these TCD patterns indirectly indicate increased ICP.[145] The major advantages of this device are its portability and the growing expertise of attending neurointensivists and neurosurgeons who may perform this study without being dependent on other technical resources.

Cerebral scintigraphy or nuclear scan is a widely available test. A single-detector rotating gamma camera is used with capabilities for monitoring and mechanical ventilation. A tracer isotope is injected intravenously 15 to 30 minutes before scanning.[27,40,50,61,72,120,126,141,164,169,182,209,218] Serial pictures are taken as part of a dynamic study, followed by lateral and anterior static images and a three-dimensional image with good spatial resolution. In patients clinically diagnosed as brain dead, arrest of cerebral circulation is found in 96% of cases;[68,78] in the remaining cases, perfusion may persist in the thalamus and brain stem, particularly in children. Absent uptake

produces a characteristic "hollow skull" or "empty light bulb" sign. Increased external flow may result in enhancement of the nose ("hot nose sign"). Absent uptake is a
reflection of absent intracranial flow due to a marked terminal rise in ICP, which was
confirmed in 22 patients with concomitant ICP recording.[116,117] Correlation with
cerebral angiogram and TCD is excellent.[145]

Tracer injection may be inaccurate, but it can be checked with imaging of
spleen uptake or assessment of the nuclear activity of the carotid arteries. Nuclear
scanning requires a specialist in nuclear medicine for interpretation and quality
control. It is not often available on an urgent basis, and both false negatives and
false positives have been noted.[92,106]

The EEG has been used in the determination of brain death in many countries,
and it remains an important ancillary test.[22] Usually, a 16- or 18-channel instrument
is used, and recordings are obtained for at least 30 minutes. Typically, electrical
activity is absent above 2 μV.[8,108] There are, however, several examples of abnormal
but existing EEG activity that continued for several hours to days.[47,203] In one
consecutive study of patients who fulfilled the clinical criteria of brain death, 20%
of 56 patients had residual EEG activity that lasted up to 168 hours. In general,
the sensitivity as well as the specificity of EEG is 90%. It should be noted that
artifacts from devices used in the ICU are common as a result of the high gain
amplification.[99] The EEG, because of its wide availability, remains a preferred
ancillary test.

Both brain stem auditory evoked potentials (BAEP) and somatosensory evoked
potentials (SSEP) have been studied as potential confirmatory tests in brain
death.[9,31,35,36] Initial enthusiasm was fostered by examples of patients in a drug-
induced coma, appearing clinically to be brain dead, who had isoelectric EEGs but
no change in the individual evoked components. Evoked potentials became a
possible indicator of brainstem function in patients with major head trauma and
barbiturate use.

Brainstem auditory evoked potentials are generated by means of bedside
equipment with click intensity set at 65 dB with a 10/second stimulus repetition
rate provided by earphones.[77,192] It is necessary to identify wave I from the ipsilat-
eral ear electrode to prove an intact auditory nerve, which can be destroyed as a
result of cochlear trauma. Waves II and III identify the cochlear nucleus and
superior olivary complex, and waves IV and V locate the upper pons; therefore,
absence of waves II through V indicates profound brainstem dysfunction.[77,132]

Brainstem auditory evoked potentials are generated within the pons and do
not measure tracts in the medulla oblongata. They do not correlate well with the
severity of brain injury.[66,73] Patients in a persistent vegetative state have normal
BAEPs, and brain-dead patients may have identifiable waveforms. Patients have
been noted to have absent waves II to V after severe traumatic brain injury or
devastating anoxic-ischemic encephalopathy yet intact brainstem reflexes.
Another concern is the limited number of studies with detailed clinical and
laboratory correlation.

Somatosensory evoked potentials are recorded at several sites, including the
cervical spine and centroparietal areas, with stimulation of the median nerve at the
wrist at a rate of 5 Hz. Typically, approximately 2000 responses are averaged, and

the evoked potentials are amplified and filtered between 5 and 1500 Hz.[193] The recorded potentials most likely travel through the proprioceptive pathway in the spinal cord dorsal column to the medial lemniscus and to the primary somatosensory cortex. The cortical wave N20 is typically absent in brain death but is also bilaterally undetectable in approximately 15% to 20% of patients who are comatose but not brain dead.[93] Recent studies suggest that disappearance of the P14 wave (at the bulbomedullary junction or cuneate nucleus) may be helpful. Distinction from artifacts is difficult, and a nasopharyngeal electrode recording of P14 may enhance its detection, only to disappear when brain death occurs.[201,202] Experience is limited.

Others have directed attention to the value of the N18 potential possibly generated in the cuneate nucleus, but it was also absent in 3 of 20 comatose patients who were not brain dead.[190] The relatively poor predictive value of the N18 potential casts doubt on the use of BAEP or SSEP as a standard ancillary test for brain death.[170,183]

The increased ease of use of magnetic resonance imaging (MRI) has resulted in a few single-case reports of patients who met the criteria for brain death. Axial T_1- and T_2-weighted MRI with spin-echo techniques, including three-dimensional time-of-flight fast imaging, have been reported. The MR findings include transtentorial or tonsillar herniation, lack of intracranial flow void, poor gray matter–white matter differentiation, and marked contrast enhancement of the nose and scalp.[139,150] Proton density and T_2-weighted MRI can show dissociated intensity changes between gray and white matter.[101,107,113,127,136] MR angiography in a patient who meets the criteria of brain death does not show intracranial vessels above the skull base similar to a conventional angiogram. There is very limited experience with MRI, and often studies have been interpreted retrospectively.

The practical problems with the use of ancillary tests are discussed in more detail in Chapter 6.

■ THE CLINICAL DETERMINATION OF BRAIN DEATH IN CHILDREN

Traumatic brain injury and anoxic-ischemic injury from asphyxia are the main causes of brain death in children.[76] Abuse is a common occurrence in neonates who become brain death and, as expected, in adolescence motor vehicle accidents in young drivers are prevalent. Pediatric brain death was carefully defined by a multidisciplinary task force in 1987[2,87,143] and has been currently updated in 2011 by the Society of Critical Care Medicine (SCCM) and the American Academy of Pediatrics (AAP) (Table 2-7). The SCCM/AAP guidelines for determination of brain death in children are very similar to adults (i.e., neurologic examination beyond 2 months) but also very different from those in adults (i.e., time of observation and number of examinations).

The neurologic examination in neonates and children is comparable to that in adults, but there are differences in preterm infants.[12-17,18,20,52,62,138,152,174,184] The landmarks of neurologic examination in newborns are shown in Figure 2-10. Moreover, any pediatrician or pediatric neurologist or neurosurgeon should be aware of the

TABLE 2-7 *New Pediatric Brain Death Guidelines as Proposed by the Society of Critical Care Medicine and the American Academy of Pediatrics*[143]

Newborn up to 30 days	Two separate examinations 24 hours apart, two different examiners
From 30 days to 18 years	Two separate examinations 12 hours apart, two different examiners
Ancillary tests	There might be indications to do ancillary tests (e.g., uncertainty or inability to complete exam/apnea testing). EEG/CBF studies are suggested, with preference given to CBF.

Abbreviations: CBF, cerebral blood flow; EEG, electroencephalogram.
Used with permission of SCCM.

difficulty of visualizing pupil responses (smaller size in newborns), corneal reflexes (less responsive due to dehydration), and caloric testing (narrow ear canal). Generally, corneal reflexes can be obtained, but some neonates have a small palpebral fissure, making it difficult to obtain the reflex. Facial trauma or swelling may be substantial, virtually prohibiting accurate assessment of these reflexes. Testing of brain stem reflexes also includes assessment of sucking and rooting reflexes. The rooting and sucking reflexes are present in normal neonates. The rooting reflex consists of turning the head to bring the mouth toward the finger of the examiner, alternately placed at both corners of the mouth and at the top and bottom lips. Infants typically demonstrate a traction response after grasping the examiner's fingers, but none is present. The Moro reflex with arm extension to a loud noise or a blow to the surface where the infant lies is absent. The tonic neck reflex requires intact labyrinthal control and is absent. The apnea test is similar to that in adults, and the PaCO$_2$ targets are comparable (questions about an increased apnea threshold are addressed in Chapter 6).[29,197] Hypotension and diabetes insipidus are not very different from those in adults.[152]

The criteria for the determination of brain death diverge from adult guidelines when it comes to the number of examinations. Most similarities are found in

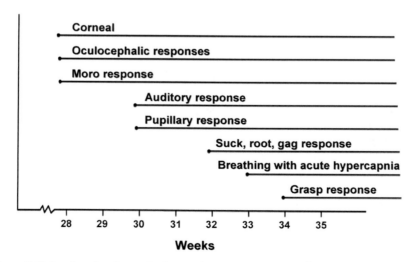

Figure 2-10 Landmarks of neurologic examination in preterm infants.

children 1 year of age or older and adults. In this time bracket the SCCM/AAP guidelines, however, require two examinations 12 hours apart by two different attending physicians although the apnea test may be performed by the same physician. The first examination determines brain death, the second examination, according to the SCCM/AAP guidelines, proves irreversibility.[143] The SCCM/AAP guideline also stipulates a 24-hour waiting period before examination when "there are concerns or inconsistencies in the examination." The SCCM/AAP states that physicians should be competent to perform examinations in infants and neonates; it also recommends that these examinations should be performed by pediatric intensivists and neonatologists, pediatric neurologists and neurosurgeons, pediatric trauma surgeons, and pediatric anesthesiologists with critical care training. In addition, the SCCM/AAP guidelines state that adult specialists should have appropriate neurologic and critical care training to diagnose brain death when caring for patients from birth to 18 years of age.[143]

Experience with electrodiagnostic tests and flow studies in children have been widely published.[3,6,14,18,19,175,180] There is a trend toward the use of cerebral blood flow studies rather than electrodiagnostic tests.[98,185] TCD and evoked potentials have also been used in infants.[175] Few studies have been published on children alone and most studies have incorporated children, making it difficult to separate the findings in children from those in adults.

As in tests involving adults, false-positive and false-negative results have been noted. A false-negative test is more common in children (estimated at 30%) and false negative studies are less common after cerebral blood flow studies (estimated at 15%). The sensitivity of an ancillary test is lowest in neonates. Moreover, a considerable proportion of neonates may have suffered anoxic-ischemic injury without cerebral edema maintaining cerebral blood flow. In one recent single photon emission computed tomography (SPECT) study in newborns, the EEG was isoelectric with perfusion on SPECT in 2 of 8 patients. The SPECT study was without flow after a second test several days later.[148] A recent study found that fontanelle compression with TCD could produce typical reverberating flow.[198]

The SCCM/AAP guidelines on pediatric brain death correctly emphasizes clinical evaluation. Most concerning in the SCCM/AAP recommendations is the inclusion of adolescents (13–18 years) in the 12 hour observation time bracket. Two examinations may unnecessarily prolong the declaration of brain death. Loss of organ donation is possible due to premature cardiac arrest from prolonged waiting for the second examination. Some families want closure and do not want to wait any longer and will refuse organ donation. The SCCM/AAP guideline however allows ancillary tests when it supports the clinical diagnosis of brain death to reduce the time of observation but 2 examinations are still needed. The SCCM/AAP recommendations including certain physician specialties are arguably restrictive.

For years, physicians have been wary of even diagnosing brain death in neonates and children (in fact, until fairly recently, it was not allowed in Japan). The concern was simple; it involved uncertainty by the physician about the plasticity of the young child's brain and difficulty with accepting the irreversibility of a combination of certain signs after a major insult. Similarly, families may have much more reluctance emotionally in accepting the death of a child compared to an adult, and some may not understand the clinical situation at all. To illustrate that further acceptance rates for both DCD and DBD protocols and organ donation are generally lower in children than in adults, although conversion rates are higher in hospitals with level 1 trauma programs or pediatric critical care fellowship programs.[208] The organ short fall in pediatric transplantation is more pronounced than in adults with loss of donors due to lack of referral (approximately 10%) and medical examiner denial.[208]

■ DOCUMENTATION

The time of brain death is documented in the medical records.[111,135,206] When patients meet all criteria, the time of death is the time when the arterial PCO_2 reached the target value. In patients with an aborted apnea test, the time of death is when the ancillary test has been officially interpreted. A checklist is filled out, signed, and dated. Federal and state laws require the physician to contact an organ procurement organization following determination of brain death. Accurate and time-sensitive brain death diagnosis by the neurologist may impact the availability of much-needed organs available for transplantation.

■ ERRORS AND ALLEGED RECOVERIES

Now and then, reports in the media surface suggesting that a patient recovered from brain death. These spurious reports become even more problematic if the involved health care providers proclaim it as a "miracle." Possible explanations for "recoveries" from brain death are shown in Table 2-8.[167,211]

Most commonly, family members are told that the patient may be brain dead and organ donation is considered. Occasionally, there may be a premature discussion to inquire about consent on the patient's driver's license. When the patient then improves, families may have assumed that the patient was brain dead. Proclaiming the patient's improvement to be a miraculous recovery would also relieve the health care team from the need to provide an explanation.

No cases of recovery from brain death in adults have been published since the publication of a single report of improvement after midbasilar artery occlusion. The clinical features did not fit the criteria for brain death.[115] A recent study summarized 11 cases of "purported reversal of findings of brain death" from 1972

TABLE 2-8 *Explanations for "Recoveries" from Brain Death*

- Premature discussion of brain death by the treating physician or premature discussion with OPOs.
- Inadequate assessment of confounding factors (e.g., unresuscitated shock, lingering drugs).
- Incomplete examination (e.g., failure to perform the apnea test).
- Reliance on a (false-positive) laboratory test.
- Misinterpretation of recovery (e.g., return of respiratory drive not recognized as ventilator self-cycling).

OPO: organ procurement organization.

to 2009[105] involving 3 adults and 8 children (the latter mostly neonates and all under 10 months of age). In all cases, the neurologic examination was incomplete (no documentation of the apnea test), major confounders were present (therapeutic hypothermia in combination with sedative drugs),[207] or no details at all were given other than the general statement that the patients met the clinical criteria. A recent report of two patients in Canada with "recovered respiration" may have involved ventilator autocycling. However, other major confounders (septic shock and severe metabolic acidosis) were present.[167] In two infants (3 and 10 months old), respiration (regular or hiccups) returned several hours or days after the determination of brain death until withdrawal of support.[105,147] In both infants, ancillary tests showed low-amplitude activity on the EEG or retained isotope uptake on the nuclear scan.

Since the publication of the detailed 1995 American Academy of Neurology (AAN) practice parameter and its use as a benchmark to detect errors, recovery of neurologic function after the clinical diagnosis of brain death has not been demonstrated in adults. The reported cases in infants remain exceptional and not fully understood. Physician errors cannot be excluded.[217]

■ LEGAL DEFINITIONS AND OBLIGATIONS

After a comprehensive discussion of brain death examination, it is important to briefly consider the legal obligations when this examination is performed. The brain death laws in the United States are based on the Uniform Determination of Death Act (UDDA; Table 2-9).[195] The main consequence of the UDDA is that

TABLE 2-9 *Uniform Determination of Death Act (UDDA)*

Text of Act: "An individual who has sustained either (1) irreversible cessation of circulatory and respiratory functions, or (2) irreversible cessation of all functions of the entire brain, including the brain stem, is dead. A determination of death must be made in accordance with accepted medical standards."

Alabama: Ala.Code 1975 § 22-31-1 (2000); Alaska: Alaska Stat. § 09.68.120 (West 1995); Arizona: *State v. Fierro*, 603 P.2d 74 (Ariz. 1979); Arkansas: Ark. Code. Ann. § 20-17-101 (West 1985); California: Cal. Health & Safety Code § 7180 (West 1982); Colorado: Colo. Rev. Stat. Ann. § 19a-279h (West 1988); Delaware: 24 Del. C. § 1760 (West 2005); District of Columbia: D.C. Code § 7-601 (1982); Florida: Fla. Stat. Ann. § 382.009 (West 1987); Georgia: Ga. Code Ann., § 31-10-16 (West 1992); Hawaii: Haw. Rev. Stat. § 327C-1 (West 1998); Idaho: Idaho Code § 54-1819 (West 1981); Illinois: 755 Ill. Comp. Stat. Ann. 50/1-10 (West 2004); Indiana: Ind. Code Ann. 1-1-4-3 (West 1986); Iowa: Iowa Code Ann. § 702.8 (West 2001); Kansas: Kan. Stat. Ann. § 77-205 (West 1984); Kentucky: Ky. Rev. Stat. Ann. § 446.400 (West 1986); Louisiana: La. Rev. Stat. Ann. 9:111 (2001); Maine: Me. Rev. Stat. Ann. tit. 22, § 2811 (1983); Massachusetts: *Commonwealth v. Golston*, 366 N.E.2d 744; Maryland: MD. Code Ann., Code, Health – Gen. § 5-202 (West 1998); Michigan: Mich. Comp. Laws. Ann. § 333.1033 (West 1992); Minnesota: Minn. Stat. Ann. § 145.135 (West 1989); Mississippi: Miss. Code Ann. § 41-36-3 (West 1981); Missouri: Mo. Ann. Stat. § 194.005 (West 1982); Montana: Mont. Code Ann. § 50-22-101 (1983); Nebraska: Neb. Rev. Stat. § 71-7202 (1992); Nevada: Nev. Rev. Stat. Ann. § 141.007 (West 1985); New Hampshire: N. H. Rev. Stat. Ann. § 141-D:2 (1987); New Jersey: N.J. Stat. Ann. § 26:6A-3 (West 1991); New Mexico: N.M. Stat. Ann. § 12-2-4 (West 2007); New York: N.Y. Comp. Codes R. & Regs. tit. 10, § 400.16 (1987); North Carolina: N.C. Gen. Stat. Ann. § 90-323 (West 1979); North Dakota: N.D. Cent. Code § 23-06.3-01 (West 1989); Ohio: Ohio Rev. Code Ann. § 2108.30 (West 1981); Oklahoma: Okla. Stat. Ann. tit. 63, § 3122 (West 1986); Oregon: OR. Rev. Stat. Ann. § 432.300 (West 1997); Pennsylvania: 35 Pa. Stat. Ann. § 10203 (West 1982); Rhode Island: R.I. Gen. Laws 1956, § 23-4-16 (1982); South Carolina: S.C. Code Ann. § 44-43-460 (2006); South Dakota: S.D. Codified Laws § 34-25-18.1 (1990); Tennessee: Tenn. Code An. § 68-3-501 (West 1982); Texas: Tex. Health & Safety Code Ann. § 671.001 (Vernon 1995); Utah: Utah Code Ann. § 26-34-2 (West 2007); Vermont: Vt. Stat. Ann. tit. 18, § 5218 (West 1981); Virginia: Va. Code Ann. § 54.1-2972 (West 2004); Washington: *In re Welfare of Bowman*, 617 P.2d 731 (Wash. 1980); West Virginia: W.Va. Code Ann. § 16-10-1 (West 1989); Wisconsin: Wis. Stat. Ann. § 146.71 (Wet 1982); Wyoming: Wyo. Stat. Ann. § 35-19-101 (1985).

a patient can be declared dead, and wills and insurance proceeds become acti-
vated. No civil or criminal liability will result from removing the body from life
support except in New York and New Jersey, where physicians are required to
honor religious objections. The UDDA was approved by the American Medical
Association, the American Bar Association, and the President's Commission on
Medical Ethics. The UDDA has been adopted by all 50 states and the District of
Columbia. (Arizona, Massachusetts, and Washington adopted the concept of
brain death judicially.) The adjustments in the language in many states are simple
and involve the qualifications of the examiner and the number of determinants
(Table 2-10).[37] The simple designation "in accordance with accepted medical
standards" may have been deliberate to avoid revisions when the practice of
medicine changes. Some states have added the term "generally" 'to "accepted
medical standards." Guidelines may serve as accepted standards of practice,
because the UDDA does not spell out the details of the neurologic examination.[217]
The U.S. law therefore differs substantially from the laws in all other countries
of the world. These laws clearly have incorporated medical judgments and
tests into their legal statutes.[212] Variability of hospital protocols is expected and
considerable.[83]

Participation in organ and tissue screening and the organ recovery process is
regulated by the Centers for Medicare and Medicaid Services. Hospitals must
contract with their federally designated organ procurement organization
(OPO). The key points are: (1) hospitals must report all deaths to the OPO in a
timely manner, (2) the OPO determines medical suitability, and (3) only an
OPO staff member may approach the family of a potential donor for consent for
organ, tissue, or eye donation (42 CFR 487.45). The Uniform Anatomical Gift
Act (UAGA) grants individuals the power to donate organs and tissues. The
2006 revision of the UAGA, which has been recently criticized, states that there

TABLE 2-10 *Variations in Qualifications and Number of Brain Death Examiners*

States	Qualification of Examiner	Number of Examiners
Alabama	Physician	2
Alaska	Physician or Registered Nurse	1
California	Physicians	2
Connecticut	Physicians	2
Florida[*]	Physicians	2
Georgia	Physician or registered nurse	1
Iowa	Physicians	2
Kentucky	Physicians	2
Louisiana	Physicians	2
Michigan	Physician or registered Nurse	1
New Jersey[†]	—	1
New York[†]	—	1
Virginia[‡]	Physicians	2

[*] One physician shall be the treating physician and the other physician shall be a board-eligible or board certified neurologist, neurosurgeon, internist, pediatrician, surgeon, or anesthesiologist.

[†] Requires physician to honor religious objection to brain death.

[‡] A physician who shall be duly licensed and a specialist in the field of neurology, neurosurgeon, or electroencephalography.

Source: Adapted from Choi et al.[37]

is no reason to seek consent from the donor's family when the individual has stated unequivocal wishes about organ and tissue donation (42 USC §1320B-8). Organ procurement organizations may require that life-sustaining interventions in order to preserve organs are continued.[100] Other legal issues surfacing in courtrooms are discussed in Chapter 6.

■ CONCLUSIONS

The clinical diagnosis of brain death in adults, children, and neonates requires a stepwise approach, with over 25 verifications and tests, and thus is a complex undertaking. The clinical diagnosis of brain death requires skill and, ideally, a neurologist or neurosurgeon. Any examiner should be aware of the state's statute and abide by it.

The clinical examination prevails over any technologic investigation. Its reliability has been tested over many decades and errors in interpretation are exceptional if competent physicians examine the patient,. Errors may be multifactorial and there may be a lapse of clinical neurologic skills in a technology-driven hospital practice. Failure to recognize confounders, and more generally, failure to perform a complete evaluation—most notoriously no apnea test—are common pitfalls. Most of the time should be spend in finding out if there is a major confounder. Once the test is completed the diagnostic accuracy is perfect. Ancillary testing has lost some of its luster due to unacceptably high false-positive and false-negative rates. Ultimately the physician who determines brain death will have to make his own best judgment.

■ REFERENCES

1. Aarabi B, Hesdorffer DC, Simard JM, et al. Comparative study of decompressive craniectomy after mass lesion evacuation in severe head injury. *Neurosurgery* 2009;64:927–939.
2. Ad-Hoc Committee on Brain Death, The Children's Hospital Boston. Determination of brain death. *J Pediatr* 1987;80:15–19.
3. Ahmann PA, Carrigan TA, Carlton D, et al. Brain death in children: characteristic common carotid arterial velocity patterns measured with pulsed Doppler ultrasound. *J Pediatr* 1987;110:723–728.
4. Alderete JF, Jeri FR, Richardson EP Jr, et al. Irreversible coma: a clinical, electrographic and neuropathologic study. *Trans Am Neurol Assoc* 1968;93:16–20.
5. al Jumah M, McLean DR, al Rajeh S, et al. Bulk diffusion apnea test in the diagnosis of brain death. *Crit Care Med* 1992;20:1564–1567.
6. Alvarez LA, Moshe SL, Belman AL, et al. EEG and brain death determination in children. *Neurology* 1988;38:227–230.
7. Ameratunga B, Jefferson NR, Ragapakse S. Further aspects of angiographic brain death. *Aust Radiol* 1976;20:291–295.
8. American Electroencephalographic Society. Guideline three: minimum technical standards for EEG recording in suspected cerebral death. *J Clin Neurophysiol* 1994;11:10–13.
9. Anziska BJ, Cracco RQ. Short latency somatosensory evoked potentials in brain dead patients. *Arch Neurol* 1980;37:222–225.
10. Araullo ML, Frank JI, Goldenberg FD, et al. Transient bilateral finger tremor after brain death. *Neurology* 2007;68:E22.

11. Arnold H, Kunhe D, Rohr W, et al. Contrast bolus technique with rapid CT scanning. A reliable diagnostic tool for the determination of brain death. *Neuroradiology* 1981;22:129–132.
12. Ashwal S. Brain death in early infancy. *J Heart Lung Transplant* 1993;12:S176–S178.
13. Ashwal S. Brain death in the newborn. Current perspectives. *Clin Perinatol* 1997;24: 859–882.
14. Ashwal S, Schneider S. Failure of electroencephalography to diagnose brain death in comatose children. *Ann Neurol* 1979;6:512–517.
15. Ashwal S, Schneider S. Brain death in children: Part I. *Pediatr Neurol* 1987;3:5–11.
16. Ashwal S, Schneider S. Brain death in children: Part II. *Pediatr Neurol* 1987;3: 69–77.
17. Ashwal S, Schneider S. Brain death in the newborn. Clinical, EEG and blood flow determinations. *Pediatrics* 1989;84:429–437.
18. Ashwal S, Serna-Fonseca T. Brain death in infants and children. *Crit Care Nurse* 2006;26:117–124.
19. Ashwal S, Smith AJ, Torres F, et al. Radionuclide bolus angiography: a technique for verification of brain death in infants and children. *J Pediatr* 1977;91:722–727.
20. Banasiak KJ, Lister G. Brain death in children. *Curr Opin Pediatr* 2003;15:288–293.
21. Beckmann YY, Ciftci Y, Secil Y et al. Fasciculations in brain death. *Crit Care Med* 2010:38:2377–2378.
22. Bennett DR. The EEG in determination of brain death. *Ann NY Acad Sci* 1978;315: 110–120.
23. Benzel EC, Mashburn JP, Conrad S, et al. Apnea testing for the determination of brain death: a modified protocol. *J Neurosurg* 1992;76:1029–1031.
24. Berenguer CM, Davis FE, Howington JU. Brain death confirmation: comparison of computed tomography with nuclear medicine perfusion scans. *J Trauma* 2010;68: 553–559.
25. Bergquist E, Bergstrom K. Angiography in cerebral death. *Acta Radiol* 1972;12: 282–288.
26. Bolger C, Bojanic S, Phillips J, et al. Ocular microtremor in brain stem death. *Neurosurgery* 1999;44:1201–1206.
27. Bonetti MG, Ciritella P, Valle G, et al. ^{99m}Tc-HMPAO brain perfusion SPECT in brain death. *Neuroradiology* 1995;37:365–369.
28. Bradac GB, Simon RS. Angiography in brain death. *Neuroradiology* 1974;7:25–28.
29. Brilli RJ, Bigos D: Altered apnea threshold in a child with suspected brain death. *J Child Neurol* 1995;10:245–246.
30. Bruce EN, Cherniack NS. Central chemoreceptors. *N Appl Physiol* 1987;62:389–402.
31. Brunko E, Delecluse F, Herbaut AG, et al. Unusual pattern of somatosensory and brain-stem auditory evoked potentials after cardiorespiratory arrest. *Electroencephalogr Clin Neurophysiol* 1985;62:338–342.
32. Buchner H, Schuchardt V. Reliability of electroencephalogram in the diagnosis of brain death. *Eur Neurol* 1990;30:138–141.
33. Bueri JA, Saposnik G, Maurino J, et al. Lazarus' sign in brain death. *Mov Disord* 2000;15:583–586.
34. Cantu RC. Brain death as determined by cerebral arteriography. *Lancet* 1973;1: 1391–1392.
35. Chancellor AM, Frith RW, Shaw NA. Somatosensory evoked potentials following severe head injury: loss of the thalamic potential with brain death. *J Neurol Sci* 1988;87: 255–263.
36. Chiappa KH, ed. *Evoked Potentials in Clinical Medicine.* 3rd ed. Philadelphia: Lippincott-Raven; 1997.
37. Choi EK, Fredland V, Zachodni C, et al. Brain death revisited: the case for a national standard. *J Law Med Ethics* 2008;36:824–836.
38. Christie JM, O'Lenic TD, Cane RD. Head turning in brain death. *J Clin Anesth* 1996;8:141–143.

39. Coimbra CG. Implications of ischemic penumbra for the diagnosis of brain death. *Braz J Med Biol Res* 1999;32:1479–1487.
40. Coker SB, Dillehay GL. Radionuclide cerebral imaging for confirmation of brain death in children: the significance of dural sinus activity. *Pediatr Neurol* 1986;2:43–46.
41. Combes J-C, Chomel A, Ricolfi F, et al. Reliability of computed tomographic angiography in the diagnosis of brain death. *Transplant Proc* 2007;39:16–20.
42. Conci F, Procaccio F, Arosio M, et al. Viscero-somatic and viscero-visceral reflexes in brain death. *J Neurol Neurosurg Psychiatry* 1986;49:695–698.
43. de Freitas GR, Andre C. Absence of the Babinski sign in brain death. *J Neurol* 2005;252:106–107.
44. de Freitas GR, André C. Sensitivity of transcranial Doppler for confirming brain death: a prospective study of 270 cases. *Acta Neurol Scand* 2006;113:426–432.
45. de Groot YJ, Jansen NE, Bakker J, et al. Donor conversion rates depend on assessment tools of the potential organ donor. *Intensive Care Med* 2011, in press.
46. de Groot YJ, Jansen NE, Bakker J, et al. Imminent brain death: point of departure for potential heart-beating organ donor recognition. *Intensive Care Med* 2010 36;1488–1494.
47. Deliyannakis E, Ioannou F, Davaroukas A. Brain stem death with persistence of bio-electric activity of the cerebral hemispheres. *Clin Electroencephalogr* 1975;6:75–79.
48. Díaz-Regañón G, Miñambres E, Holanda M, et al. Usefulness of venous oxygen saturation in the jugular bulb for the diagnosis of brain death: report of 118 patients. *Intensive Care Med* 2002;28:1724–1728.
49. Dickerson J, Valadka AB, LeVert T, et al. Organ donation rates in a neurosurgical intensive care unit. *J Neurosurg* 2002;97:811–814.
50. Donohoe KJ, Frey KA, Gerbaudo VH, et al. Procedure guideline for brain death scintigraphy. *J Nucl Med* 2003;44:846–851.
51. Dosemeci L, Dora B, Yilmaz M, et al. Utility of transcranial Doppler ultrasonography for confirmatory diagnosis of brain death: two sides of the coin. *Transplantation* 2004;77:71–75.
52. Drake B, Ashwal S, Schneider S. Determination of cerebral death in the pediatric intensive care unit. *Pediatrics* 1986;78:107–112.
53. Draper WB, Whitehead RW. Diffusion respiration in dog anesthetized by pentothal sodium. *Anesthesiology* 1944;5:262–273.
54. Ducrocq X, Braun M, Debouverie M, et al. Brain death and transcranial Doppler: experience in 130 cases of brain dead patients. *J Neurol Sci* 1988;160:41–46.
55. Ducrocq X, Hassler W, Moritake K, et al. Consensus opinion on diagnosis of cerebral circulatory arrest using Doppler-sonography: Task Force Group on Cerebral Death of the Neurosonology Research Group of the World Federation of Neurology. *J Neurol Sci* 1998;159:145–150.
56. Dupas B, Gayet-Delacroix M, Villers D, et al. Diagnosis of brain death using two-phase spiral CT. *Am J Neuroradiol* 1998;19:641–647.
57. Eger EI, Severinghaus JW. The rate of rise of $PaCO_2$ in the apneic anesthetized patient. *Anesthesiology* 1961;22:419–425.
58. Engel GL, Ferris EB, Webb JP, et al. Voluntary breath holding: the relation of the maximum time of breath holding to the oxygen tension of the inspired air. *J Clin Invest* 1946;25:729–733.
59. Escudero D, Otero J, Marques L, et al. Diagnosing brain death by CT perfusion and multislice CT angiography. *Neurocrit Care* 2009;11:261–271.
60. Escudero D, Otero J, Muñiz G, et al. The bispectral index scale: its use in the detection of brain death. *Transplant Proc* 2005;37:3661–3663.
61. Facco E, Zucchetta P, Munari M, et al. ^{99m}Tc-HMPAO SPECT in the diagnosis of brain death. *Intensive Care Med* 1998;24:911–917.
62. Fackler JC, Troncoso JC, Gioia FR. Age specific characteristics of brain death in children. *Am J Dis Child* 1998;142:999–1003.
63. Feery JJ, Waller GA, Solliday N. The use of apneic-diffusion respiration in the diagnosis of brain death. *Respir Care* 1985;30:328–333.

64. Feri M, Ralli L, Felici M, et al. Transcranial Doppler and brain death diagnosis. *Crit Care Med* 1994;22:1120–1126.
65. Ferris EB, Engel GL, Stevens CD, et al. Voluntary breath holding; the relation of the maximum time of breath-holding to the oxygen and carbon dioxide tensions of arterial blood, with a note on its clinical and physiological significance. *J Clin Invest* 1946;25:734–743.
66. Firsching R. The brain-stem and 40 Hz middle latency auditory evoked potentials in brain death. *Acta Neurochir* 1989;101:52–55.
67. Fischgold H, Mathis P. Obnubilations, Comas et Stupeurs. Etudes Electroencephalographiques. *Electroencephalogr Clin Neurophysiol* 1959;Suppl 11:27–68.
68. Flowers WM Jr, Patel BR. Radionuclide angiography as a confirmatory test for brain death: a review of 229 studies in 219 patients. *South Med J* 1997;90:1091–1096.
69. Forster FM, Nims LF. Electroencephalographic effects of acute increases of intracranial pressure. *Arch Neurol Psychiatry* 1942;47:449–453.
70. Frampas E, Videcoq M, de Kerviler E, et al. CT angiography for brain death diagnosis. *Am J Neuroradiol* 2009;30:1566–1570.
71. Friedman Y, Lee L, Wherrett JR, et al. Simulation of brain death from fulminant de-efferentation. *Can J Neurol Sci* 2003;30:397–404.
72. Furgiuele TL, Frank LM, Riegle C, et al. Prediction of cerebral death by cranial sector scan. *Crit Care Med* 1984;12:1–3.
73. Garcia-Larrea L, Bertrand O, Artru F, et al. Brain-stem monitoring. II. Preterminal BAEP changes observed until brain death in deeply comatose patients. *Electroencephalogr Clin Neurophysiol* 1987;68:446–457.
74. Gerard RW. Anoxia and neural metabolism. *Arch Neurol Psychiatry* 1938;40:985–996.
75. Goetting MG, Contreras E. Systemic atropine administration during cardiac arrest does not cause fixed and dilated pupils. *Ann Emerg Med* 1991;20:55–57.
76. Goh AY-T, Mok Q. Clinical course and determination of brainstem death in a children's hospital. *Acta Paediatr* 2004;93:47–52.
77. Goldie WD, Chiappa KH, Young RR, Brooks EB. Brainstem auditory and short-lacency somatosensory evoked responses in brain death. *Neurology* 1981;31:248–256.
78. Goodman JM, Mishkin FS, Kyken M. Determination of brain death by isotope angiography. *JAMA* 1969;209:1869–1872.
79. Goudreau JL, Wijdicks EFM, Emery SF. Complications during apnea testing in the determination of brain death: predisposing factors. *Neurology* 2000;55:1045–1048.
80. Goulon M, Nouailhat F, Babinet P. Irreversible coma. *Ann Med Interne* (Paris) 1971;122:479–486.
81. Gray AT, Krejci ST, Larson MD. Neuromuscular blocking drugs do not alter the pupillary light reflex of anesthetized humans. *Arch Neurol* 1997;54:579–584.
82. Greer DM, Strozyk D, Schwamm LH. False positive CT angiography in brain death. *Neurocrit Care* 2009;11:272–275.
83. Greer DM, Varelas PN, Haque S, et al. Variability of brain death determination guidelines in leading U.S. neurologic institutions. *Neurology* 2008;70:284–289.
84. Greitz T, Gordon E, Kolmodin G, et al. Aortocranial and carotid angiography in determination of brain death. *Neuroradiology* 1973;5:13–19.
85. Grigg MM, Kelly MA, Celesia GG, et al. Electroencephalographic activity after brain death. *Arch Neurol* 1987;44:948–954.
86. Gros C, Vlahovitch B, Roilgen A. Circulatory arrest in hyperacute intracranial hypertension. *Presse Med* 1959;67:1065–1067.
87. Guidelines for the determination of brain death in children. *Pediatrics* 1987;80:298–300.
88. Guidelines for the determination of death. Report of the medical consultants on the diagnosis of death to the President's Commission for the Study of Ethical Problems in Medicine and Biochemical and Behavioral Research. *JAMA* 1981;246:2184–2186.
89. Hadani M, Bruk B, Ram Z, et al. Application of transcranial Doppler ultrasonography for the diagnosis of brain death. *Intensive Care Med* 1999;25:822–828.

90. Hanks EC, Ngai SH, Fink BR. The respiratory threshold for carbon dioxide in anesthetized man. Determination of carbon dioxide threshold during halothane anesthesia. *Anesthesiology* 1961;22:393–397.
91. Hanna JP, Frank JI. Automatic stepping in the pontomedullary stage of central herniation. *Neurology* 1995;45:985–986.
92. Hansen AVE, Lavin PJM, Moody EB, et al. False-negative cerebral radionuclide flow study, in brain death, caused by a ventricular drain. *Clin Nucl Med* 1993;18:502–505.
93. Hansotia PL. Persistent vegetative state. Review and report of electrodiagnostic studies in eight cases. *Arch Neurol* 1985;42:1048–1052.
94. Hassler W, Steinmetz H, Gawlowski J. Transcranial Doppler ultrasonography in raised intracranial pressure and in intracranial circulatory arrest. *J Neurosurg* 1988;68:745–751.
95. Haun SE, Tobias JD, Deshpande JK. Apnea testing in the determination of brain death: is it reliable? *Clin Intensive Care* 1991;2:182–184.
96. Hazratji SM, Singh BM, Strobos RJ. Angiography in brain death. *NYS J Med* 1981;81:82–83.
97. Herrick MK, Agamanolis DF. Displacement of cerebellar tissue into spinal canal. A component of the respirator brain syndrome. *Arch Pathol* 1975;99:565–571.
98. Holzman BH, Curless RG, Sfakianakis GN, et al. Radionuclide cerebral perfusion scintigraphy in determination of brain death in children. *Neurology* 1983;33:1027–1031.
99. Hughes JR. Limitations of the EEG in coma and brain death. *Ann NY Acad Sci* 1978;315:121–136.
100. Iltis AS, Rie MA, Wall A. Organ donation, patient's rights, and medical responsibilities at the end of life. *Crit Care Med* 2009;37:310–315.
101. Ishii K, Onuma T, Kinoshita T, et al. Brain death: MR and MR angiography. *Am J Neuroradiol* 1996;17:731–735.
102. Jefferson NR, Ameratunga B, Rajapakse S. Angiographic evidence of brain death. *Australas Radiol* 1975;19:289–296.
103. Jeret JS, Benjamin JL. Risk of hypotension during apnea testing. *Arch Neurol* 1994;51:595–599.
104. Joels N, Samueloff M. The activity of the medullary centres in diffusion respiration. *J Physiol* 1956;133:360–372.
105. Joffe AR, Kolski H, Duff J, et al. A 10-month-old infant with reversible findings of brain death. *Pediatr Neurol* 2009;41:378–382.
106. Joffe AR, Lequier L, Cave D. Specificity of radionuclide brain blood flow testing in brain death: case report and review. *J Intensive Care Med* 2010;25:53–64.
107. Jones KM, Barnes PD. MR diagnosis of brain death. *Am J Neuroradiol* 1992;13:65–66.
108. Jorgensen EO. Technical contribution. Requirements for recording the EEG at high sensitivity in suspected brain death. *Electrocephalogr Clin Neurophysiol* 1974;36:65–69.
109. Joshi MC, Azim A, Gupta GL, et al. Guillain-Barré syndrome with absent brainstem reflexes—a report of two cases. *Anaesth Intensive Care* 2008;36:867–869.
110. Jung KY, Han SG, Lee KH, et al. Repetitive leg movements mimicking periodic leg movement during sleep in a brain-dead patient. *Eur J Neurol* 2006;13:e3–e4.
111. Kafrawy U, Stewart D. An evaluation of brainstem death documentation: the importance of full documentation. *Paediatr Anaesth* 2004;14:584–588.
112. Kainuma M, Miyake T, Kanno T. Extremely prolonged vecuronium clearance in a brain death case. *Anesthesiology* 2001;95:1023–1024.
113. Karantanas AH, Hadjigeorgiou GM, Paterakis K, et al. Contribution of MRI and MR angiography in early diagnosis of brain death. *Eur Radiol* 2002;12:2710–2716.
114. Klingelhofer J, Conrad B, Benecke R, et al. Evaluation of intracranial pressure from transcranial Doppler studies in cerebral disease. *J Neurol* 1988;235:159–162.
115. Koberda JL, Clark WM, Lutsep H, et al. Successful clinical recovery and reversal of midbasilar occlusion in clinically brain dead patient with intra-arterial urokinase. *Neurology* 1997;48:A154.

116. Korein J, Braunstein P, George A, et al. Brain death: I. Angiographic correlation with the radioisotopic bolus technique for evaluation of critical deficit of cerebral blood flow. *Ann Neurol* 1977;2:195–205.

117. Korein J, Braunstein P, Kricheff I, et al. Radioisotopic bolus technique as a test to detect circulatory deficit associated with cerebral death. 142 studies on 80 patients demonstrating the bedside use of an innocuous IV procedure as an adjunct in the diagnosis of cerebral death. *Circulation* 1975;51:924–939.

118. Kricheff II, Pinto RS, George AE, et al. Angiographic findings in brain death. *Ann NY Acad Sci* 1978;315:168–183.

119. Kuo J-R, Chen C-F, Chio C-C, et al. Time dependent validity in the diagnosis of brain death using transcranial Doppler sonography. *JNeurol Neurosurg Psychiatry* 2006;77:646–649.

120. Kurtek RW, Lai KK, Tauxe WN, et al. Tc-99m hexamethylpropylene amine oxime scintigraphy in the diagnosis of brain death and its implications for the harvesting of organs used for transplantation. *Clin Nucl Med* 2000;25:7–10.

121. Lampl Y, Gilad R, Eschel Y, et al. Diagnosing brain death using the transcranial Doppler with a transorbital approach. *Arch Neurol* 2002;59:58–60.

122. Lang CJ. Apnea testing by artificial CO_2 augmentation. *Neurology* 1995;45:966–969.

123. Lang CJ, Heckmann JG. Apnea testing for the diagnosis of brain death. *Acta Neurol Scand.* 2005;112:358–369.

124. Lang CJ, Heckmann JG, Erbguth F, et al. Transcutaneous and intra-arterial blood gas monitoring—a comparison during apnea testing for the determination of brain death. *Eur J Emerg Med* 2002;9:51–56.

125. Langfitt TW, Kassell NF. Non-filling of cerebral vessels during angiography: correlation with intracranial pressure. *Acta Neurochir* 1966;14:96–104.

126. Laurin NR, Driedger AA, Hurwitz GA, et al. Cerebral perfusion imaging with technetium-99m HM-PAO in brain death and severe central nervous system injury. *J Nucl Med* 1989;30:1627–1635.

127. Lee DH, Nathanson JA, Fox AJ, et al. Magnetic resonance imaging of brain death. *Can Assoc Radiol J* 1995;46:174–178.

128. Leestma J, Hughes J, Diamond E. Temporal correlates in brain death. EEG and clinical relationships to the respirator brain. *Arch Neurol* 1984;41:147–152.

129. Levesque S, Lessard MR, Nicole PC, et al. Efficacy of a T-piece system and a continuous positive airway pressure system for apnea testing in the diagnosis of brain death. *Crit Care Med* 2006;34:2213–2216.

130. Löfstedt S, von Reis G. Diminution or obstruction of blood flow in the internal carotid artery. *Opuse Med* 1959;4:345–360.

131. López-Navidad A, Caballero F, Domingo P, et al. Early diagnosis of brain death in patients treated with central nervous system depressant drugs. *Transplantation* 2000;70:131–135.

132. Machado C, Valdés P, García-Igera J, et al. Brain-stem auditory evoked potentials and brain death. *Electroencephalogr Clin Neurophysiol* 1991;80:392–398.

133. Marks SJ, Zisfein J. Apneic oxygenation in apnea tests for brain death. A controlled trial. *Arch Neurol* 1990;47:1066–1068.

134. Martí-Fàbregas J, López-Navidad A, Caballero F, et al. Decerebrate-like posturing with mechanical ventilation in brain death. *Neurology* 2000;54:224–227.

135. Mathur M, Petersen L, Stadtler M, et al. Variability in pediatric brain death determination and documentation in southern California. *Pediatrics* 2008;121:988–993.

136. Matsumura A, Mequero K, Tsurushima H, et al. Magnetic resonance imaging of brain death. *Neurol Med Clin Chir* 1996;36:166–171.

137. McNair NL, Meador KJ. The undulating toe flexion sign in brain death. *Mov Disord* 1992;7:345–347.

138. Mejia RE, Pollack MM. Variability in brain death determination practices in children. *JAMA* 1995;274:550–553.

139. Mishkin FS, Dyken JL. Increased early radionuclide activity in the nasopharyngeal area in patients with internal carotid artery obstruction: "hot nose." *Radiology* 1970;96:77–80.

140. Moseley JI, Molinari GF, Walker AE. Respirator brain: report of a survey and review of current concepts. *Arch Pathol Lab Med* 1979;100:61–64.

141. Munari M, Zucchetta P, Carollo C, et al. Confirmatory tests in the diagnosis of brain death: comparison between SPECT and contrast angiography. *Crit Care Med* 2005;33:2068–2073.

142. Muralidharan R, Wijdicks EFM, Rabinstein AA. Cervicomedullary injury causing quadriplegia after fulminant meningitis. *Arch Neurol* 2011, in press.

143. Nakagawa TA, Ashwal S, Mathur M, Mysore M and the Committee for Determination of Brain Death in Infants and Children: an update of the 1987 task force recommendations. *Crit Care Med* 2011, in press.

144. Nebra AC, Virgós B, Santos S, et al. Clinical diagnosis of brain death and transcranial Doppler, looking for middle cerebral arteries and intracranial vertebral arteries: agreement with scintigraphic techniques. *Rev Neurol* 2001;33:916–920.

145. Newell DW, Grady MS, Sirotta P, et al. Evaluation of brain death using transcranial Doppler. *Neurosurgery* 1989;24:509–513.

146. Oehmichen M. Brain death: neuropathological findings and forensic implications. *Forensic Sci Int* 1994;69:205–219.

147. Okamoto K, Sugimoto T. Return of spontaneous respiration in an infant who fulfilled current criteria to determine brain death. *Pediatrics* 1995;96:518–520.

148. Okuyaz C, Gucuyener K, Karabacak NI, et al. Tc-99m-HMPAO SPECT in the diagnosis of brain death in children. *Pediatr Int* 2004;46:711–714.

149. Orliaguet GA, Catoire P, Liu N, et al. Transesophageal echocardiographic assessment of left ventricular function during apnea testing for brain death. *Transplantation* 1994;58:655–658.

150. Orrison WW Jr, Champlin AM, Kesterson OL, et al. MR "hot nose sign" and "intravascular enhancement sign" in brain death. *Am J Neuroradiol* 1994;15:913–916.

151. Ostermann ME, Young B, Sibbald WJ, et al. Coma mimicking brain death following baclofen overdose. *Intensive Care Med* 2000;26:1144–1146.

152. Outwater KM, Rockoff MA. Diabetes insipidus accompanying brain death in children. *Neurology* 1984;34:1243–1246.

153. Palmer S, Bader MK. Brain tissue oxygenation in brain death. *Neurocrit Care* 2005;2:17–22.

154. Parker BL, Frewen TC, Levin SD, et al. Declaring pediatric brain death: current practice in a Canadian pediatric critical care unit. *CMAJ* 1995;153:909–916.

155. Pearson J, Lorein J, Braunstein P. Morphology of defectively perfused brains in patients with persistent extracranial circulation. *Ann NY Acad Sci* 1978;315:265–271.

156. Peter JV, Prabhakar AT, Pichamuthu K. In-laws, insecticide—and a mimic of brain death. *Lancet* 2008;371:622.

157. Petty GW, Mohr JP, Pedley TA, et al. The role of transcranial Doppler in confirming brain death: sensitivity, specificity, and suggestions for performance and interpretation. *Neurology* 1990;40:300–303.

158. Powers AD, Graeber MC, Smith RR. Transcranial Doppler ultrasonography in the determination of brain death. *Neurosurgery* 1989;24:884–889.

159. Practice parameters for determining brain death in adults (summary statement). The Quality Standards Subcommittee of the American Academy of Neurology. *Neurology* 1995;45:1012–1014.

160. Prechter GC, Nelson SB, Hubmayr RD. The ventilatory recruitment threshold for carbon dioxide. *Am Rev Respir Dis* 1990;141:758–764.

161. Quesnel C, Fulgencio J-P, Adrie C, et al. Limitations of computed tomographic angiography in the diagnosis of brain death. *Intensive Care Med* 2007;33:2129–2135.

162. Rangel RA. Computerized axial tomography in brain death. *Stroke* 1978;9:597–598.

163. Rappaport ZH, Brinker RA, Rovit RL. Evaluation of brain death by contrast-enhanced computerized cranial tomography. *Neurosurgery* 1978;2:230–232.

164. Reid RH, Gulenchyn KY, Ballinger JR. Clinical use of technetium-99m HM-PAO for determination of brain death. *J Nucl Med* 1989;30:1621–1626.

165. Report of the American Academy of Neurology, Therapeutics and Technology Assessment Subcommittee. Assessment: transcranial Doppler. *Neurology* 1990;40: 680–681.

166. Richard IH, LaPointe M, Wax P, et al. Non-barbiturate, drug-induced reversible loss of brainstem reflexes. *Neurology* 1998;51:639–640.

167. Roberts DJ, MacCulloch KAM, VersnickEJ, et al. Should ancillary brain blood flow analysis play a larger role in the neurologic determination of death? *Can J Anesth* 2010;57:927–935.

168. Rohling R, Wagner W, Mühlberg J, et al. Apnea test: pitfalls and correct handling. *Transplant Proc* 1986;18:388–390.

169. Roine RO, Launes J, Lindroth L, et al. ^{99m}Tc-hexamethylpropyleneamine oxime scans to confirm brain death. *Lancet* 1986;2:1223–1224.

170. Roncucci P, Lepori P, Mok MS, et al. Nasopharyngeal electrode recording of somatosensory evoked potentials as an indicator in brain death. *Anaesth Intensive Care* 1999;27:20–25.

171. Ropper AH. Unusual spontaneous movements in brain-dead patients. *Neurology* 1984;34:1089–1092.

172. Ropper AH, Kehne SM, Wechsler L. Transcranial Doppler in brain death. *Neurology* 1987;37:1733–1735.

173. Ropper AH, Kennedy SK, Russel L. Apnea testing in the diagnosis of brain death: clinical and physiological observations. *J Neurosurg* 1981;55:942–946.

174. Ruiz-Garcia M, Gonzalez-Astiazaran A, Collado-Corona MA, et al. Brain death in children: clinical, neurophysiological and radioisotopic angiography findings in 125 patients. *Childs Nerv Syst* 2000;16:40–45.

175. Ruiz-López MJ, Martínez de Azagra A, Serrano A, et al. Brain death and evoked potentials in pediatric patients. *Crit Care Med* 1999;27:412–416.

176. Salim A, Velmahos GC, Brown C, et al. Aggressive organ donor management significantly increases the number of organs available for transplantation. *J Trauma* 2005;58:991–994.

177. Santamaria J, Orteu N, Iranzo A, et al. Eye opening in brain death. *J Neurol* 1999;246:720–722.

178. Saposnik G, Bueri JA, Maurino J, et al. Spontaneous and reflex movements in brain death. *Neurology* 2000;54:221–223.

179. Savard M, Turgeon AF, GariépyJL, et al. Selective 4 vessel angiography in brain death: a retrospective study. *Can J Neurol Sci* 2010;37:492–497.

180. Scher MS, Barabas RE, Barmada MA. Clinical examination findings in neonates with the absence of electrocerebral activity: an acute or chronic encephalopathic state? *J Perinatol* 1996;16:455–460.

181. Schmidt JE, Tamburro RF, Hoffman GM. Dilated nonreactive pupils secondary to neuromuscular blockade. *Anesthesiology* 2000;92:1476–1480.

182. Schwartz JA, Baxter J, Brill DR. Diagnosis of brain death in children by radionuclide cerebral imaging. *Pediatrics* 1984;73:14–18.

183. Sharbrough FW. Unique contributions of short-latency auditory and somatosensory evoked potentials to neurologic diagnosis. *Prog Clin Neurophysiol* 1980; 7:231–263.

184. Shemie SD. Diagnosis of brain death in children. *Lancet Neurol* 2007;6:87–88.

185. Shimizu N, Shemie S, Miyasaka E, et al. [Preliminary report: use of clinical criteria for the determination of pediatric brain death and confirmation by radionuclide cerebral blood flow]. *Masui* 2000;49:1126–1132.

186. Shulgman D, Parulekar M, Elston JS, et al. Abnormal pupillary activity in a brainstem-dead patient. *Br J Anaesth* 2001;86:717–720.

187. Silverman D, Saunders MG, Schwab RS, et al. Cerebral death and the electroencepha-logram. Report of the Ad Hoc Committee of the American Electroencephalographic Society on EEG Criteria for Determination of Cerebral Death. *JAMA* 1969;209: 1505–1510.

188. Silverman D, Masland RL, Saunders MG, Schwab RS. Irreversible coma associated with electrocerebral silence. *Neurology* 1970;20:525–33.

189. Snavely SR, Hodges GR. The neurotoxicity of antibacterial agents. *Ann Intern Med* 1984;101:92–104.

190. Sonoo M, Tsai-Shozawa Y, Aoki M, et al. N18 in median somatosensory evoked poten-tials: a new indicator of medullary function useful for the diagnosis of brain death. *J Neurol Neurosurg Psychiatry* 1999;67:374–378.

191. Sprung CL, Cohen SL, Sjokvist P, et al. End-of-life practices in European intensive care units: the Ethicus Study. *JAMA* 2003;290:790–797.

192. Starr A. Auditory brain-stem responses in brain death. *Brain* 1976;99:543–554.

193. Stohr M, Riffel B, Trost E, et al. Short-latency somatosensory evoked potentials in brain death. *J Neurol* 1987;234:211–214.

194. Stojkovic T, Verdin M, Hurtevent JF, et al. Guillain-Barré syndrome resembling brain-stem death in a patient with brain injury. *J Neurol* 2001;248:430–432.

195. Uniform Determination of Death Act, 12 uniform laws annotated 589 (West 1993 and West supp (1997)).

196. Van Velthoven V, Calliauw L. Diagnosis of brain death. Transcranial Doppler sonogra-phy as an additional method. *Acta Neurochir* 1988;95:57–60.

197. Vardis R, Pollack MM. Increased apnea threshold in a pediatric patient with suspected brain death. *Crit Care Med* 1998;26:1917–1919.

198. Vicenzini E, Pulitano P, Cicchetti R, et al. Transcranial Doppler for brain death in infants: the role of the fontanelles. *Eur Neurol* 2010;63:164–169.

199. Vivien B, Marmion F, Roche S, et al. An evaluation of transcutaneous carbon dioxide partial pressure monitoring during apnea testing in brain-dead patients. *Anesthesiology* 2006;104:701–707.

200. Vivien B, Paqueron X, Le Cosquer P, et al. Detection of brain death onset using the bispectral index in severely comatose patients. *Intensive Care Med* 2002;28:419–425.

201. Wagner W. SEP testing in deeply comatose and brain dead patients: the role of nasopharyngeal, scalp and earlobe derivations in recording the P14 potential. *Electroencephalogr Clin Neurophysiol* 1991;80:352–363.

202. Wagner W. Scalp, earlobe and nasopharyngeal recordings of the median nerve soma-tosensory evoked P14 potential in coma and brain death. *Brain* 1996;119:1507–1521.

203. Walker AE, Feeney DM, Hovda DA. The electroencephalographic characteristics of the rhombencephalectomized cat. *Electroencephalogr Clin Neurophysiol* 1984;57: 156–165.

204. Walker AE. Pathology of brain death. *Ann NY Acad Sci* 1978;315:272–280.

205. Walker AE, Diamond E, Moseley J. The neuropathological findings in irreversible coma. A critique of the "respirator." *J Neuropathol Exp Neurol* 1975;34:295–323.

206. Wang M, Wallace P, Gruen JP. Brain death documentation: analysis and issues. *Neurosurgery* 2002;51:731–736.

207. Webb A, Samuels O. Reversible brain death following cardiopulmonary arrest. *Crit Care Med* 2010;38(suppl):723. Abstract.

208. Webster PA, Markham L. Pediatric organ donation: a national survey examining consent rates and characteristics of donor hospitals. *Pediatr Crit Care Med* 2009;10: 500–504.

209. Wieler H, Marohl K, Kaiser KP, et al. Tc-99m HMPAO cerebral scintigraphy: a reliable, noninvasive method for determination of brain death. *Clinl Nucl Med* 1993;18:104–109.

210. Wijdicks EFM. In search of a safe apnea test in brain death: is the procedure really more dangerous than we think? *Arch Neurol* 1995;52:338–339.

211. Wijdicks EFM. What anesthesiologists should know about what neurologists should know about declaring brain death. *Anesthesiology* 2000;92:1203–1204.

212. Wijdicks EFM. Brain death worldwide: accepted fact but no global consensus in diagnostic criteria. *Neurology* 2002;58:20–25.
213. Wijdicks EFM. The case against confirmatory tests for determining brain death in adults. *Neurology* 2010;75:77–83.
214. Wijdicks EFM, Manno EM, Holets SR. Ventilator self-cycling may falsely suggest patient effort during brain death determination. *Neurology* 2005;65:774.
215. Wijdicks EFM, Pfeifer EA. Neuropathology of brain death in the modern transplant era. *Neurology* 2008;70:1234–1237.
216. Wijdicks EFM, Rabinstein AA, Manno EM, et al. Pronouncing brain death: contemporary practice and safety of the apnea test. *Neurology* 2008;71:1240–1244.
217. Wijdicks EFM, Varelas PN, Gronseth GS, et al. Evidence-based guideline update: determining brain death in adults: report of the Quality Standards Subcommittee of the American Academy of Neurology. *Neurology* 2010;74:1911–1918.
218. Yatim A, Mercatello A, Caronel B, et al. ^{99m}Tc-HMPAO cerebral scintigraphy in the diagnosis of brain death. *Transplant Proc* 1991;23:2491.
219. Yee AH, Mandrekar J, Rabinstein AA, et al. Predictors of apnea test failure during brain death determination. *Neurocrit Care* 2010;12:352–355.
220. Yoneda S, Nishimoto A, Nukada T, et al. To-and-fro movement and external escape of carotid arterial blood in brain death cases: a Doppler ultrasonic study. *Stroke* 1974;5:707–713.
221. Young GB, Shemie SD, Doig CJ, et al. Brief review: the role of ancillary tests in the neurological determination of death. *Can J Anaesth* 2006;53:620–627.
222. Zubkov AY, Wijdicks EFM. Plantar flexion and flexion synergy in brain death. *Neurology* 2008;70:e74.
223. Zurynski Y, Dorsch N, Pearson I, et al. Transcranial Doppler ultrasound in brain death: experience in 140 patients. *Neurol Res* 1991;13:248–252.

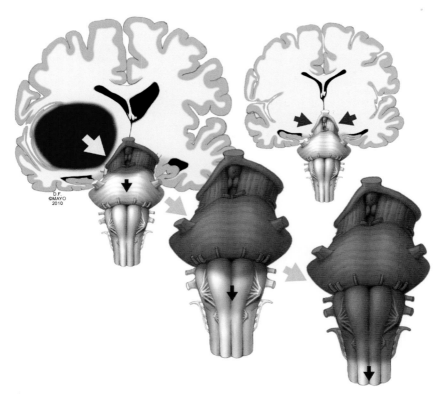

Figure 2-1 Drawing of the brain and brainstem showing rostrocaudal progression leading to brain death.

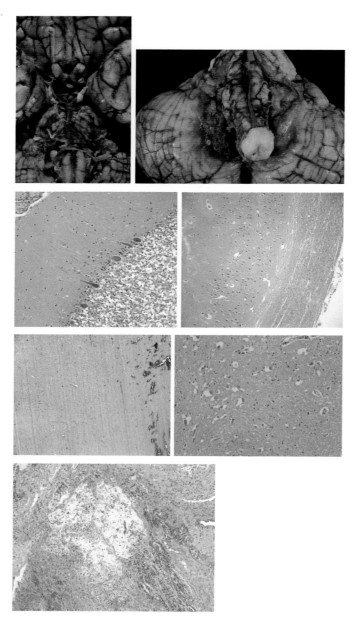

Figure 2-2 Neuropathology in brain death. *Upper row*: Macroscopy: diffuse brain swelling, tonsillar herniation, and third nerve grooving; necrotic tip of the cerebellar tonsil. *Second row*: Microscopy: preserved Purkinje cells, hippocampus. *Third row*: Preserved occipital area next to hemorrhage, but severe neuronal injury to the brainstem. *Fourth row*: necrotic areas in the pituitary gland.

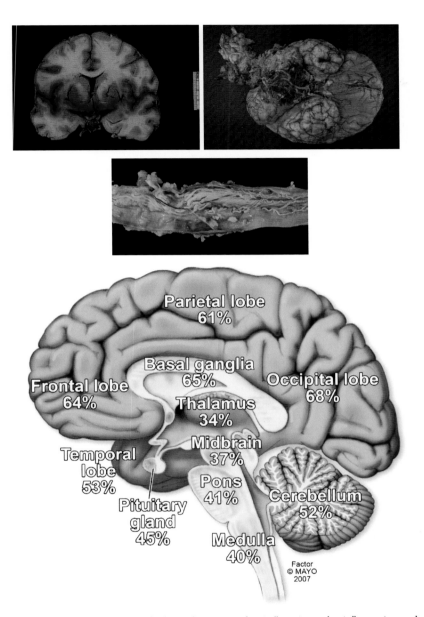

Figure 2-2 (Continued) Musky brain known as classic "respirator brain" seen in modern times only with prolonged support showing fragmentation and cerebellar remnants in spinal cord. Illustration shows distribution of severe neuronal injury to the brain. From Wijdicks and Pfeifer.[215] Used with permission from *Neurology*.

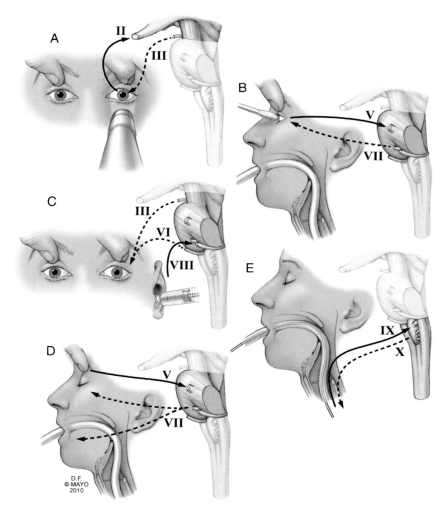

Figure 2-4 (A) Pupil size and light response. (B) Corneal reflexes. (C) Oculovestibular reflexes. (D) No facial movement to pressure on supraorbital nerve. (E) Cough and gag reflex. Roman numerals refer to cranial nerves.

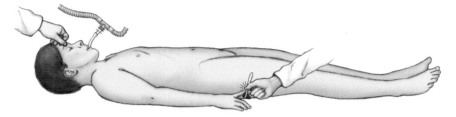

Figure 2-5 Motor responses to stimuli is absent (nailbed and supraorbital nerve compression).

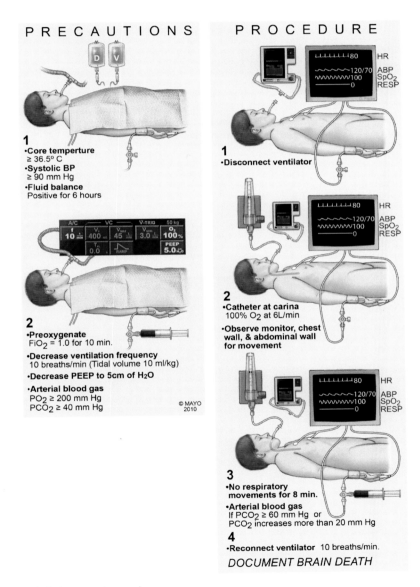

PRECAUTIONS

1
- **Core temperture**
  ≥ 36.5° C
- **Systolic BP**
  ≥ 90 mm Hg
- **Fluid balance**
  Positive for 6 hours

2
- **Preoxygenate**
  FiO$_2$ = 1.0 for 10 min.
- **Decrease ventilation frequency**
  10 breaths/min (Tidal volume 10 ml/kg)
- **Decrease PEEP to 5cm of H$_2$O**
- **Arterial blood gas**
  PO$_2$ ≥ 200 mm Hg
  PCO$_2$ ≥ 40 mm Hg

© MAYO 2010

PROCEDURE

1
- **Disconnect ventilator**

2
- **Catheter at carina**
  100% O$_2$ at 6L/min
- **Observe monitor, chest wall, & abdominal wall for movement**

3
- **No respiratory movements for 8 min.**
- **Arterial blood gas**
  If PCO$_2$ ≥ 60 mm Hg or
  PCO$_2$ increases more than 20 mm Hg

4
- **Reconnect ventilator** 10 breaths/min.

DOCUMENT BRAIN DEATH

Figure 2-6 Apnea test procedure.

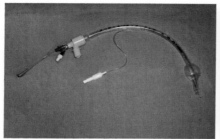
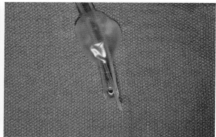

Figure 2-7 Oxygen insufflation catheter. Note the tip of the catheter just out of the endotracheal tube. The port jet ventilator adaptor has an insufflation catheter that is measured from the distal tip approximately 1 cm beyond the end of the endotracheal tube and is estimated to be just above the carina. This will prevent injury and a sandblasting effect.

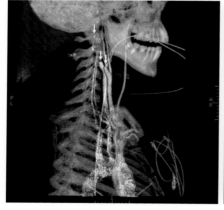
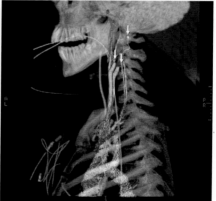

D

Figure 2-9 Examples of electrophysiologic tests and flow studies. (D) CTA showing absent intracranial flow in both vertebral and carotid circulation (arrows).

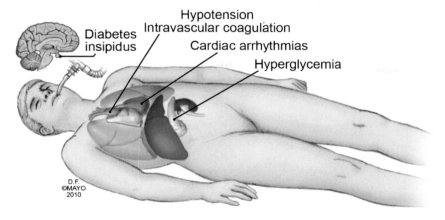

Diabetes
insipidus

Hypotension
Intravascular coagulation
Cardiac arrhythmias
Hyperglycemia

D.F.
©MAYO
2010

Figure 5-4 Organ donor and medical complications.

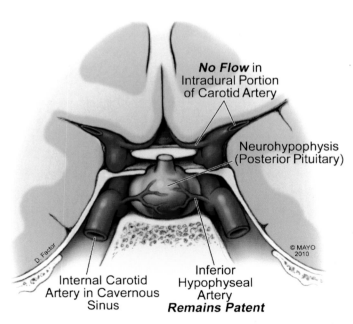

No Flow in
Intradural Portion
of Carotid Artery

Neurohypophysis
(Posterior Pituitary)

Internal Carotid
Artery in Cavernous
Sinus

Inferior
Hypophyseal
Artery
Remains Patent

D. Factor

© MAYO
2010

Figure 5-5 Blood supply to the pituitary gland and its relation to the dura, emphasizing
the extradural locations.

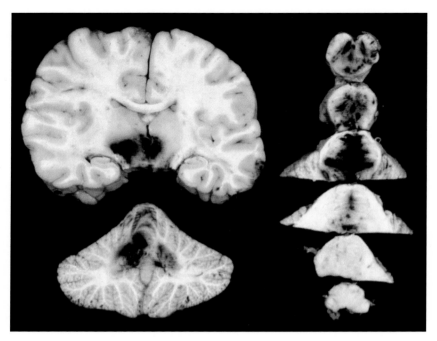

Figure 6-3 Traumatic head injury and epidural hematoma. The patient had a normal breathing drive and cough responses, but all pontomesencephalic reflexes remained absent. After 1 week of full support and no clinical change, the family decided to withdraw support. Neuropathologic examination showed thalamic, cerebellar, and upper brainstem lesions but sparing of the medulla. From Wijdicks et al.[7] with permission of the publisher.

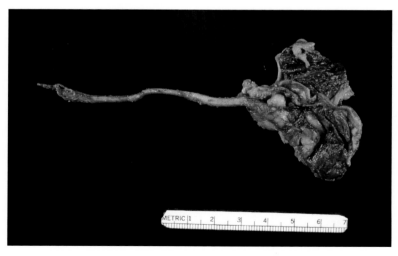

Figure 6-7 Gross macroscopic view showing some preservation of the brainstem structures but amorf cerebrum.

3   Beliefs and Brain Death

Globalization has increased cultural diversity and with it physician exposure to families with different views of death and dying. Spiritual reflections may play a role in end-of-life decisions prompted by the sadness of unexpected brain death in a loved one. Cultural attitudes and traditional beliefs may also affect the decision of the patient's proxy to proceed with organ donation. When there is opposition it may be framed by moral objections of removing organs from the dead, but also by the definition of death. In some, the conversion from life to death is simply loss of breath (Hinduism)[17,37] or is defined more radically as decomposition (Tibetan Buddhism).[35] Moreover, certain religions are more concerned about the afterlife and reincarnation. At the present time, major Western religions support organ and tissue donation, and only in a limited sense does objection to donation continue. There are a few contestants of brain death in Judaism and Christianity, and some of these scholars demand a vitalist approach.

This chapter presents a general overview of religious and cultural beliefs and how they may pertain to the acceptance of brain death and organ donation. A comprehensive discussion of the theology of death or funeral rites is outside the scope of this chapter. This chapter also touches on the role of the clergy in the intensive care unit. Although religious views about the concept of brain death are complex enough to attract our attention, religious affiliation is not an overriding concern for most Americans, British, and Europeans when confronted with brain death and organ donation. In other parts of the world, the role of faith in these decisions is apparent.[36]

■ RELIGIOUS BELIEFS

The major religions in the United States are Christianity, Islam, and Judaism. These three religions are divided into various denominations. Both Islam and Judaism have long traditions of defining death as the absence of respiration, but brain death has become an accepted definition of death in these religious traditions. Many mainstream religions in the United States have official policy statements in their doctrines in support of donation. However, certain aspects and moral objections need attention. It is important to review these positions in detail, because online Web sites may be biased toward controversy, and a recent study found opinions contradicting major religious positions at various sites.[4]

Among Christian denominations, beliefs are rooted in the Bible. Jesus says that He is the resurrection and the life and that those who believe in him will never die. The dominant emphasis in Christianity is belief in the resurrection of Christ and his followers. Several scriptures in the Bible may guide Christian thinking (e.g., Luke 6:37–38: "Give and it shall be given unto you"; Revelation 214–215: "In eternity we will not need our earthy bodies: former things will pass away, all things will be made new"). Christians do accept the neurologic criteria of death, and many also acknowledge that irreversible coma may lead to withdrawal of intensive care support if nothing more can be done.

For Catholics, most of the ethical questions concerning the signs of death have been discussed in working groups of the Pontifical Academy of Sciences. Proceedings were held in 1985 (the artificial prolongation of life and the determination of the exact moment of death) in 1989 (the determination of brain death and its relationship to human death) and most recently in 2006 (the signs of death) (Figure 3-1). These documents stressed the fact that brain death is a true criterion for death. The position last held in 2006 has remained unchanged, but it is theoretically possible that new uncertainties over the signs of death could lead to reassessment by the Holy See of the practice of organ transplantation. The Roman Catholic Church legitimizes organ donation by the principle of solidarity and charity. The pope continues to stress academic rigor and research in this field and emphasizes the principle of defending life at all times. (According to Bruzzone, Pope Benedict XVI has been a registered potential organ donor since he was a cardinal, and he has considered it an act of love toward a person in need.[5])

Islam asks Muslims to submit to the one and only God (Allah) and His will. People have been created to worship Allah. The family system in an Islamic community is strong and includes neighbors and friends. When hardships come,

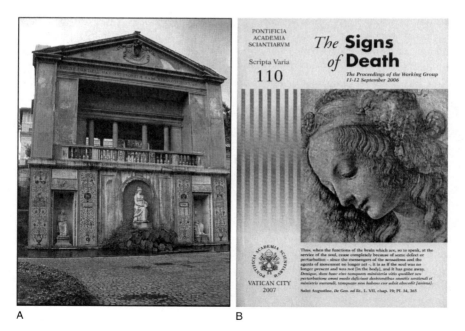

A   B

Figure 3-1 (A) Seat of the Pontifical Academy of Sciences in Vatican City. (B) Proceedings of the working group in 2006. (www.vatican.va)

the Muslim should not give up and has no right to determine anyone's time to die (i.e., to terminate life support). Nonetheless, the third International Conference of Islamic Jurists was resolute in favor of defining brain death as the death of a person.[1] A person is considered legally dead, and all the principles of Sharia can be applied when (1) complete stoppage of the heart and breathing occurs and doctors decide that the condition is irreversible and (2) complete stoppage of all the vital functions of the brain occurs, doctors decide that the condition is irreversible, and the brain has started to degenerate.[25,27] Islamic law after death requires shrouding the body with white cloth, and a funeral prayer is offered. The body should be washed by a pious person. Some Muslim muftis oppose any form of donation (live or deceased) simply because the body should not be desecrated, but some concerns have also involved the potential for trading in organs.

Traditionally in Judaism, life begins and ends with breathing. Absence of breathing has major significance in the determination of death; thus, apneic brain death is an acceptable criterion for many prominent rabbis. The essence of Judaism is unconditional belief in God and objection to desecration of the body. Many different groups with different rabbinic views of the Jewish law (Halacha) exist. In the United States, Orthodox, Reform, Conservative but also reconstructionist and secular denominations are prevalent. Orthodox Jews accept the Torah as the textual "word of God." Other groups accept the Torah as the work of man "inspired by God," and reform rabbis reject a literal interpretation. Although Orthodox Jews accept the whole Torah, word for word, with its restrictive traditions, modern Orthodoxy is more moderate. Other denominations within Judaism believe that the Torah laws, although sacrosanct, can be interpreted differently, paving the way for independence of individual congregations. Reform and Conservative Jews have accepted brain death after analysis of traditional writings by their rabbis. The sources for such a decision by the chief rabbinate were the Gemara and other rabbinic opinions (the Gemara teaches that cessation of breathing—no air through the nostrils and no movement of the umbilicus— defines death).[20] In contrast, Orthodox rabbis David Bleich and Joseph Soloveitchik in the United States and former Chief Rabbi Lord Jakobovits in England interpreted the ancient teachings as cardiac arrest and the defining moment of death. An explanatory reading of the Talmudic tract published by Moses Tendler has compared and equated brain death with (physiologic) decapitation and thus accepts its premise of death. The most notable act was a change in New York State law initiated by the Orthodox Jewish community to include a religious exemption for declaring death and subjecting the physician, if this is ignored, to a possible malpractice lawsuit if death is declared (Chapter 2). A recent comprehensive study in 2010 by the Vaad Halacha of the Rabbinical Council of America has summarized major reservations with the diagnosis of brain death and emphasized cardiac death as being definitive (www.rabbis.org). The report has caused a stir in these circles after Lord Jonathan Sacks, chief rabbi of Orthodox Jews in London, agreed publicly. Its impact is not yet fully known.[36]

Nonetheless, the overwhelming majority of Jews support the concept of brain death. In fact, synagogues may encourage congregrants to register as donors. Eventually all would need to consult with their rabbi first.

Buddhism is the world's fourth largest religion, with an estimated 1.5 million Buddhists living in the United States. Buddhists teach that "to be is to suffer" and that all life is filled with suffering. They also teach eight noble paths to relieve suffering and that there is virtue to relief of suffering. Buddhists see death as a process leading to rebirth on the path to Nirvana.[36] They accept brain death when all the "reflexes" of the brain are absent. Mettanando Bhikkhu, the venerable monk from Thailand, has accepted that withdrawal of life support is permissible when brain death has been diagnosed. Others have defined death as loss of vitality and sentiency.

The religious views on organ donation can be found in a reference guide for clergy (www.organtransplant.org/understanding/religion) edited by Cooper and Taylor in 2000. All Christian denominations do accept organ donation for transplantation. Jehovah's Witnesses demand that all blood be removed from organs and state that the organ donor should not receive a blood transfusion. Many positions, particularly those of the Eastern religions, are unknown. Specific statements about a cardiocentric view of death or brain death as a prerequisite for possible organ donation are not always available. Unless views are specifically stated, we cannot assume, by implication, that the definition of death for a layperson is simply a medical issue and is to be left to the discretion of the physician.

■ CULTURAL VIEWS

Culture and religion influence and impact each other in many ways. For example, a Catholic may be aware that the Catholic Church supports organ donation, but he may also be a member of a Hispanic community that puts great emphasis on the importance of the heart. Occasionally, families may be hesitant to donate their loved one's heart but would allow the donation of other organs.

Data provided by the United Network of Organ Sharing (UNOS) on ethnicity and donors consistently shows a persistent trend of African-American, Hispanic, and Asian organ donation rates below that of whites.[41,42] Organ donation is much less approved of among these groups.[15] Some believe that this is due to poor understanding, poor education, or mistrust of the messenger. Barriers that complicate the decision to donate may include lack of faith in the success of transplantation, hostility toward physicians, or problems with communication. African-Americans usually are members of religious denominations, such as Baptists or Methodists, that are very supportive of donation. However, perceived mistreatment by the medical community may influence decisions on donation and some fear that whites are more helped than blacks.[32,33,34] African-Americans report mistrust in many surveys, and in one survey often agreed with the statement "Doctors would not try as hard to save me if they knew I was an organ donor." Callender et al. championed many of the organ donor campaigns in the African-American community, and identified five common reasons for unwillingness to donate among the African American population of the District of Columbia.[6] First, there is a documented lack of awareness of renal disease and transplantation. Second, religious myths, misperceptions, and superstitions prevail among persons at all income levels. Third, trust in health care providers and the health administration process is fragile, as is evident in many interactions with families. Fourth, there is a perception that signing an organ donor card might change the emphasis from lifesaving to organ donation. Finally, there is a perceived fear that racism, which African-Americans experience daily, would remain after death, resulting in all black-donated organs going to white people. Moreover, many minorities, especially African-Americans, wait twice as long for kidneys as do whites. This is a result of human leukocyte antigen (HLA) typing duration allocation and difficulty finding matches between persons of different races.[9,21] This longer waiting time has been misinterpreted as racial prejudice by some. However, despite the prevailing sense among some African-Americans that organ donation is not fair, 9 out of 10 African-Americans receive a graft from a white donor.

Similar apprehension is seen among Native Americans. Most Native Americans believe in a Creator or Master Spirit. However, Native American cultures are wary of organ donation, based on their spiritual beliefs about the afterlife. In addition, some fear ghosts and also fear that they may become sick when touching a dead body. Organ donation is a concern of great debate in these communities, but no official position is known.[3] Native tribes in the upper Midwest with traditional powwows to formulate opinions showed increased willingness to donate when approached by health care workers of their own culture. Another survey identified hesitation prompted by the possibility of donating unhealthy organs, but also by a desire to keep the body intact. Here again, the pietistic role of the body comes into play.

Hispanic populations encompassing people of Mexican, Puerto Rican, and Cuban heritage cite mutilation of the body as a common concern. Some immigrants from the Caribbean countries believe that disturbing the body may anger the spirit of the body. To what extent these superstitions permeate the Hispanic community is unknown, but they are quite unlikely to be the norm. Nonetheless, a recent evaluation of a Hispanic population in southern California found that opposition to organ transplantation was related in some cases to fear, taboo, misperception, and misinformation. Many felt that to know that the loved one's heart beats in someone else's body is particularly noteworthy. There was also a desire to meet the recipient.[13,14]

Roma (gypsies) are a people of distinct ethnicity with a set of folk beliefs. Virtually all of them oppose organ and tissue donation. Approximately 12 million Roma live in Europe, Russia, and the Middle East. Their traditional belief is that, for 1 year after death, the soul retraces its steps. The soul maintains its physical shape, and the body must remain intact. Many Roma adopt the faith of the countries they reside in, including Roman Catholicism, Eastern Orthodoxy, and Islam. Strong family traditions exist, and families may create clans. Roma believe in healing rituals and practice fortune-telling and supernatural ways to cure disease. After death, some Roma believe, evil spirits can enter the body, which is reflected by a desire to plug the nostrils with wax or pearls.

Both the Chinese and Japanese have different cultural value systems and do not—as in Western Cultures—emphasize self determination. Many spiritual movements including Taoism, prevalent in China, have not expressed opinions on brain death and a considerable diversity is expected. Organ transplantation is practiced, but not after brain death diagnosis (Chapter 1). Whether the major ideologies are going play a role in constructing a brain death law in China remains unclear. Japanese thinking is influenced by Confucian homilies, Buddhist traditions of care for the infirm, and Shinto beliefs,[18,23] as well as other religious views, western cultural influences, and pageantry. Confucian philosophy emphasizes that the body is a parental gift and cannot be given away. The Buddhist view emphasizes continuation of life after physical death (impermanence or *mujo*).[38] A cardiocentric view may be prevalent in some Japanese certainly because the word *heart* (*kanji*) is deeply ingrained in the written symbols for the words, *think*, *love*, and *center* (Figure 3-2). More likely, the reluctant acceptance by the Japanese of brain death may have its roots in a tendency to mistrust physicians and lingering tensions between physicians, nurses, and families in dealing with these sentimentalities rather than in Japanese culture.[19]

The situation in Japan is unique, with an extremely complicated protocol for assessment of the brain-dead patient and very slow progress in organ donation (Chapter 1). Japan has been struggling with methods of integrating brain death into medical practice; currently, nearly 65% of the Japanese accept brain death. However, few wish to have a donor card and few want organ donation after brain death. The latest tally at the end of 2009—after the lower Diet of the

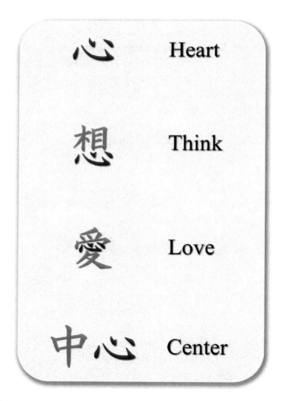

Figure 3-2 The letter Kanji (*heart*) appears in the words *think, love,* and *center.*

Japanese parliament approved legalized organ transplants—was 82 cases of organ transplantation. Currently, the Japan Organ Transplantation systems (JOTs) manage the national waiting list, which includes approximately 15,000 patients waiting for kidney transplants.

Organ donation in India is infrequent, but the consent rate is not much lower than in Western countries if transplant programs are carefully planned. Surprisingly, over 80% of live donors were female, which is considered to be a result of bias by a male-dominated society. Ethnic minorities in India have a much lower acceptance rate of organ donation.[30]

All of these cultural attitudes, superstitions, and prejudices may be separate from original religious beliefs in families and may negatively impact on care, brain death acceptance, and possible organ procurement.[31,35] Regardless of the race, cultural background, or religion of the health care team, it is imperative to approach the family in a manner that is sensitive to their culture and religion. Several studies providing direction have been published.[2,7,8,10,11,16,22,24,26,28,29,31,40]

Clergy can play a crucial role in the mediation between family and physician, and it is important to be able to view them as supportive and neutral allies. Some hospitals entrust the request for donation to the hospital chaplain, but chaplains do not have consent rates as high as those of trained organ procurement coordinators.[28,39] As was mentioned earlier, many religious leaders do not fully understand the concept of brain death and may confuse it with other comatose states such as a vegetative state. When a family is divided, the chaplain can explain the major benefits of organ donation, try to heal mistrust, if any, and explain the urgency of the decision.[12,16]

Hospital chaplains can be instrumental in offering final prayers or last rites. It can be difficult for family members, as well as clergy and medical personnel, to fully realize the finality of brain death. Having specific prayers and other "good-bye" rituals performed at the bedside can be very comforting.

■ RELIGIOUS CONFLICT RESOLUTION

Religion and spirituality affect the majority of Americans and members of other societies, but rarely fully determine the decision to donate organs and tissue. The reasons for refusal to donate involve private beliefs or possible concern about disfigurement, but most commonly they are due to the proxy's unfamiliarity with the prior wishes of the brain-dead person. When religious or cultural objections are put forward by family members, it is important to have families hold a conference with their own religious leader. In our experience, local clergy have been very helpful in clarifying the meaning of brain death and the process of donation. It is important to emphasize that organ donation can save many lives, not just one.

Miracles may be at the center of discussions with families because most religious traditions were founded on the basis of healing miracles. Some families request a prayer for a healing miracle, and others wish to pray for a resurrection. Christians, for example, may have faith in miracles. The Bible provides examples of raising the dead through Elijah and Elisha (1 Kings 17; 2 Kings 4). However, miracles are not for the asking and Jesus was generally reluctant to perform

Position	Christian	Judaic	Islamic	Buddhist	Confucian	Hindu	Shinto
Death by neurologic criteria	Accept	Accepted by most Rabbis	Accept	Accept	Accept	Accept	Mostly unacceptable
Ritual	Sacrament of prayer for sick/wake	Final prayer of forgiveness	Cover body, fasten jaws with cloth	Body rest for 2 hr	Certain customs	Prayers	Prayers
Autopsy	Allowed	Allowed	Allowed if mandated by law	Rarely allowed	Unclear	Allowed if mandated by law	Unacceptable
Burial	Open casket (orthodox Christian)	<24 hr if possible	<24 hr	Prolonged service	Closed casket	<24 hr	Multiple ceremonies

Figure 3-3 Positions of major religions on brain death, autopsy, and funeral.

miracles. Jesus performed miracles only to make someone believe that He was the Christ (John 20). Raising Lazarus (from the Hebrew *Eleazar*, which means "God has helped") from the dead after he had been entombed for several days made many Jews believe in Jesus as the Christ (John 11). Generally, divine intervention creating miracles is an uncommon belief among families. However, rather than showing skepticism, continuous communication of the hopeless situation is the best approach.

Some families question whether an incomplete body may go to heaven or preclude resurrection. Some people state that God has promised to make all things whole in death. To resolve this matter, physicians have emphasized that many persons die by fire or destructive accidents, and cremations are commonly performed. Other families have questioned whether you are really dead if your organs are going to be functioning in someone else's body.

Nonetheless, families with certain beliefs may object to the determination of brain death and express a desire to try all possible care. Typically, all available options are requested, including pharmaceutical support, prolonged cardiac resuscitation, and continuous stay in the intensive care unit with comprehensive nursing care. Consultation with ethics committees may be useful, but they may not take away ambivalence and discomfort with the attending physician. When no resolution can be achieved, brief continuation of care (but anticipating cardiac arrest) is one option. More likely it is necessary to involve the legal department of the hospital (more details are found in Chapter 6).

■ **CONCLUSION**

There is support from Western and Eastern religions for both organ donation and the clinical state of brain death, particularly among Christians and increasingly among Jews and Muslims (Figure 3-3). Although initially unexpected, ultraconservative Christian denominations have made a very strong statement in favor of organ donation. The main impediment is that many religious leaders and their congregants are unaware of this support and lack some degree of medical knowledge. Opposition by some theologians remains, and these strong opinions are displayed on the Internet. The fact is that in many religions, concern about desecration of the body after death is overridden by the obligation to save lives by organ donation. By working with physicians and organ procurement organizations, clergy may help to increase the number of organ donors throughout the world.

■ **REFERENCES**

1. Al-Mousawi M, Hamed T, al-Matouk H. Views of Muslim scholars on organ donation and brain death. *Transplant Proc* 1997;29:3217.
2. Anonymous. Altruism and confidentiality in organ donation. *Lancet* 2000;355:765.
3. Blagg CR, Helgerson SD, Warren CW, et al. Awareness and attitudes of Northwest Native Americans regarding organ donation and transplantation. *Clin Transplant* 1992;46:436–442.

4. Bresnahan MJ, Mahler K. Ethical debate over organ donation in the context of brain death. *Bioethics* 2010;24:54–60.
5. Bruzzone P. Religious aspects of organ transplantation. *Transplant Proc* 2008;40: 1064–1067.
6. Callender CO, Hall LE, Yeager CL, et al. Organ donation and Blacks. A critical frontier. *N Engl J Med* 1991;325:442–444.
7. Chabalewski F, Norris MKG. The gift of life: talking to families about organ and tissue donation. *Am J Nurs* 1994;94:28–33.
8. Christmas AB, Burris GW, Bogart TA, et al. Organ donations: family members not honoring patient wishes. *J Trauma* 2008;65:1095–1097.
9. Ciancio G, Burke GW, Gomez C, et al. Organ donation among Hispanics: a single-center experience. *Transplant Proc* 1997;29:37–45.
10. DeJong W, Franz HG, Wolf SM, et al. Requesting organ donation: an interview study of donor and nondonor families. *Am J Crit Care* 1998;7:13–23.
11. Envanisko MJ, Beasley CL, Brigham LE, et al. Readiness of critical care physicians and nurses to handle requests for organ donation. *Am J Crit Care* 1998;7:4–12.
12. Franz HG, DeJong W, Wolfe SM, et al. Explaining brain death: a critical feature of the donation process. *J Transplant Coord* 1997;7:14–21.
13. Frates J, Bohrer GG. Hispanic perceptions of organ donation. *Transplantation* 2002;12:169–175.
14. Frates J, Bohrer GG, Thomas D. Promoting organ donation to Hispanics: the role of the media and medicine. *J Health Commun* 2006;11:683–698.
15. Gentry D, Brown-Holbert J, Andrews C. Racial impact: increasing minority consent rate by altering the racial mix of an organ procurement organization. *Transplant Proc* 1997;29:3758–3759.
16. Gortmaker SL, Beasley CL, Sheehy E, et al. Improving the request process to increase family consent for organ donation. *J Transplant Coord* 1998;8:210–217.
17. Green J. Death with dignity: Hinduism. *Nurs Times* 1989;85:50–51.
18. Green J. Death with dignity: Buddhism and Shinto on the issue of brain death and organ transplant. *Camb Q Healthcare Ethics* 1994;3:585–601.
19. Kinura R. Japan's dilemma with the definition of death. *Kennedy Inst Ethics* 1991;1: 123–131.
20. Kunin J. Brain death: revisiting the rabbinic opinions in light of current medical knowledge. *Tradition* 2004;38:48–62.
21. McNamara P, Beasley CL. In: Cecka JM, Terasaki P, eds. *Clinical Transplants 1997*. Los Angeles: UCLA Tissue Typing Laboratory, 1997.
22. Morton J, Blok GA, Reid C, et al. The European Donor Hospital Education Programme (EDHEP): enhancing communication skills with bereaved relatives. *Anaesth Intensive Care* 2000;28:184–190.
23. Namihira E. Shinto concept concerning the dead human body. *Transplant Proc* 1990;22:940–941.
24. Niles PA, Mattice BJ. The timing factor in the consent process. *J Transplant Coord* 1996;6:84–87.
25. Rasheed HZA. Organ donation and transplantation—a Muslim viewpoint. *Transplant Proc* 1992;24:2116–2117.
26. Rudy LA, Leshman D, Kay NA, et al. Obtaining consent for organ donation: the role of the healthcare profession. *J S C Med Assoc* 1991;87:307–310.
27. Sachedina AA. Islamic views on organ transplantation. *Transplant Proc* 1988;20: 1084–1088.
28. Salim A, Brown C, Inaba K, et al. Improving consent rates for organ donation: the effect of an in-house coordinator program. *J Trauma* 2007;62:1411–1415.
29. Seth AK, Nambiar P, Joshi A, et al. First prospective study on brain stem death and attitudes toward organ donation in India. *Liver Transplant* 2009;15:1443–1447.

30. Siminoff LA, Gordon N, Hewlett J, et al. Factors influencing families' consent for donation of solid organs for transplantation. *JAMA* 2001;286:71–77.
31. Siminoff LA, Lawrence RE. Knowing patients' preferences about organ donation: does it make a difference?. *J Trauma* 2002;53:754–760.
32. Siminoff LA, Lawrence RH, Arnold RM. Comparison of black and white families' experiences and perceptions regarding organ donation requests. *Crit Care Med* 2003;31: 146–151.
33. Siminoff L, Mercer MB, Graham G, et al. The reasons families donate organs for transplantation: implications for policy and practice. *J Trauma* 2007;62:969–978.
34. Stouder DB, Schmid A, Ross SS, et al. Family, friends, and faith: how organ donor families heal. *Progress Transplant* 2009;19:358–361.
35. Sugunasiri SHJ. The Buddhist view concerning the dead body. *Transplant Proc* 1990;22:947–949.
36. The Lancet. Religion, organ transplantation and the definition of death. *Lancet* 2011; 377:271.
37. Trivedi HL. Hindu religious view in context of transplantation or organs from cadavers. *Transplant Proc* 1990;22:942.
38. Tsuji KT. The Buddhist view of the body and organ transplantation. *Transplant Proc* 1988;20:1076–1078.
39. von Pohle WR. Obtaining organ donation: who should ask? *Heart Lung* 1996;25: 304–309.
40. Wheeler MS, O'Friel M, Cheung AHS, et al. Cultural beliefs of Asian Americans as barriers to organ donation. *J Transplant Coord* 1994;4:146–150.
41. Yuen CC, Burton W, Chiraseveenuprapund D, et al. Attitudes and beliefs about organ donation among different racial groups. *J Natl Med Assoc* 1998;90:13–18.

4   Critics and Brain Death

For some scholars, the whole notion of brain death does not seem right. Even after more than 40 years of clinical practice in diagnosing brain death in numerous countries, essays have been published by bioethicists and theologians—but also by some physicians questioning the accuracy of the concept of brain death.[37,38]

It may be difficult to understand why such criticism exists and what drives the persistent motivation to emphasize the supposed fallacies of brain death—a neurologic condition that, for neurologists and neurosurgeons practicing in intensive care units (ICUs), is an accepted certitude and death. The main philosophy that sustains the critique is often a pro-sanctity of life position. Some critics are troubled by the practice of organ retrieval for organ transplantation. Even more blatantly some have stated that organ donation is a form of physician-assisted death and have insinuated that organ procurement coordinators may change ("erode") the care of the critically ill neurologic patient.[41] Many critics believe that physicians have simply convinced themselves and families that brain dead is dead, whereas in fact, patients have only lost consciousness, are alive, and are not even supported with complex means. The prevailing argument for those who object is that all 3 bodily systems—cardiovascular, respiratory and nervous system[45,55]—must be destroyed for death to occur.[38]

The responses to these critiques have been appropriately muted, but no one has condescendingly argued that these opinions should not be given a forum or that discussion of the alleged controversy is unworthy of the effort. There is a responsibility to categorically refute these ideas. Physicians[10,21,46,48] who oppose the concept of brain death and may be involved in these determinations should be taken more seriously than nonmedical professionals. This chapter therefore concentrates on their viewpoints and motivations. Opinions of philosophers and bioethicists can be found elsewhere.[16,24,37,38,60]

■ THE UNCERTAINTY OF DEATH

Even before bioethicists criticized the concept of brain death—in particular, the medical decision of equating it with death—many physicians struggled with the certainty of the clinical signs of death.[9] For centuries, books were published in Europe that questioned the certitude of death (Figure 4-1) and putrefaction after a "death watch" was considered the only infallible sign of death. It took several decades before Laennec's invention of the stethoscope allowed physicians to diagnose reliably the absence of an audible heartbeat in an apneic patient.

In the twentieth century, signs of death were not initially a topic of controversy, but they became more closely scrutinized with the emergence of organ transplantation. The early transplants that took place in the late 1960s were cadaver transplants, and an arbitrary period (several minutes) of cardiac arrest was allowed

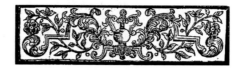

THE

UNCERTAINTY

OF THE

SIGNS of DEATH, &c.

SECT. I.

HO' Death, at fome Time or other, is the neceffary and unavoidable Portion of Human Nature in its prefent Condition, yet it is not always certain, that Perfons taken for dead are really and irretrievably deprived of Life; fince it is evident from Experience, that many apparently dead, have afterwards proved

B   themfelves

Figure 4-1 Book questioning the signs of death.

before kidney, heart, and liver recovery proceeded (e.g., in Christian Barnard's first heart transplant, after withdrawal of ventilation and cardiorespiratory arrest for 5 minutes, a forensic pathologist was called into the operating room to declare the donor dead).[3]

The required period of cessation of respiration and circulation in order to determine death has remained a topic of debate ever since. However, the need to correctly identify the moment of irreversibility of respiratory and circulatory arrest became less urgent when organ donation was linked to brain death determination. With a rekindling of the practice of donation after cardiac death (DCD), prompted by a growing and substantial shortage of organs, certain definition of the signs of irreversible circulation appeared warranted.

Modern medicine thus changed the equation, and hospital patients now could die in different ways. Respiratory arrest would lead irrevocably to hypoxemia, hypotension, circulatory arrest, and cardiac asystole. As a result, the brain injury would be severe and brain function irretrievably compromised. In another clinical scenario, catastrophic brain injury with lost brain function would lead to respiratory arrest followed by circulatory and cardiac standstill. The irreversibility of lost brain function was easily accepted; the irreversibility of respiratory and circulatory arrest was not.[31]

Quickly controversies emerged over these clinical determinations. First, *autoresuscitation* or resumption of circulation, seen as long as 30 minutes after the patient was declared dead, was observed. The explanation for this phenomenon (also known as the *Lazarus phenomenon*) is unclear and has been attributed to delayed action of intravenous epinephrine or increased venous return after ventilation is discontinued. This event has been noted exclusively after cardiopulmonary resuscitation in adults. It is a rare occurrence, transient and largely irrelevant clinically, with no patient surviving long term.[17]

Second, extracorporeal membrane oxygenation (ECMO) could replace circulation and oxygenation in a patient previously declared dead to preserve organs used for donation. Some have even suggested that in these patients ECMO may restore brain circulation and consciousness and provocatively surmise that the patient may in fact become aware and in severe distress.[7,41] The basic reality is that this scenario is implausible, but such a misdirected representation perfectly captures some of the ongoing discussion.

Third, similar to discussions of brain death, new terminology and language in DCD protocols are often unclear and mostly very confusing. Examples include *mechanical asystole, permanent versus irreversible cessation, cardiocirculatory death*, and *circulatory-respiratory determination of death*.[15]

Recently, the debate intensified after two hearts from severely injured but not brain-dead newborns were successfully transplanted after 85 seconds of circulatory arrest.[10] This apparent contradiction—nonfunctioning organs in dead bodies functioning in living bodies—fueled a new discussion of what constitutes death. In Veatch's words, cardiac donation in DCD is "reversing the irreversible."[54] Bernat suggested rewording the C in DCD as *circulatory*, in line with the Uniform Determination of Death Act (UDDA) statute that defined death as "irreversible cessation of circulatory and respiratory functions."[7] So, it was emphasized that cardiac death involved permanent respiratory and circulatory arrest, not the loss of cardiac function.

An equally debatable definition of death is to decide irreversibility as a result of a medical choice not to resuscitate. Thus, a patient with 2 minutes of circulatory and respiratory arrest is dead when not resuscitated and alive if circulation can be restored. It is easy to appreciate that placing the threshold at several minutes may blur the distinction between irreversible and reversible circulatory arrest.[49,50]

It is hard to believe that anyone observing a DCD protocol in the operating room would have difficulty pronouncing death in a cyanotic and apneic patient who became pulseless in a matter of minutes and was observed for several additional minutes. The time to permanent cessation of respiration and circulation has been set at 2 to 5 minutes, but this standard may not satisfy critics and the discussion will likely continue until—at least for them—a better evidentiary basis is available. Donation after cardiac death protocols are currently used in several countries but have remained contentious in many other countries (Chapter 5).

Some have advocated abandonment of the *dead-donor rule* in transplantation (which states that the patient must be dead before organs can be recovered), but this will create a new set of ethical quandaries.[49]

■ CREATING A CONTROVERSY

The clinical diagnosis of brain death became controversial in the United States in the years after publication of the Harvard Criteria (Chapter 1), and most of the debate has remained in this country. The themes have changed, ranging from objection to the workings of the Harvard Ad Hoc Committee (Chapter 1) to lack of prospective data.

With publication of the Harvard Criteria, most of the objection was directed to the makeup of the committee. The presence of a transplant surgeon and a transplant nephrologist was considered indicative of a conflict of interest.[60] Legally declaring a patient brain dead (and thus dead) would greatly facilitate transplantation, particularly cardiac transplantation, and remove any legal challenge to the surgeon. This early objection concerning a potential conflict of interest continues to resurface and to incorrectly imply that transplant organizations have a hidden agenda.

Dissatisfaction was also noted with the term *brain death*. This term was first suggested by Schwab in a paper on the role of EEG, followed by the Harvard Ad Hoc Committee's use first as *brain death syndrome* and later as a subtitle of the major document (Chapter 1). *Brain death* became a deeply anchored medical term and replaced *irreversible coma* largely to allow a distinction from persistent vegetative state. Others used the term *cerebral death* to indicate cessation of function of the hemispheres[56] or *dissociated death* to emphasize death of the brain and the living heart.[29]

In like-minded critics, brain death implied death of the brain and all functioning neurons. Assuming that the brain cannot be entirely dead, other terms would better reflect the pathophysiology. Some suggested eliminated the word *death* in *brain death*. Therefore, *total brain failure* has been used (most recently by the President's Council on Bioethics) to better describe a lack of brain function.[40] *Brain arrest* was also introduced, presumably to provide a complementary term to *cardiac arrest*.[43] Other terms are lengthy, and less distinctive (e.g., *irreversible apneic coma*) (Table 4-1).[61] However, apart from bickering over the right terminology, the major issue was whether death could be defined by neurologic criteria.

TABLE 4-1 *Alternative Terms for Brain Death*

The aperceptivity, areactive, apathic and atonic syndrome[25]
Status deanimatus (dissociated death)[29]
Total brain infarction[18]
Mortal brain damage[13]
Irreversible apneic coma[60]
Brain arrest[43]
Total brain failure[40]

The definition of death as "death of the whole brain" by the President's Commission (Chapter 1) may in retrospect have been unsatisfactory. To contrast *whole brain death* with other conditions, two other formulations of brain death were introduced: *higher brain death* or *brainstem death*. The controversy began in reference to the word *whole*.

Whole brain criteria implied that the hemispheres, brainstem, and cerebellum must be all dead. Absent neuronal function may have to be demonstrated by additional ancillary tests showing encephalographic silence or absence of cerebral blood flow. Failure to find supportive documentation would deny such a conclusion.

Korein interpreted death by neurologic criteria as failure of a "critical vital system" that leads to a state of greater disorder and entropy.[27,28] Bernat defined death as "the permanent cessation of the critical organism as a whole" and emphasized loss of functional integrity of an organism similarly to Korein in earlier manuscripts.[4,6] In a 1981 article authored with a psychiatrist, Charles Culver, and a philosopher, Bernard Gert—neurologist—Bernat emphasized "the irreversible cessation of total brain function," replacing the word *whole* with the word *total*.[6] Use of the terms *critical* and *whole* or *total* has resulted in numerous rebuttals by bioethicists.

The higher brain criteria of death include a permanently comatose state (e.g., spontaneously breathing patients in a persistent vegetative state). Many scholars argue that absence of hemispheric function is more or less the philosophical equivalent to the absence of hemispheric and brainstem function. The higher brain criterion argues that personal identity is essential for a human organism; when personal identity is absent, the person ceases to exist.[30,33,47,51,52,53]

The brainstem formulation of death implies that without a functioning brainstem, the person is irreversibly unconscious and apneic. The formulation of brainstem death is largely pragmatic. In Pallis' words, "Brainstem death is the physiologic kernel of brain death, the anatomical substratum of its cardinal signs (apneic coma with absent brainstem signs)."[35,36] The line of thinking here—and scientifically the most convincing one—is that the brainstem in evolutionary biology has been the major structure preceding the development of the neocortex. When clinical examination in a comatose patient without confounders shows absence of brainstem reflexes and apnea, the presence of normal brain tissue elsewhere is not relevant. Brainstem formulation of death stipulates that the brainstem is, in fact, an indispensibly necessary system and not just part of a group of important neuronal systems.

As expected, therefore, most of the earlier arguments in the 1970s and 1980s against brain death concentrated on finding ways to show that the whole brain is not dead and thus that the person has not died. Over the years, multiple essays and a number of textbooks including multiple contributors with diverse specialties have appeared. The many other arguments further developed in this chapter are summarized in Table 4-2.[11,12,13,20,22,26,44,46,53]

In the critiques, significant attention has been directed to a possible presence of integrated neuroendocrine function. Some early studies (but not later ones) found no evidence of diabetes insipidus and no evidence of a deficiency of pituitary

TABLE 4-2 *Main Critiques Against Brain Death by Physicians*

Author	Specialty	Critique
Byrne[11]	Pediatrician	• No consensus; multiple criteria; brain death by one but not by another. • The brain may be "stunned," not dead. • There is no valid science. • The Harvard Committee had an agenda.
Evans[13,14]	Cardiologist	• Too many protocols, indicating that brain death is not a scientifically based entity. • Tests in the United Kingdom (brainstem only) are insufficient. • There is no test of cranial nerves I and II ("patient is in a visual nightmare"). • A sufficient criterion could only be no blood/oxygen to the entire brain for a considerable amount of time.
Coimbra[12]	Neurologist	• Apnea test is unethical (because it is dangerous), and hypercapnia-acidosis may cause cerebral vasoconstriction. Hypoxemia during the test may cause further necrosis.
Shewmon[44-46]	Pediatric neurologist	• The body may remain alive without brain function, and there is no cardiac arrest in several cases.
Joffe[19-23]	Pediatric intensivist	• "Recovery" of brain function has been reported.

Others have used similar arguments or combinations (i.e., Karakatsanis, a nuclear medicine physician[26]; Rady, an anesthesiologist[41]; Zamperetti, an anesthesiologist[61]).

hormones such as prolactin, human growth hormone, luteinizing hormone, and thyrotropin (thyroid stimulating hormone), all suggesting an intact hypothalamus and pituitary axis despite absence of flow to the brain on a cerebral angiogram.[1]

Other critics could not live with the idea that in a considerable proportion of patients electroencephalographic activity remained, suggesting in their mind important neuronal function. In other patients, uptake of radioactive material found on cerebral blood flow studies was preserved in several areas of the brain. Cerebral angiograms could document flow in the posterior circulation and slow flow beyond the siphon, providing blood to many areas of the brain that were supposedly dead.

Several physicians maintain a strong opposing voice. Paul Byrne, a neonatologist and past president of the Catholic Medical Association, has lectured extensively against clinical testing for brain death and against organ transplantation.[11] Byrne's main arguments are that (1) spontaneous movements cannot be spinal reflexes and thus are not compatible with death, (2) the apnea test causes more brain swelling due to acidosis and hypercarbia, (3) recovery of patients occurs when an apnea test is not performed, (4) the appearance of brain death is different from the appearance of a corpse, (5) the heart rate and blood pressure increase during recovery of organs and imply a response of a living patient, and (6) organ donation is "legal killing of vulnerable patients" or "defenseless comatose patients" and, therefore, all organ donation in brain-dead patients should be rejected. In another paper coauthored with cardiologist, Weaver, entitled "'Brain Death Is Not Death,'" Byrne claims that the observed loss of brain function could in fact be only "stunning" of brain tissue. The authors also suggest that procurement may prevent recovery of the brain.[11]

Karakatsanis, a nuclear medicine physician, has formulated four more or less similar arguments against brain death.[26] The arguments are, again, against the concept of complete and total brain destruction. First, the spinal reflexes could well be generated from the brainstem and not the cervical or thoracic cord. These movements cannot be clinically distinguished from movements seen in brainstem injury and are never seen in patients with an acute cervical spinal cord lesion, suggesting that these movements are generated from intact (or perhaps partly intact) diencephalon and brainstem. Second, physicians are unable to test the neocortex clinically because all reflexes go through the brainstem and the brainstem reflexes are absent. Patients may be "locked in" and cannot express themselves. Third, many electrophysiologic tests and blood flow studies show activity demonstrating that neurons are intact. Fourth, often the posterior circulation perfusing the brainstem is intact, and pathologic studies have shown no changes in the brainstem.

These arguments lingered for years, but the controversy over brain death became definitively more interesting after a pediatric neurologist, Shewmon, published a provocative paper titled "Chronic 'Brain Death.'"[46] In the paper, he gathers 56 previously published documented cases of survival for 1 week or more. Cardiac arrest in other cases was presumed to be due to prior injury (i.e., severe brain injury leading to sympathetic storm or disseminated intravascular coagulation) rather than a direct consequence of brain death. These examples of prolonged support in persons after brain death occurred because of certain beliefs, because of pregnancy, and because physicians were giving in to the unreasonable demands of emotionally distraught family members who refused to accept the death of a loved one.

Shewmon's charge has been fundamental. Patients who have fulfilled the clinical criteria of brain death do not necessarily progress to what he called somatic disintegration. The full panoply of modern life-prolonging machinery may not be needed for stabilization of the rest of the body. These integrative functions— observed in two personal cases—included wound healing, fighting off infection, development of a febrile response to infection, maturation in children, and improvement in clinical condition (withdrawal of vasopressors).

Shewmon concludes, "The phenomenon of chronic brain death implies that the body's integrative unity derives from mutual interaction among its parts, not from a top-down imposition of one 'critical' organ upon an otherwise mere bag of organs and tissues. If brain death is to be equated with human death, therefore, it must be on some basis more plausible than that the body is dead."[46] Shewmon credited his recent conversion to theism as being responsible for his change in position and his moral obligation to speak out, but his earlier writings include an article on a mathematical calculation on the impossibility of validating criteria for brain death.[47]

His definition of brain death is deep coma in a dying patient but not death. He stated the following: "a probable valid criterion close to the mode of death might be something like cessation of circulation of blood for a sufficient time, depending on blood temperature, depending on body temperature, to produce irreversible damage to a critical number of organs and tissue throughout the body so that irrevocable process of disintegration has begun. At normothermia, the minimum sufficient time is probably somewhere around 20 minutes, although there is insufficient data to support the precise duration with certainty. I do not believe that the critical number of organs and tissues can be universally specified as it will no doubt vary from case to case. Surely the brain is included but not only the brain."[46]

Thus, the view expressed is that the ICU can be seen as "the surrogate brain stem."[48] If we are able to maintain integrated somatic function for many months, critics claim, the ICU treatment (ventilator, vasopressors, vasopressin, nutrition) maintains life.

The controversy has continued, with the critics challenging the defenders. The defenders of brain death have a few spokespersons who have tried to debunk the critics,[5] only to leave open the discussion of why the defense is not good enough. None of the critics feel that any of the arguments presented are sufficient to change their minds. Shewmon stated recently that the defenders have an "apologetic task" and should explain why they still feel that brain death is death.[59]

Joffe, pediatric intensivist, recently emerged as another critic of the clinical state of brain death by publishing a series of provocative articles.[19-22] In one recent commentary, he summarized the inadequate defenses of the brain death concept.[21] This was buttressed by a recent survey of neurosurgeons and pediatric intensivists in Canada.[22] Approximately one-third of physicians would continue life support if the family insisted on it for a patient who met the clinical criteria of brain death. In addition, the survey exposed lack of understanding among physicians concerning the concept of brain death. When asked whether brain death and cardiac death were the same, 45% of Canadian neurosurgeons answered no, meaning that they did not consider both to signify the death of a patient. Joffe also criticized prior statements, particularly by Bernat, saying that brain death might be a "compromise or approximation" in order to maintain public confidence in organ procurement. Joffe also pointed out that if brain death is the loss of brain function in the entire brain, including the brainstem, he has great difficulty accepting that 20% of patients have EEG activity, 50% have evidence of hypothalamic function, and none have evidence of excessive brain destruction in many areas of the brain. Finally— and most provocatively—Joffe published the case of a newborn diagnosed as brain dead who developed "hiccups" that were interpreted as return of a respiratory drive (the examination was markedly confounded by the prior use of sedatives). In addition, Joffe claimed to have identified cases of "recoveries," but he acknowledged that the examinations in the published articles were incomplete.[23]

In 2008, a white paper by the President's Council on Bioethics was published (Figure 4-2).[40] This Council was chaired by Edmond Pellegrino, emeritus professor of Medicine and Medical Ethics. It consisted mostly of professors of medical ethics law, social and political ethics, metaphysics, political economy, government, and international studies, among other fields. One pediatric neurosurgeon and one neurologist participated. The Council invited Shewmon to present his case. He introduced his presentation with multiple examples alleging that even experts in this area write confusing texts, claiming that some use the word *comatose* when referring to brain death (implying a living organism) and others use the term *mode of death* when writing about brain death, also suggesting that another event is needed to die. Shewmon also compared the clinical manifestations of acute spinal cord transsection and bilateral vagotomy with the clinical manifestations of brain death, showing that the only difference is the presence of consciousness and thus

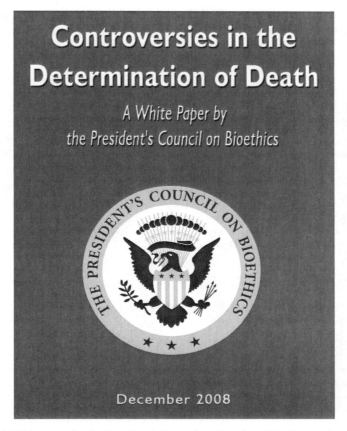

Figure 4-2 White paper by the President's Council on Bioethics (2008).

arguing that the systemic manifestations in brain death are not sufficiently dis-
criminatory.[45] Moreover, his prior examples of prolonged support suggest that the
body is integrated with the ability to survive with support and recover from intermittent illnesses such as infections. In his opinion, one could only conclude that
these are living organisms.

The Council used his arguments to formulate a divided conclusion. "The
Council has concluded that the neurologic standard remains valid. A few Council
members argue that there is sufficient uncertainty about the neurologic standard
to warrant an alternative approach to the 'brain dead' human being and the
question of organ procurement." The Council further concluded that "if there
are no signs of consciousness and if spontaneous breathing is absent and if
the clinical judgment is that these neurophysiological facts cannot be reversed . . .
a once living patient has now died."[39] The white paper also included three personal
statements (including that of the chairman of the Council) that dis-
agreed with the final letter. In a more recent critique of the Council's manuscript,
Shewmon bluntly stated that the time has come to add a footnote to signing a

donor card and he suggested the following language: "Warning: It remains controversial whether you will actually be dead at the time of removal of your organs. . . . You should study the President's Council on Bioethics white paper carefully and decide for yourself before signing an organ donor card."[46]

The Council was abruptly dissolved by the Obama administration. The council accepted the dismissal but speculation that its bias may have played a role abound (the Council had just prepared a document on "the ethics of transplantation" but the document was not finalized before dismissal).

So, the selection and interpretation of single cases by several critics, taking a few inconsistencies and blowing them out of proportion, may succeed in creating some doubt. Certain organizational bodies may become persuaded, and the issue could become a matter of debate. The next step is to place the onus on the "defenders of brain death." Then, if the defenders are unconvincing or, worse ambiguous, in their answers, critics will argue that both positions (supporting vs. opposing) will need to be taken into account and allowed to participate in the discussion on this topic. And so a "controversy" is created.

■ CRITIQUE

There is no disagreement that brain death is a separate clinical neurologic state. The clinical findings in brain death are different from those in any other comatose patients. Brain death has been understood medically as loss of all brain function, and its unique clinical presentation—an apneic comatose, poikilothermic, polyuric, and hypotensive patient with no brainstem reflexes—may be the best that physicians can diagnose. It has been argued that brain death is death and is close enough for practical medical purposes.[2] It is impossible to have a better medical standard. (Functional magnetic resonance imaging—perhaps the closest test showing activation of the brain—shows the absence of functional connectivity.[8]) Brain death is unsustainable. Patients who meet the criteria of brain death without any further intensive care support would de facto progress to apnea, hemodynamic collapse, and cardiac standstill.

Brain death can be reliably diagnosed and when it is present, the findings are irreversible in adults. In children—mostly neonates—"return of respiration or respiratory-like hiccups" have been reported, but a recovery such as a permanent vegetative state is not known or expected. All "recovered" cases reported in the literature—recently compiled by Joffe—are suspect (due to the presence of confounders) or incomplete (with no detailed description of testing and no mention of the apnea test). To claim that the brain is "stunned" is a grave misreading of the neurobiology of a catastrophic injury.[11] Brain death has a sound physiologic basis and is mostly the end stage of destruction of the thalamus, mesencephalon, pons, and medulla, in that order. To claim that the apnea test causes further brain injury (hypercarbia causes a rise in ICP) ignores the absence of cerebral autoregulation with this degree of injury and also ignores the significantly elevated ICP that led to brain death in the first place.[12] Hypoxemia resulting in additional brain injury could theoretically occur with a poorly performed apnea test, but our findings argue otherwise. In a correctly performed apnea test, hyperoxemia is a common finding at the completion of the test.[58]

The repeated claim that patients during organ recovery "squirm" (Byrne's term[11]) and develop tachycardia and hypertension at the time of recovery is false and is not seen in the experience of transplant surgeons. Anesthesia is never used, but neuromuscular blocking agents are used in some instances to relax the abdominal musculature in order to assess the organs for procurement.

Long-term hemodynamic support of brain death patients for weeks is not feasible and the overwhelming majority of cases show a hemodynamic instability or relentless progressive decline in blood pressures despite increase in vasopressors. If brain death diagnosis takes too long, patients are lost for organ procurement as a result of circulatory arrest (Chapter 6).

How can this possibly agree with Shewmon's case of prolonged support? It is therefore important to summarize the breakdown of these cases.[46] The 56 cases of prolonged support consisted of 28 cases from four series of patients with brain death (from a total of 143 cases) and 28 isolated cases from letters to the editor, case reports, and newspaper articles. Of the latter 28 isolated cases, 15 involved a "brain-dead" pregnant mother. Imprecision in the study sample is introduced by excluding all reportedly brain-dead patients in whom cardiac arrest developed within 1 week.

These cases almost certainly represent incomplete brain death determinations. First, in only 2 of the 56 cases were apnea tests done, with documentation of absent respiratory effort at a $PaCO_2$ of 60 mm Hg. Most cases included brief (minutes) disconnection of the ventilator alone. Second, many cases did not have sufficient documentation of the details of the neurologic examination, coughing to tracheal suctioning was not mentioned, and examination of the patients by at least one neurologist was inconsistent. Most disturbingly, the cited material provided with the paper included a neurosurgeon's telling note: "We knew she was brain dead but we did not do any tests to formally establish this because a death certificate would have to be completed. We were conscious of the stigma attached to a child born to a dead mother." The questionable literature associated with prolonged support of maternal death is further discussed in Chapter 6 and I have not come across a single convincing case.[39] To illustrate this further, a case of a "brain-dead" adult patient with 5½ months of successful support has recently been published.[32] The case is questionably accurate because of failure to perform the apnea test (the case demonstrates the challenges that physicians in Japan face, with continuous threat of criminal charges when the ventilator is removed).[32] The apnea test remains an important test not because it assesses lack of a breathing drive, but because it is an indicator of significant medulla-pontine injury; conversely, patients who have a persistent breathing drive almost always have hemodynamic stability.

Most of this new argument—lack of top-down function of the brain and largely autonomic, coordinated multisystem organ function—is based on the extraordinary Repertinger case. Repertinger and associates, from the Department of Pathology at Creighton University Medical Center, published a pathology report of a 4½-year-old boy with a fulminant *Hemophilus influenzae* type B meningitis.[42] Few details are provided about his medulla oblongata function and breathing drive.

The boy was able to survive without vasopressors, resulting in maturation to adulthood. At autopsy, a calcified and mummified brain was found with no recognizable neurons. Unfortunately, the cervical cord was not examined, leaving open the possibility that the cervical medullary junction and medulla oblongata were not subjected to microscopy. One is inclined not to accept this case as meeting the criteria of brain death.

Whether patients are biologically dead when the brain irrevocably stops functioning is purely a philosophical and perhaps spiritual issue. In Shewmon's words, most neuroscientists are brain (mind) reductionists, in contrast to traditional philosophical anthropologists, who may see a human organism—without a brain—as biologically unified and alive. His basic premise is thus quite simple. The determination of death is not based on brain function, and he—seemingly paradoxically, as a neurologist—rejects any neurologic criteria of death.

It may come down not only to a neurologic-versus-vitalist argument, but also to a logical-versus-implausible argument. In the practice of medicine, certain signs suffice for a diagnosis; in the practice of philosophy, none are definitive. Not one recent essay written by a philosopher has declared solidarity with the neurologic determination of death, and all have noncritically accepted alternative explanations.

Not the introduction of death by neurologic criteria, but more likely the discussion about whole brain, higher brain, or brainstem definitions, provoked controversy. Pallis considered it "terminologic quagmires."[36] Speculation on how patients might be living (in heaven or hell) with no functioning brainstem alone is useless, and simplifies the catastrophic injury and the clinical context. Precisely such issues are at the heart of the misconceptions about defining irreversible loss of brain function.

■ CONCLUSIONS

Over the years, the commentaries against the clinical diagnosis of brain death or the concept of brain death have shifted their focus. These range from criticisms of the Harvard Committee (alleging conflict of interest, as shown by the presence of transplant physicians), to clinical examination (alleging injury with the apnea test), to critiques of the total brain necrosis criteria (alleging intact pituitary and hypothalamic function), to critiques on the difficulty of support (alleging long-term support in pregnant "brain-dead" women and children) and, most recently, to critiques on irreversibility (alleging possible recoveries). Critics can demand an alternative explanation but as yet they have no original data on large series of patients. All have been using previously published data and interpret them wholly otherwise (i.e., variability in brain death protocols becomes dead in one hospital, alive in another; total brain necrosis at autopsy is rare and becomes minimal neuronal damage is found in some areas in supposedly brain-dead patients).[55]

Is there nothing disconcerting? Going back to the Harvard Criteria, a committee without transplantation representatives would have been more ideal, but a carefully detailed evaluation of the deliberation has not found a major influence or attempted bias toward the writers of the document.[57] Brain death determination and organ procurement are two totally different procedures but are linked closely, with 70% of brain death declarations converting into organ donors. Intermingling of transplant surgeons in brain death determination is avoided carefully in most practices and in fact most transplant surgeons want nothing to do with it.

There is no questioning the early arguments that (1) the brain is totally necrotic, (2) cardiac arrest always occurs within hours after clinical diagnosis, and (3) invariably supporting electrophysiology or blood flow studies confirming the clinical condition have been weak. We now know that neuropathologic examination of brains coming to autopsy soon after the diagnosis of brain death may show normal areas of the brain in patients with and without complete circulatory arrest on blood flow testing. This suggests that no study can reliably exclude cerebral perfusion. Arguments that brain death is similar to physiologic decapitation thus are incorrect,[34] but this does not mean that with the presence of seemingly intact regions of the brain, the brain did not irreversibly stop functioning.[57] Hemodynamic instability is common in most patients, but hypertension (likely due to unopposed sympathetic spinal cord activity or by lingering effects of caudal medulla oblongata pressor areas) requiring antihypertensives may occur. Nothing here should invalidate the diagnosis.

Since the original description of brain death more than 40 years ago (as well as enormous clinical experience), the certitude of a brain death diagnosis has not been questioned by expert physicians in the field. The scientific foundation underlying the argument of lack of somatic disintegration is simply mistaken, and the President's Council on Bioethics could be faulted for taking selected sources— by way of published documents in the ethics realm—and for gathering selected information—by interviewing those who object and then interpreting the data the way they appear to be. It would be improbable to find patients—or should we say supported organs—that could be sustained for a prolonged period of time.

These criticisms are also indirectly a comment on our practice of judging irreversible neurologic injury and the use of organ donation, and perhaps even insinuating that those involved in these decisions may have less respect for the patient's life. There may be a serious attempt to delegitimize the practice or organ donation.[41] Physicians in the neurosciences who are closely and frequently involved in brain death determination will be vexed and less intrigued by the disputations outlined in this chapter, and some may be greatly struck by the fact that such vast literature even exists. It will be hard to find one who would concede that these potential organ donors are not dead.

■ REFERENCES

1. Arita K, Uozumi T, Oki S, et al. The function of the hypothalamo-pituitary axis in brain dead patients. *Acta Neurochir* 1993;123:64–75.
2. Barnard CN. A human cardiac transplant: an interim report of a successful operation performed at Groote Schuur Hospital, Cape Town. *S Afr Med J* 1967;41:1271–1274.
3. Battro A, Bernat JL, Bousser N, Cabibbo N, Card G, Cottier G, Daroff RB, Davis L, Deecke L, Estol CJ, Hacke W, Hennerici MG, Huber JC, Lopez Trujillo-Card A , Martini CM, Masdeu J, Mattle H, Posner JB, Puybasset L, Raichle M, Ropper AH, Rossini PM, Sanchez Sorondo M, Schambeck H, Sgreccia E, Tandon PN, Vicuna R, Wijdicks EFM, Zichini A. Why the concept of brain death is valid as a definition of brain death. The Pontifical Academy of Sciences, Scripta Varia 110, 2006.
4. Bernat JL. How much of the brain must die in brain death? *J Clin Ethics* 1992;3:21–26.

5. Bernat JL. In defense of the whole-brain concept of death. *Hastings Center Rep* 1998;28:14–23.
6. Bernat JL, Culver CM, Gert B. On the definition and criterion of death. *Ann Intern Med* 1981;94:389–394.
7. Bernat JL, Capron AM, Bleck TP, et al. The circulatory-respiratory determination of death in organ donation. *Crit Care Med* 2010;38:963–970.
8. Boly M, Tshibanda T, Vanhaudenhuyse A, et al. Functional connectivity in the default network during resting state is preserved in a vegetative state but not in a brain dead patient. *Hum Brain Mapp* 2009;30:2393–2400.
9. Bondeson J. *Buried Alive: The Terrifying History of Our Most Primal Fear*. New York: W.W. Norton; 2001.
10. Boucek MM, Mashburn C, Dunn SM. Pediatric heart transplantation after declaration of cardiocirculatory death. *N Engl J Med* 2008;359:709–714.
11. Byrne PA, Weaver WF. "Brain death" is not death. In: Machado C, Shewman DA, eds. *Brain Death and Disorders of Consciousness*. New York: Kluwer Academic Press/ Plenum; 2004:43–60.
12. Coimbra CG. Implications of ischemic penumbra for the diagnosis of brain death. *Braz J Med Biol Res* 1999;32:1479–1487.
13. Evans DW. The demise of "brain death" in Britain. In: Potts M, Nilges RG. eds. *Beyond Brain Death*. London: Kluwer Academic; 2000:139–158.
14. Evans DW. Brainstem tests not adequate to diagnose brain death in organ donors. *Nature* 2009;461:1198.
15. Fugate JE, Rabinstein AA, Wijdicks EFM. Variability in language of DCD protocols: a national survey. *Transplantation* 2011;91:386–389.
16. Green MB, Wikler D. Brain death and personal identity. *Philos Public Aff* 1980;9: 105–133.
17. Hornby K, Hornby L, Shemie SD. A systematic review of autoresuscitation after cardiac arrest. *Crit Care Med* 2010;38:1246–1253.
18. Ingvar DH. Brain death—total brain infarction. *Acta Anaesthesiol Scand Suppl* 1971;45:129–140.
19. Joffe AR. Brain death is not death: a critique of the concept, criterion, and tests of brain death. *Rev Neurosci* 2009;20:187–198.
20. Joffe AR. Are recent defenses of the brain death concept adequate? *Bioethics* 2010;24: 47–53.
21. Joffe AR, Anton N. Brain death: understanding of the conceptual basis by pediatric intensivists in Canada. *Arch Pediatr Adolesc Med* 2006;160:747–752.
22. Joffe AR, Anton N, Mehta V. A survey to determine the understanding of the conceptual basis and diagnostic tests used for brain death by neurosurgeons in Canada. *Neurosurgery* 2007;61:1039–1047.
23. Joffe AR, Kolski H, Duff J, et al. A 10-month-old infant with reversible findings of brain death. *Pediatr Neurol* 2009;41:378–382.
24. Jonas H. Against the stream. In: *Philosophical Essays: From Ancient Creed to Technological Man*. Englewood Cliffs, NJ: Prentice-Hall; 1974.
25. Jouvet M. Coma and other disorders of consciousness. In: Vinken PJ, Bruyn GW, eds. *Handbook of Clinical Neurology. Vol. 3: Disorders of Higher Nervous Activity*. Amsterdam: North-Holland; 1969:62–79.
26. Karakatsanis KG. Brain death: should it be reconsidered?. *Spinal Cord* 2008;46: 396–401.
27. Korein J. The problem of brain death: development and history. *Ann NY Acad Sci* 1978;315:19–38.
28. Korein J. Ontogenesis of the brain in the human organism: definitions of life and death of the human being and person. *Adv Bioethics* 1997;2:1–74.
29. Kramer W. From reanimation to deamination (intravital death of the brain during artificial respiration). *Acta Neurol Scand* 1963;39:139–153.

30. Lizza JP. The conceptual basis for brain death revisited: loss of organic integration or loss of consciousness? *Adv Exp Med Biol* 2004;550:51–59.
31. Marquis D. Are DCD donors dead?. *Hastings Center Rep* 2010;40:24–31.
32. Maruya J, Nishimaki K, Nakahata J-I, et al. Prolonged somatic survival of clinically brain-dead adult patient-case report. *Neurol Med Chir* 2008;48:114–117.
33. Miller FG, Truog RD. Rethinking the ethics of vital organ donations. *Hastings Center Rep* 2008;38:38–46.
34. Miller FG,Truog RD.Decapitation and the definition of death. *J Med Ethics* 2010;36: 632–634.
35. Pallis C. Whole brain death reconsidered: physiological facts and philosophy. *J Med Ethics* 1983;9:32–37.
36. Pallis C. Brainstem death. *Med Leg J* 1987;55:84–107.
37. Pernick MS. Back from the grave: recurring controversies over defining and diagnosing death in history. In: Zaner RM, ed. *Death: Beyond Whole-Brain Criteria*. Dordrecht: Kluwer Academic; 1988:17–24.
38. Potts M, Byrne PA, Nilges RG, eds. *Beyond Brain Death: The Case Against Brain-Based Criteria for Human Death*. Dordrecht: Kluwer Academic, 2000.
39. Powner DJ, Bernstein IM. Extended somatic support for pregnant women after brain death. *Crit Care Med* 2003;31:1241–1249.
40. President's Council on Bioethics: *Controversies in the Determination of Death: A White Paper by the President's Council on Bioethics*. Washington, DC, 2008. Available at http://www.bioethics.gov/reports/death/index.htm.
41. Rady MY, Verheijde JL, McGregor JL. Scientific, legal and ethical challenges of end-of-life organ procurement in emergency medicine. *Resuscitation* 2010;81:1069–1078.
42. Repertinger S, Fitzgibbons WP, Omojola MF, et al. Long survival following bacterial meningitis–associated brain destruction. *J Child Neurol* 2006;21:591–595.
43. Shemie SD, Doig C, Dickens B, et al. Severe brain injury to neurological determination of death: Canadian forum recommendations. *CMAJ* 2006;174:S1–S13.
44. Shewmon DA. Chronic "brain death": meta-analysis and conceptual consequences. *Neurology* 1998;51:1538–1545.
45. Shewmon DA. Hypothesis: spinal shock and "brain death": somatic pathophysiological equivalence and implications for the integrative-unity rationale. *Spinal Cord* 1999;37:313–324.
46. Shewmon DA. Brain death: can it be resuscitated?. *Issues Law Med* 2009;25:3–14.
47. Shewmon DA. The probability of inevitability: the inherent impossibility of validating criteria for brain death or 'irreversibility' through clinical studies. *Stat Med* 1987;6: 535–553.
48. Truog RD. Brain death: too flawed to endure, too ingrained to abandon. *J Law Med Ethics* 2007;35:273–281.
49. Truog RD, Miller FG. The dead donor rule and organ transplantation. *N Engl J Med* 2008;359:674–675.
50. Troug RD, Miller FG. Counterpoint: are donors after circulatory death really dead and does it matter? No and not really. *Chest* 2010;138:16–18.
51. Veatch RM. Brain death and slippery slopes. *J Clin Ethics* 1992;3:181–187.
52. Veatch RM. The impending collapse of the whole-brain definition of death. *Hastings Center Rep* 1993;23:18–24.
53. Veatch RM. The death of whole brain death: the plaque of the disaggregators, somaticists and mentalists. *J Med Philos* 2005;4:353–378.
54. Veatch RM. Donating hearts after cardiac death: reversing the irreversible. *N Engl J Med* 2008;359:672–673.
55. Verheijde JL, Rady MY, McGregor JL. Brain death, states of impaired consciousness, and physician-assisted death for end-of-life organ donation and transplantation. *Med Health Care Philos* 2009;12:409–421.
56. Walker EA.*Cerebral Death*. Baltimore and Munich: Urban & Schwarzenberg; 1985.

57. Wijdicks EFM. The neurologist and Harvard Criteria for brain death. *Neurology* 2003;61:970–976.
58. Wijdicks EFM, Rabinstein AA, Manno EM, et al. Pronouncing brain death: contemporary practice and safety of the apnea test. *Neurology* 2008;71:1240–1244.
59. Working Group on the Signs of Death, ed HE Msgr. *Marcelo Sanchez Sorondo*. Vatican City: Pontificia Academia Scientiarum; 2007:292–333.
60. Youngner SJ, Arnold RM, Schapiro R, eds. *The Definition of Death: Contemporary Controversies*. Baltimore: Johns Hopkins University Press; 1999.
61. Zamperetti N, Bellomo R, Defanti CA, et al. Irreversible apneic coma 35 years later: towards a more rigorous definition of brain death? *Intensive Care Med* 2004;30: 1715–1722.

5 Procurement after Brain Death

After the determination of brain death, the family gathers for a conference. This conversation takes place in a room where the next of kin can sit down quietly and meet the attending physician or consulting neurologist. The exchange centers on letting the family know that their loved one has died and the body exists merely on support. Another purpose of this meeting is to discuss important decisions the family will have to make on organ donation. In the United States, hospitals have a legal requirement to involve organ procurement agencies. It is customary for the organ transplant coordinator will have a separate discussion with the family about the possibility of organ and tissue donation.

Well-managed organ transplantation organizations exist in many countries. In the United States, organ procurement is administered and medically managed by the United Network of Organ Sharing (UNOS), and participation of hospitals in organ donation requires certification. The number of patients on the waiting list to receive organs remains distressingly high (currently, it exceeds 110,000). Although there are over 7000 donors in the United States each year, and globally more than 15,000 organ donors after brain death these numbers are far from meeting demand.[90] Great benefit could come from organ donation and upto 7 lives may be saved (lungs, heart, kidney [2], liver [split in 2] and pancreas). Tissue donation adds another dimension (e.g., bone, cornea, heart valves, and skin).

After the family has consented to donation, a skillful organization will procure organs in the best possible condition and will match recipients. Organ donation following catastrophic neurologic injury may follow two pathways: donation after cardiac death (DCD) or donation after brain death (DBD). This chapter discusses the practice of organ procurement.

■ TRANSITIONING TO ORGAN DONATION

Early identification of potential organ donors among patients with an irreversible catastrophic brain injury not only is essential to maintain the practice of organ donation and transplantation but also may increase the pool of potential donors. The number of lost opportunities is not precisely known but there is a concern it may be substantial.

The UNOS and the organ procurement and transplantation network have defined criteria under the term *imminent neurologic death*. These criteria identify a comatose patient younger than 70 years old with a need for mechanical ventilation and loss of at least three brainstem reflexes (e.g., pupil reflexes, corneal reflexes, and cough reflex). In addition, a recent study has found that a sum FOUR score of 0 (no eye opening to pain; no motor response to pain; absent pupil, corneal, and cough reflexes; and no obvious respiratory drive) not only identifies potential donors but also may increase conversion rates.[21,22] Without early identification of patients with imminent brain death, the organ donors will decrease over time. This simply may be a consequence of ultra early withdrawal of care when the situation looks dire. Thus, in day-to-day intensive care unit (ICU) practice, the nursing staff may contact organ donation agencies when such patients are admitted. These referrals are merely anticipatory and do not activate any protocols to secure consent for procurement. Only after the clinical diagnosis of brain death is made or withdrawal of support is decided upon by the attending staff do these agencies become involved.

Medical decisions are totally independent of decisions to consider organ donation, and every ICU staff member understands the separation of these two clinical pathways. Physicians have to make the decision that any therapeutic intervention (medical or neurosurgical) is futile. The diagnostic knowledge used to do that accurately is outside the scope of this book but is discussed in another work.[95]

Once a patient with imminent brain death with no therapeutic options has been identified, several clinical pathways are possible. This applies to hospitals with both DCD and DBD operational protocols. If the patient meets brain death criteria, the options are withdrawal of support or organ donation. If the patient does not meet the brain death criteria, the choice is prolonged care after tracheostomy and percutaneous gastrostomy placement, palliative care after withdrawal of life support, or organ donation through DCD protocol (Figure 5-1). If DCD protocols are not available, only two choices remain.

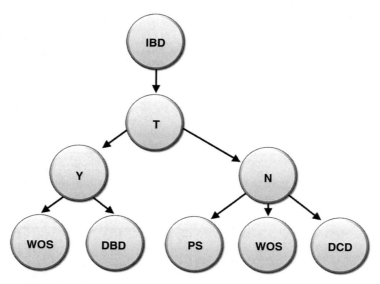

Figure 5-1 Clinical pathway in patients with imminent brain death (IBD). T, clinical testing; Y, meets clinical criteria for brain death; N, does not meet clinical criteria for brain death; PS, prolonged ICU support; WOS, withdrawal of life support; DBD, donation after brain death; DCD, donation after cardiac death.

■ ORGAN PROCUREMENT ORGANIZATIONS

The UNOS (www.unos.org) administers over 58 federally regulated organ procurement organizations (OPOs). These OPOs are independent, private, non-profit organizations, and a specific geographic area for each OPO has been assigned by the Health Care Financing Authority (HCFA). Independent OPOs are governed by a board of directors comprised of transplant surgeons from each transplant center in their service area, a neurosurgeon or neurologist, a histocompatibility representative, and members of the public. All OPOs are funded by HCFA and by transplant centers that receive organs recovered by the OPO. The OPOs bill a standard acquisition charge (SAC) to the receiving transplant center for every organ transplanted. In simplified terms, the SAC calculates the cost per organ by adding up all expenses incurred to recover each organ and dividing by the number of organs transplanted. Services provided by OPOs generally include 24-hour availability, immediate response to organ donor referrals, organ donor case management, public and professional education, and donor family aftercare. The OPO coordinators generally have a background as a nurse, physician assistant, or paramedic. They receive training in all aspects of organ donation, including approach to the family, donor management, organ allocation policy, and operating room recovery procedures, and competency is measured by a national standard.

Until recently, the United States was unique in using transplant coordinators in the organ donation process. But many other countries are now recruiting coordinators who offer the option of organ donation to families of potential organ donors. In addition, public and professional education programs and better administration of organ donor potential are becoming more prevalent.

Spain has long been a recognized worldwide leader in organ donation, with approximately 31 organ donors per million population annually. This rate (82%) is twice as high as those of other European countries and higher than that of the United States, with an estimated 24 organ donors per million. Spain's utilization of hospital-based coordinators who are either specially trained physicians or nurses may explain their superb consent rate.

EuroTransplant (www.eurotransplant.nl), which includes Austria, Belgium, Germany, the Netherlands, and Luxembourg, is one of the oldest transplant consortiums in the world. Other well-established programs include Scandiatransplant (Denmark, Finland, Iceland, Norway, and Sweden) and the United Kingdom Transplant Service (the United Kingdom and Ireland).

Asian countries have developed transplantation programs with brain-dead organ donors instead of living donors and non-heart-beating cadaveric donors. Nonetheless, only Malaysia, the Philippines, Singapore, Taiwan, and Thailand have repeatedly recovered organs from brain-dead patients. New programs and organ donation initiatives are also rapidly expanding in Latin America and the Baltic states. However, laws concerning organ donation and brain death vary drastically. Some countries (e.g., Austria, Sweden, and Spain) have so-called presumed (implied) consent to organ donation. Others require informed consent (e.g., the United States, Germany, the Netherlands). Table 5-1 presents a complete list of international organ donation organizations.

TABLE 5-1 *Major Transplantation Organizations in the World*

Country	Organization
Argentina	INCUCAI
Australia	Australia and New Zealand Organ Donation Registry
Austria	OEBIG
Bangladesh	Kidney Foundation
Belgium	Eurotransplant
Bolivia	Grupo Punta Cana
Brazil	Associação Brasileira de Transplantes de Órgãos
Bulgaria	Bulgarian Executive Agency of Transplantation
Canada	Canadian Institute for Health Information
Chile	Grupo Punta Cana
Colombia	Red de Donación y Trasplantes
Croatia	Ministry of Health and Social Welfare
Cuba	Centro Nacional de Urgencias Médicas
Cyprus	Paraskevaidio Surgical and Transplant Center
Czech Republic	Transplantation Coordinating Centre
Denmark	Scandiatransplant
Dominican Republic	Instituto Nacional de Coordinación de Trasplantes
Estonia	Tartu University Clinics
Finland	Scandiatransplant
France	Agence de la Biomédecine
Georgia	Georgian Association of Transplantologists
Germany	Deutsche Stiftung Organtransplantation
Greece	Hellenic Transplant Organization
Hong Kong	Hospital Authority
Hungary	HNBTS, Organ Coordination Office
Iceland	Scandiatransplant
Iran	Management Center for Transplantation and Special Diseases
Ireland	NHS Blood and Transplant
Israel	Israel Transplant Center
Italy	Centro Nazionale Trapianti
Japan	Japan Organ Transplant Network
Latvia	BaltTransplant–Latvian subdivision
Libya	National Organ Transplantation Program
Lithuania	National Transplantation Bureau
Luxembourg	Eurotransplant
Malaysia	National Transplant Resource Centre
Malta	Mater Dei Hospital
Mexico	Centro Nacional de Trasplantes
Netherlands	Dutch Transplant Foundation
New Zealand	Australia and New Zealand Organ Donation Registry
Norway	Scandiatransplant
Pakistan	Sindh Institute of Urology and Transplantation–SIUT
Poland	Poltransplant
Portugal	Autoridade para os Serviços de Sangue e Transplantação
Puerto Rico	Programa de Trasplante Renal–Hospital Auxilio Mutuo
Qatar	Organ Transplant Committee–Hamad Medical Corporation
Romania	National Transplant Agency
Russia	Research Center of Transplantology and Artificial Organs

(Continues)

TABLE 5-1 (Continued)

Country	Organization
Saudi Arabia	Saudi Center for Organ Transplantation
Slovak Republic	Slovak Centre of Organ Transplantation
Slovenia	Slovenija Transplant
Spain	Organización Nacional de Trasplantes
Sweden	Scandiatransplant
Switzerland	Swisstransplant
Taiwan	Chia-Chi Liu
Trinidad and Tobago	National Organ Transplant Unit
Tunisia	Centre pour la Promotion de la Transplantation d'Organes
Turkey	UKM
Ukraine	National Institute of Surgery and Transplantology, Bioimplant
United Kingdom	NHS Blood and Transplant
United States	UNOS
Uruguay	Instituto Nacional de Donación y Trasplante
Venezuela	Grupo Punta Cana

Presumed consent increases organ donation rates.[68] This construct presumes that patients want to donate organs after death; if they do not, they have to sign an official document stating that they refuse. The default position is organ donation, which may be helpful in facilitating decisions by family members. However, in most countries, the families would still have veto power, and such a law does not preclude a sensitive discussion. In countries with presumed consent, the percentage of refusals is less than 10%. Nonetheless, it is difficult to tease out the effect of presumed consent, and some countries with presumed consent (e.g., Austria) do not have much higher rates of consent. Proponents of presumed consent state that in every survey in the United States, more than 90% support organ donation.

The process after the diagnosis of brain death is multilayered and stepwise and the separate elements of organ procurement are shown in Figure 5-2. In the United States, all patients, regardless of age, past medical history, or current organ function, who have been declared brain dead or in whom brain death is imminent are referred to the hospital's designated OPO. All patients less than 60 years old with acute, devastating neurologic disease, with no hope of any improvement and a final decision to withdraw support should also be seen by an OPO coordinator for a possible DCD protocol.

The responsibility to determine medical suitability for organ donation has been assigned to the OPO. After review of the medical history and current organ function of the potential organ donor on site or by phone, the OPO coordinator may determine, in conjunction with local transplant surgeons or the OPO medical director, whether the patient is a suitable candidate for organ donation. This determination is ultimately based on the probability of successfully transplanting at least one organ. The final decision on suitability is often left to the transplant surgeon.

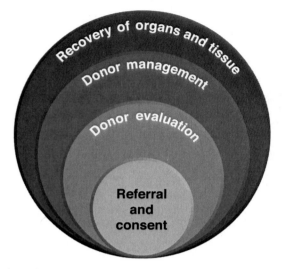

Figure 5-2 Multifaceted approach to organ procurement.

■ ORGAN DONATION REQUESTS

Once the prognosis is established, communication of the hopeless clinical situation to the family is the first step in preparing the family for the patient's end-of-life care. The announcement of brain death should not come as a surprise to the family and with intermittent contacts, they should become aware of the patient's imminent death from a catastrophic brain injury. Rarely is the progression so quick that there is no time to discuss the clinical course. Ideally, families should be told that brain death testing may be performed and that they will be informed when the clinical examination will start. Although it has been argued that family observation of brain death testing may be helpful for those families who are having difficulty understanding the concept of brain death, there are no data showing that their actual presence will convince them.

After brain death testing is complete, a meeting with all present family members should be arranged. The family is usually gathered in a room, and the charge nurse, clergy, and fellows or residents should be present. When appropriate, before brain death and organ donation are discussed, the physician should have inquired with clergy about possible cultural or religious objections (Table 5-2).

The family should be told in unequivocal and nontechnical terms that the patient is dead. Despite preparatory discussions with the family, this devastating news is still unexpected and the response is often a heartbreaking outburst of grief. The physician should anticipate this reaction, and time should be allowed for grieving. Understandably, families who have just suddenly lost a loved one are powerless, helpless, and confused, and their perception of events may be skewed. Some families dissolve into collective grieving that significantly interferes with

TABLE 5-2 *Systematic Approach to Families of Patient with Brain Death*

- Identification of next of kin (decedent's spouse, decedent's adult child, either of decedent's parents, decedent's adult brother or sister, or legal guardian of the decedent)
- Explanation of the irreversibility of neurologic injury and Brain death determination
- Explanation of the time of death
- Introduction of organ donation coordinator to the family
- Verification of family's understanding of the death of the family member
- Requesting organ donation and providing extensive information
- Allowing time for discussion
- Obtaining informed consent

communication. Considerable time should be allowed to have the family members compose themselves and regain a sense of realism. The physician may opt for further reconstruction of the illness and clinical course, and often it is comforting for the family to know that nothing could have been to done to change the outcome. Families may also want to hear that some devastating illnesses or accidents are overwhelmingly severe and that patients in similar situations may not even survive before they reach the hospital.

The physician then explains that certain decisions will have to be made. There would be no need to maintain any form of support of a dead person, and the family is told that the ventilator will be disconnected and all medication will be stopped. At this time, the family can be told that the only reason to maintain ICU support is possible organ donation. Frequently, families do understand that organ donation will be discussed, and it may become quickly clear whether the family is willing to donate or if the driver's license of their loved one has indicated consent. Even if they are initially opposed, the family is still invited to speak with an OPO coordinator to discuss the option of organ and tissue donation (Chapter 6).

Organ donation should not be discussed with the family until their loved one is brain dead. However, as public education and experience with organ donation and transplantation increase, more families approach physicians or nurses about their donation options, often before brain death is declared. We believe that if a family asks questions about donation, it is better to postpone a detailed discussion and explain the present condition of the patient. But when the physician is pressed by the family, time should be allowed to answer specific questions about the process of organ donation. Once the family is ready for a discussion of donation (soon after notification of brain death), the types of organs (kidney, heart, liver and pancreas) and tissues that can be donated should be discussed.

After the family conference with the attending physician, the OPO usually meets with the family 1–2 hours later. Often this brief delay has already provided the family with some time to recuperate from the initial shock.

The OPO then systematically discusses the time of death (when the diagnosis of brain death was made) and the benefit of organ donation, with its high success rate ("there are people in need of a transplant dying every day, and this would truly be the gift of life"), the time it takes to assess for donor suitability, and the tests needed to do so. It is appropriate to tell the family that 24–36 hours is typical and organ procurement is thus a lengthy process and not the rush of organ harvesting seen on TV. When donation is allowed, the OPO coordinator will assume care of the patient, but the nursing staff will remain involved and available. The family says their last goodbyes before the patient goes to the operating room, but they may leave earlier if they wish—many do. The organ donation process should be explained in two parts, the evaluation and placement phase and organ recovery in the operating room. The family should understand that all of the organs will be tested to determine suitability for transplantation, and testing may include blood tests, chest x-rays, echocardiograms, coronary angiography and liver biopsy. After the organs are evaluated, they are matched with recipients on the waiting list. The family should be informed that the recovery process is done by trained transplant surgeons. The OPO then proceeds with a discussion of the operation and explains that it involves one incision, exactly as it does with heart or abdominal surgery. The deceased then goes to the hospital morgue and the funeral home.

The consent will apply to all possible organs, and this should be clarified. The family is also asked if there are specific indications of intention; a driver's license designation is an important example. (Unfortunately, in the United States, the percentage of driver's license indicators of willingness to donate organs is not exactly known and likely small.[83]) After this explanation, the OPO will have the next of kin sign a consent form, with a nurse as witness, and then will go over the medical history.

There are several reasons why families decline organ donation.[80,81] It may matter who asks and when (Table 5-3). Studies of the process of obtaining consent for organ donation have shown that when the request for organ donation occurs simultaneously with the communication of brain death, the consent rate is 20% to 40% lower than if the request is separated from the explanation of brain death (decoupling). One study of 71 families approached for organ donation found a similar increase in consent rate with decoupling.[92] A more recent study reviewed 177 requests for organ donation over a 1-year period. The consent rate for OPO coordinators who approached the family alone was substantially higher than the consent rate for a hospital staff member. Simultaneous requests (by the patient's physician and the organ procurement coordinator) did not increase organ donation consent rates in one randomized, controlled trial in the United Kingdom.[2] With a growing number of neurointensivists experienced in supporting these unfortunate families, the differences may not be that large, but to allow separate

TABLE 5-3 *Factors that Increase the Chance of Declining Organ Donation*

- Race or ethnic group (African American, Hispanic)
- Culture supporting a cardiocentric view or reincarnation
- Desire to keep the body whole
- Desire for immediate closure
- Unexperienced discussant
- Discussion about organ donation occurs hours after declaration of brain death

discussions (the brain death discussion and the request for organ donation) may continue to be helpful and certainly more compassionate.

A recent study in central and south Texas found that 43% of families declined organ donation, and multiple reasons were given.[10] Persons of Hispanic descent were four times more likely and African Americans were seven times more likely than whites to decline. Important new findings other than the known objections— all modifiable factors—include the way the health care team approached the family, a long delay in discussing organ donation, and a preconceived notion by family members that organs from older patients would not qualify.[10] In countries other than the United States, providing insufficient information in discussions on organ donation is also a major later complaint.[4]

Conversely, one study found that families that had more specific conversations about organ donation were more likely to donate. The factors discussed included the cost of donation, the impact of donation on the funeral, the choice of which body part to donate, and concerns about disfigurement, among others.[81] As expected, this study also noted that most health care providers cannot predict accurately who would want to donate. Most recently, one study in the United States found that a number of organ donations were missed when families were not asked about the driver's license consent status.[16]

Declining or accepting organ or tissue donation may be a result of personal and cultural values or fear of mutilation of the body. In the end, it may simply indicate lack of interest in making this decision in the first place. Many families may never have thought that this could happen to them and do not want to make the situation even more complicated. Families may not always be persuaded by altruistic arguments.

Families with an interest in donation often have two additional concerns about organ donation: timing and disfigurement. While the timing varies due to the geographic location of the hospital and the number of organs evaluated for transplant, the family should be given an approximate time for the entire process. On average, it takes 36 hours from the time of consent until the start of the recovery of organs in the operating room. As noted earlier, a single incision is made from below the navel to just above the sternum. After the surgery, the incision is closed and the donor is transferred to the medical examiner (if an autopsy is planned) or to the funeral home. The utmost respect and dignity are guaranteed. The family should be reassured that organ donation generally does not interfere with the type of funeral service planned (such as an open-casket funeral). The family and the physician will receive a letter after the donation telling them what organs were transplanted and providing some information about the recipients. The letter sent to the family also states how long the recipient was on the waiting list (often several years) (Figure 5-3). However, organ donation is an anonymous process, and every effort is made to ensure the anonymity of both the donor and the organ recipients.

The issue of correspondence and contact between donor families and recipients has been the subject of debate. While policies vary nationwide, anonymous correspondence between donor families and transplant recipients could be facilitated through the OPO. Contact with the recipients has been granted when

LifeSource
Organ & Tissue Donation

August 27, 2010

Mr. David Alexander
2100 Great Acres Pass
Rochester, MN 55901

Dear Mr. Alexander,

Please accept our heartfelt sympathy on the death of your son, Jacob. Our greatest hope is that you can find peace in remembrances of special times together and in the warmth of lasting memories. Also, we would like to express our deepest gratitude to you for your decision to help others through donation. Your compassion for others has given many a second chance at a quality life.

Donation celebrates life: Jacob's life and the lives of those who benefit from your decision to give the gift of life. We hope the following information comforts you as you learn about the outcome of your son's donation.

Nationally, over 81,000 people are currently waiting for a kidney transplant. Those awaiting a kidney transplant must sustain their health with a time intensive and tiring medical treatment called dialysis. When they receive the call of transplant they have an improved quality of life, free from the rigors of dialysis. Two people received that call because of Jacob's generosity.

A forty-three-year-old man from South Dakota received the gift of Jacob's right kidney. This recipient is married, has three children and three sisters. He suffered from hypertension, which resulted in his need for a transplant. He is a college math professor, who enjoys fishing and hunting. Following his transplant, he is doing well and is recovering at home.

A fifty-four-year-old man from Delaware received a double gift from Jacob, his left kidney and a portion of his liver. This gentleman suffered from a genetic disorder resulting in cysts in his kidneys and liver, which slowly lead to organ failure. He is a father of three, has four step-children, and works in the automotive industry. This recipient is grateful for this second chance at a healthy life and is looking forward to being able to garden and go fishing again.

A nine-year-old girl, who underwent surgery in Illinois, received the left lobe of Jacob's liver. This young lady will soon have the opportunity to return to school because of the graciousness of your family.

A Donate Life Organization

Figure 5-3 Follow-up letter to the family of an organ donor. (In order to respect patient confidentiality, the names and locations in this letter do not represent actual situations.)

approved by the recipient, and some encounters have been successful. Other questions surrounding organ donation are discussed in Chapter 6.

◼ PREPARATION FOR DETERMINING ORGAN SUITABILITY

After consent has been obtained from the family, and in some cases from the medical examiner, a detailed medical and social history should be obtained from the family. Absolute contraindications are shown in Table 5-4. Contraindications to organ

August 27, 2010
Page 2

A fifty-year-old woman from Nebraska received the double gift of Jacob's lungs. A restrictive lung disease had progressively caused her breathing to become very difficult. This recipient worked at a medical center. She is a widow with two children and is expecting her first grandchild very soon. Following the surgery, she is doing very well, recuperating at home in the care of her friends and family.

A 65-year-old Minnesota man received the gift of Jacob's heart. This recipient, a retired school teacher, is married and has three adult children. He suffered from a disease that caused weakness and loss of tissue in his heart muscle. He is doing extremely well following his transplant and, thanks to Jacob's gift, will be able to look forward to the activities he enjoys, including sports and photography. He wishes to say thank you to his donor and family for this wonderful gift.

Your son also gave the gift of tissue. Jacob's connective tissue may be used to repair ligaments or facial deformities which help restore a patient's independence. Through the donation of bone, others may experience relief from pain and restored mobility, through the repair of bone damage or loss. Fascia, the membrane surrounding the thigh muscle, may be used for uterine or bladder reconstruction. Donated tissue might help many individuals. Because tissue can be saved for up to five years from the time of recovery, it may take some time before Jacob's donations are ultimately used. Please be assured that your son's gifts are deeply appreciated.

Jacob's pancreas was gratefully accepted by researchers studying the disease of diabetes. This research helps in the understanding of the regulation and production of insulin. One day this research may further the process of islet cell transplantation. This type of transplant holds real promise of helping those who suffer from the complex disease of diabetes. These researchers were grateful for this opportunity to help others.

During the next few weeks, you will hear from LifeSource Donor Family Advocate, Joyce Williams. LifeSource will continue to maintain contact with you, if you wish, to provide support and to pay tribute to the memory of your son.

On behalf of these recipients, their families and LifeSource, thank you again for helping us enable your son to give the precious Gift of Life through donation. Jacob is truly a hero to those he has helped. These grateful transplant recipients and their families will long remember Jacob's generosity.

We hope the information in this letter provides comfort and peace to you. If you have any questions, or if you just need to talk, please do not hesitate to call us at LifeSource at 1-888-536-6283.

Sincerely,   Sincerely,

Suzanne Nelson   Dawn Rydell
Donation Coordinator   Donation Coordinator

Figure 5-3 (Continued).

donation may include infectious diseases (notably HIV and hepatitis C), potentially transmissible malignancies and, most commonly, organ failure, which will result in primary nonfunction of the organ in the recipient. Another concern is the transmission of a primary high grade CNS tumor of a donor to a recipient and multiple single cases with fatal outcome have been reported. A recent study evaluated the risk in liver transplantation and found it to be very low (less than 3%). Nonetheless, molecular chimera studies have proven malignant brain tumors came from a donor.[44] Prior manipulation by biopsy or ventriculostomy are

TABLE 5-4 *Contraindications to Organ Donation*

Infections

Bacterial

- Tuberculosis
- Gangrenous bowel or perforated bowel and/or intra-abdominal sepsis
- Multisystem organ failure (MSOF) due to overwhelming sepsis or MSOF without sepsis, defined as three or more systems in simultaneous failure for a period of 24 hours or more with no response to treatment or resuscitation

Viral

- HIV infection by serologic or molecular detection
- Rabies
- Reactive hepatitis B surface antigen
- Retroviral infections
- Viral encephalitis or meningitis
- Active herpes simplex, varicella zoster, or cytomegalovirus viremia or pneumonia
- Acute Epstein-Barr virus (mononucleosis)
- West Nile virus infection
- Severe acute respiratory syndrome

Fungal

- Active infection with *Cryptococcus, Aspergillus, Histoplasma,* or *Coccidioides*
- Active candidemia or invasive yeast infection

Parasitic

- Active infection with *Trypanosoma cruzi* (Chagas' disease), *Leishmania, Strongyloides,* or malaria (*Plasmodium* sp.)

Prion

- Creutzfeldt-Jakob disease

General Conditions

- Aplastic anemia
- Agranulocytosis
- Extreme immaturity (<500 g or gestational age of <32 weeks)
- Current malignant neoplasms except nonmelanoma skin cancers such as basal cell and squamous cell cancer and primary central nervous system tumors without evident metastatic disease
- Previous malignant neoplasms with current evident metastatic disease
- Prior melanoma
- Hematologic malignancies: leukemia, Hodgkin's disease, lymphoma, multiple myeloma

not the only factors in transmission and the graft and lymph nodes should be carefully examined. A positive HIV test disqualifies a donor, but an accurate social history for homosexual relations, intravenous drug abuse, or incarceration that placed the patient at high risk for exposure to infectious diseases is obligatory. Nonetheless, incidental cases have been reported of HIV transmission from donor to recipients despite a negative HIV test at the time of donation. The history may identify prospective donors who are in the window period (24 to 28 days) from the time of infection until the antigen or antibody can be detected by serologic testing. UNOS has recently removed the requirement of screening for HTLV-1 and HTLV-2.[41]

A blood sample should be sent to the hospital laboratory for immediate type and crossmatch because this may take up to 6 hours when the laboratory is geographically distant. Blood (or tissue) samples are subsequently sent to an OPO-directed designated lab for serologic testing and tissue typing. While organ recovery may begin without the results, serologic testing must be completed prior

TABLE 5-5 *Organ Procurement and Preparation for Transplantation*

Heart

12-lead echocardiogram
 Echocardiogram (transesophageal route preferred)
 Coronary angiography (for organ donors >40 years of age or those with cardiac risk factors
  such as hypercholesterolemia, obesity, diabetes, or a convincing family history of
  heart disease)
 Swan-Ganz readings (optional)
 Cardiology consultation

Lung

 Chest x-ray
 Arterial blood gas
 PEEP
 Bronchoscopy
 Oxygen challenge test
 Pulmonary consultation

Serologic tests

 HIV
 HCV
 HBsAg, anti-HBc, HBs/Ab
 CMV
 RPR/STS

Laboratory tests

 General (electrolytes, BUN, creatinine, glucose, CBC, calcium, magnesium, phosphorus)
 Blood cultures
 Liver tests (AST, ALT, bilirubin, GGT, alkaline phosphatase, LDH, PT, PTT)
 Kidney (urinalysis, urine culture)
 Heart (CPK, troponin)
 Pancreas (amylase, lipase)
 Lungs (sputum, Gram stain)

Abbreviations: ALT, alanine aminotransferase; AST, aspartate transaminase; BUN, blood urea nitrogen; CBC, complete blood count; CMV, cytomegalovirus; CPK, creatine phosphokinase; GGT, gamma-glutamyl transpeptidase; HBc, hemoglobin C; HBsAb, hepatitis B surface antibody; HBsAg, hepatitis B surface antigen; HIV, human immunodeficiency virus; LDH, lactic dehydrogenase; PEEP, positive end-expiratory pressure; PT, prothrombin time; PTT, partial thromboplastin time; RPR/STS, rapid plasma reagin/syphilis serology.

to transplantation of the organs. Tissue typing or identification of the human lymphocyte antigen (HLA) is less critical than serologic testing; however, the results are critical to the allocation of kidneys and the pancreas. Organ evaluation should proceed with the tests outlined in Table 5-5.

■ DONATION PROTOCOLS

This book concentrates on DBD protocols, but a few words on DCD protocols are in order.[28] The difficulty of determining irreversible cardiac arrest has been discussed in Chapter 4. Both DCD and DBD protocols exist throughout the world, but there are notable exceptions and restrictions (e.g., Germany, Austria). Organ recovery for both protocols is very similar, although there are some marked differences (Table 5-6). The similarities include exclusion of confounders and determination of proximate cause and irreversibility. Some patients destined for a DCD

TABLE 5-6 *Differences Between DCD and DBD Protocols*

	DCD	DBD
Age limit	≤60 years*	No established limit
Apnea test	Breathing sustainability test	Apneic oxygenation
Family goodbye	Operating room	ICU
Organ recovery	5 minutes of circulatory arrest	Immediately
Organs and tissue to recover	All those consented except heart (lungs possible)	All those consented
Triage	May return to ICU for palliation	Morgue

Abbreviations: DBD, donation after brain death; DCD, donation after cardiac death; ICU, intensive care unit.
*The age limit varies in DCD protocols from 55 to 70 years and may be organ specific. For many protocols, no specific age limitation is mentioned. Some protocols exclude young children and neonates. (Generally, recipient function declines with heart, lung, and renal donors after the age of 60 years; this is the cutoff age at Mayo Clinic.)

protocol may become brain dead in the course of preparation for organ procurement and then could transition to a DBD protocol.

The DBD protocol is well structured, with families saying their last good-byes in the ICU followed by transfer of the donor to the operating room, with a full transplantation team at work after arrival. In the operating room, the donor is prepared for recovery of organs. After incision of the abdomen and chest, cannulation and infusion of the preservation fluid, the organs designated for transplantation are mobilized and prepared for excision. Cross-clamping of the aorta follows, the patient is extubated, and organs are recovered. After organ recovery, the body leaves for the morgue.

The DCD protocol is less structured and varies considerably in process.[30] After the decision to withdraw support and consent of the next of kin to proceed with a possible DCD protocol, a breathing sustainability test is performed. Patients are placed on a continuous positive airway pressure (CPAP) mode of 5 cm H_2O or on a T-piece, and oxygenation and arterial PCO_2 retention are monitored with serial blood gas measurements. In many hospitals, the DCD protocol will not proceed if respiration is stable for 15–30 minutes, because this indicates that it is less likely that respiratory and circulatory arrest will occur quickly.

Most evaluations for DCD also use a combination of pulmonary and hemodynamic criteria (oxygen saturation <80%; respiratory rate <12 per minute; tidal volume <200 cc; negative inspiratory pressure <20 cm H_2O; body mass index >30; and need for vasopressors). When many of these indicators are present respiratory-circulatory arrest is likely after extubation.

Prediction of respiratory-circulatory arrest within 1 hour using neurologic criteria has been recently investigated. Absent corneal reflex, absent cough reflex, and extensor or absent motor responses predicted cardiac arrest in 83% of patients when all three clinical signs were present. When combined with an abnormal oxygenation index, the prediction increased to 93%. Each factor alone predicted respiratory-circulatory arrest in about 66% of patients. The validity of these clinical signs will need to be tested prospectively before they are uniformly used.[98] A low probability of respiratory arrest within 1 hour after extubation avoids unnecessary operating room expenses and more agony for the family.

In a DCD protocol, families are allowed to enter the operating room after the patient has been draped and the surgical team has temporarily left the room. Families are allowed to stay with the patient until respiratory and circulatory arrest occur and then are led away. The surgical team arrives and proceeds 5 minutes after documentation of circulatory arrest (measured by absence of a carotid pulse or documentation of a zero reading of the arterial catheter). The abdomen and chest is opened quickly, followed by cannulation and clamping of the abdominal aorta, infusion of preservation fluid, heparinization and large amount of ice.

In current ICU practice, the choice of a DCD or DBD protocol may seem to be based on the clinical course of the neurologic injury. Acute devastating neurologic injury may progress to brain death in several days (about one-third within day of ictus), and DBD procedures are less complicated and structured. Nevertheless, DCD protocols often involve patients with more stable injury and a final decision to withdraw all support. Proponents of a DCD protocol have claimed a significant increase in the donation rate, but the increase has been less than hoped for. Refusal of families to proceed with a DCD protocol often relates to the long time it takes to achieve closure and the possibility of return of the patient from the operating room. (If the patient still continues to breathe in the operating room 1 hour after extubation, the patient is returned to the ICU or ward for palliative care.) For these families, one extra day is incredibly long.

The DCD protocols have been subjected to substantial scrutiny, and the language in these protocols is ambiguous and confusing.[30] In a review of 64 DCD protocols in the US, only 48% stipulated a mandatory observation time from death pronouncement to organ procurement. The "5-minute death watch" was noted in only 28% of the protocols with listed time intervals.[30] There was no uniform understanding of what constituted circulatory arrest; multiple cardiac rhythms were mentioned, and many protocols still required asystole. In many of the surveyed protocols, the distinction between electrical and mechanical asystole was not always made.[30] A uniform medical standard for the determination of irreversible circulatory arrest is needed to provide consistent management.

■ MEDICAL MANAGEMENT OF THE ORGAN DONOR

Brain death affects nearly every organ system. Complications of brain death that may impact the organ donation process include hypotension, diabetes insipidus, hypothermia, electrolyte abnormalities, coagulopathy, anemia, hypoxia, cardiac arrhythmia, and cardiac arrest (Figure 5-4).[64] Medical management of the donor is aimed at anticipating the normal physiologic sequelae of brain death and achieving optimal organ perfusion and cellular oxygenation, minimizing ischemic injury. Following the declaration of brain death, care of the donor shifts to optimizing organ perfusion and protection. The initial medical management of the brain-injured patient in conjunction with cerebral resuscitation with osmotic diuresis, fluid restriction, and hyperventilation may compound many of the pathophysiologic changes associated with brain death. Hypotension initially due to vasoparesis

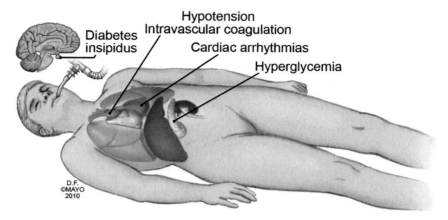

Figure 5-4 Organ donor and medical complications. *See* Figure 5-4 in the color insert.

is worsened by untreated diabetes insipidus or diuretic-induced hypovolemia, hypothermia, and electrolyte disorders.

Medical management of the organ donor is directed by one or two organ procurement coordinators (usually trained ICU nurses) (see Appendix 1 and 2). In the United States, the involvement of intensivists (or neurointensivists) has been minimal or has occurred on a "curbside" basis at best. There have been calls to change this situation, but there is insufficient reason (and data) to suggest that management is inadequate or suboptimal.[97] However, timely management of the organ donor before the OPO arrives in the ICU is critical. Potential donors may be lost if the key effects of brain death on the major organ systems are not recognized and handled accordingly.

Pathophysiologic Changes Due to Brain Death

Brain injury is known to affect multiple organ systems, and many brain-injured patients may have suffered systemic tissue injury before hospitalization.[4,19] Brain injury due to projectiles, high-speed rapid deceleration such as during motor vehicle accidents, and massive subarachnoid or intracranial hemorrhage that ultimately leads to brain death are particularly associated with systemic injuries initiated and augmented by the catecholamine surge that occurs at the time of the injury.[5,70,93] The magnitude of the force and the rate of change to the brainstem in laboratory and clinical studies of brain injury directly correlate with two profound physiologic effects.[13,86] One is apnea, which, by way of hypoxia, hypercarbia, and acidosis, significantly affects myocardial function. Ultimately, the clinical outcome is determined by the duration and degree of apnea before mechanical ventilation is provided or spontaneous ventilation returns. The other effect is a catecholamine surge, which, under laboratory circumstances, produces catecholamine levels many times those of resting baseline values.[45]

Most pronounced in the cascade of events immediately following the defining moment of brain death are loss of tone of the vascular bed, abnormal cardiac inotropy, and cardiac arrest. Physicians are challenged with the complex ventilatory management of pulmonary edema and the treatment of frequently emerging cardiac arrhythmias, disseminated intravascular coagulation, hypotension, and hypothermia. These physiologic changes should be anticipated and managed in order to successfully shepherd the donor through the critical time until tissue and organ retrieval. The potential negative impact of these physiologic changes on organ utilization is substantial, as exemplified by rejection of approximately 25% of potential donor hearts and 20% of potential donor lungs.

Understanding the pathophysiologic mechanisms after brain death may lead to effective countermeasures and, ideally, increase recovery of suitable organs. This section discusses the pathophysiologic impact of brain death on the function of the organs most relevant in organ procurement.

Systemic Inflammatory Response

A phenomenon that is poorly understood is that brain death in the donor may affect early graft rejection.[12] The injury occurs in the donor. First there is extreme hypertension with vasoconstriction and organ ischemia followed by marked hypotension from vasodilatation resulting in organ ischemia from hypoperfusion.[94] This catecholamine storm followed by hemodynamic injury of the donor's, organs leads to a generalized progressive systemic inflammatory response and potentially injures the procured organs.

Recent work has elucidated an early systemic inflammatory response with upregulation of cytokines and adhesion molecules after brain death.[7,14] Some investigators have found that serum interleukin IL-1β and IL-6 increase several hours after brain death.[84] An increase in IL-6 levels may induce expression of adhesion molecules and could promote the rejection cascade. Proapoptotic genes are also expressed, and caspases are mostly responsible for the machinery of apoptosis. The response is more pronounced in brain death caused by cardiac arrest, suggesting that the initial severity of the insult may play a role.[3]

Whether this cytokine onslaught is specific for brain death or is more a consequence of any severe neuronal injury with sympathetic overdrive is unclear. Further support for the relevance of this inflammatory response comes from the observation that administering methylprednisolone improves the outcome in liver recipients.[47]

Hypothalamic-Pituitary Function

When deprived of arterial perfusion, the neurosecretory neurons of the hypothalamus will die and disconnect the hypothalamic-pituitary axis. Though the pituitary gland may remain structurally intact, the pituitary stalk may be damaged as a consequence of brain tissue shift.[40,53] Displacement of the diencephalon, particularly in centrally located masses, compresses the pituitary stalk against the sharp edge of the sellar diaphragm. If the pituitary gland becomes damaged, the posterior lobe is most often involved, as reflected clinically by diabetes insipidus.

In more severe cases, a pituitary infarct can be found (Chapter 2). Diabetes insipidus may thus be seen more often (up to 95%) in persons suffering acute mass effects and is less commonly in persons with diffuse processes such as encephalitis, meningitis, and diffuse anoxic-ischemic injury. The posterior lobe is usually damaged directly and not likely from ischemia because it receives blood from the unaffected extradural hypophyseal arteries.

In our experience, two-thirds of the patients who meet the clinical criteria for brain death developed clinical diabetes insipidus. Diabetes insipidus became evident with sudden polyuria and leads to dehydration, hypotension, and oliguria if not treated with hormone or fluid replacement therapy. Because of the short half-life of antidiuretic hormone, the concentration of this hormone decreases to a barely detectable level within 15 minutes, and it disappears from the circulation within 4 hours.

Diabetes insipidus can be diagnosed not only by polyuria but also by an increase in plasma sodium and osmolality. A decreased urinary sodium concentration (<10 mmol/L) together with hypernatremia is diagnostic, but the use of mannitol and diuretics may be major confounders. Laboratory criteria for diabetes insipidus are a plasma osmolality of more than 300 mosm/L, hypotonic polyuria (more than 4 mL/kg/h), decreased specific gravity (<1.005), and urine osmolality of less than 300 mosm/L. Diabetes insipidus leads to dehydration, hypomagnesemia, hypokalemia, hypophosphatemia, and hypocalcemia.

The posterior part of the pituitary lobe is normally perfused through inferior hypophyseal arteries from the cavernous portion of the carotid artery. The extradural source of the blood supply to the pituitary may explain why normal hormone

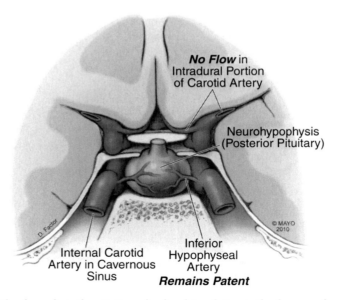

Figure 5-5 Blood supply to the pituitary gland and its relation to the dura, emphasizing the extradural locations. *See* Figure 5-5 in the color insert.

production may persist (Figure 5-5). The anterior lobe of the pituitary gland is compartmentalized in the sella turcica and perfused by the superior hypophyseal arteries that branch off after the carotid pierces the dura and could be hypoperfused in situations of increased intracranial pressure, explaining the predominance of ischemic changes in the anterior lobe of the gland. Intact pituitary function after the declaration of brain death may be due to a residual reservoir, preservation of the basal part, or the production of trophic factors from organs such as the pancreas.

Thyroid function should remain normal, and laboratory findings reveal a characteristic picture of euthyroid sick syndrome. Typically, as in many critical illnesses and during fasting, serum levels of triiodothyronine (T3), total serum thyroxine (T4), the free T4 index, and the free T4 are decreased or borderline, but the level of thyroid-stimulating hormone is normal. Increased concentration of reverse T3 is a consequence of the transformation of T4 into reverse T3. This shift occurs because, in critical illness, levels of serum proteins such as thyroid-binding globulin (TBG) decrease and binding to TBG is reduced as a result of binding-inhibiting substances. Novitzky and colleagues claim that true hypothyroidism is due to decreased free T3. Indeed, free T3 may be a better marker for disturbance of the pituitary-thyroid axis. Despite evidence of a certain degree of hypothyroidism, probably coinciding with a euthyroid sick syndrome, it is uncertain whether T3 or T4 infusions are systematically needed. Proponents of T4 infusion have justified its use on the basis of its effects on transsarcolemmal calcium entry, myocardial myosin, and adenosine triphosphatase (ATPase) activity, effects that may maintain ventricular contractility. In fact, studies by Novitzky and associates showed a dramatic effect of T3 infusion in brain-dead, hemodynamically unstable patients.[56-58] A 4-hour infusion of combined T3, cortisol, and insulin significantly improved their circulatory status, with improvement in cardiac output and reduced need for inotropic agents. A follow-up randomized study confirmed the superb hemodynamic parameters achieved with hormonal therapy. However, two other studies failed to document effects of T3 administration on myocardial contractility.[31,65] Currently, T4 infusions are part of a preservation protocol and often are reserved for hemodynamically unstable patients. Infusions of T4 may result in significantly smaller requirements for vasopressors, and in some patients none is needed during T4 infusion.

The noteworthy fact that circulating levels of prolactin, cortisol, growth hormone, and gonadal hormones (luteinizing hormone, follicle-stimulating hormone, testosterone) do not decrease appreciably confirms the clinical impression that panhypopituitarism may not be part of brain death.[33] Some studies showed that patients with severe hypotension (defined as systolic blood pressure <80 mm Hg) did not have significantly lower serum cortisol levels. These persistent hormone levels are compatible with pathologic studies of the pituitary gland, which, even in patients who are on ventilators for days, may show only a few patchy infarcts with petechial hemorrhages. Other studies showed a decreased cortisol reserve.[23] Moreover, a recent study in 31 patients with brain death found complete adrenal insufficiency, as measured by changed cortisol levels in 85%. In this study, 77% of patients were corticotropin (ACTH) responders, reflecting a hypothalamic-pituitary failure (secondary adrenal failure).[55]

Pancreatic dysfunction may occur but is not due to pituitary insufficiency.[51] Early insulin release is suppressed and this leads to hyperglycemia, but the effect may be indirectly related to exogenously administered epinephrine. Another explanation is that pancreatic dysfunction is due to resistance to insulin from impaired receptor binding.

To summarize, although rapid depletion of vasopressin, cortisol, insulin, T4, and free T3 occurs in experimental animal models of brain death, the endocrine dysfunction seems limited in clinical practice and is manifested mostly as isolated diabetes insipidus. Nonetheless, certain protocols exist for hormonal resuscitation therapy, consisting of methylprednisolone, insulin, arginine vasopressin, and T4. These measures are initiated if use of inotropes and volume loading does not result in a stable hemodynamic state.[69,72,91]

Myocardial Function

A massive outpouring of plasma catecholamines may occur after a neurologic catastrophe, a hyperdynamic response that is in a sense comparable to pheochromocytoma-associated hypertensive crisis.[18,24,43] The effect of this catecholamine surge on the myocardium is still demonstrable on the electrocardiogram (ECG) hours later.[63] Pathologically, a panoply of changes may occur, including depressed and increased ST segments, inverted T waves, widened QRS complexes, and prolonged QT intervals.[52] Multifocal myocardial contraction bands and subendocardial, intraseptal, and papillary myocytolysis can be produced in baboons and rats as a result of a massive catecholamine surge, and these changes may be ameliorated by adrenalectomy.[11] Subendocardial damage is very frequent. It may be a consequence of the shunting away of blood, which has been documented in canine heart preparations subjected to infusion of norepinephrine. In humans, similar changes occur, and these myocardial abnormalities can produce a decrease in ejection fraction and a mosaic of wall motion abnormalities. Catecholamine-induced mechanisms of myocardial injury that have been put forward include calcium overload due to modifications of sarcolemma permeability, reperfusion injury after vasoconstriction, and cytotoxic free radicals.

In our study of 66 consecutive brain deaths, 42% of potential heart donors were found to have echocardiographically confirmed myocardial dysfunction.[25] Myocardial dysfunction was not predicted by the cause of brain injury, the time from brain injury to brain death, or the need for pressor support. Similarly, ECG abnormalities were insensitive for the detection of myocardial dysfunction, and localization studies did not match. In our study, only 14% of patients with myocardial dysfunction on echocardiography had prolongation of the QTc interval (>500 milliseconds), and 14% had ST segment depression or elevation. Ventricular arrhythmias occurred more frequently in patients with myocardial dysfunction than in those with normal function. Therefore, the onset of these arrhythmias should prompt not only treatment but also evaluation of myocardial damage with echocardiographic tests.

Spontaneous intracranial hemorrhage has been associated with segmental left ventricular dysfunction, and most of these patients had sparing of the left ventricular apical region.[46] In contrast, patients with traumatic brain injury had either a segmental or a global pattern of left ventricular dysfunction. Segmental myocardial dysfunction may be related to inhomogeneous distribution of adrenergic innervation of the heart, differences in sudden preload and afterload changes during catecholamine surges, or differences in the myosubendocardial blood supply. A relative lack of innervation of the apex of the normal canine heart has been reported. Apical sparing, therefore, may indicate that the mechanism of the dysfunction is neurogenic.[20]

Echocardiographic wall motion abnormalities may reflect reversible or irreversible myocardial injury. Although contraction band necrosis has been considered a characteristic feature of neurogenic myocardial dysfunction, a poor correlation between echocardiographically demonstrated dysfunction and pathologic findings may exist. Consequently, the myocardium may not be irreversibly damaged when echocardiographic wall motion abnormalities are present. Therefore, it is conceivable that the presence of echocardiographic abnormalities may not adversely affect cardiac function after transplantation into the recipient.[9] In addition, a recent low-dose dobutamine stress echocardiography study in catastrophically injured patients found, in some, reversibility of dysfunction. In this study, 23% had a severe decrease in left ventricular fractional shortening, but in three of these patients contractility became normal after 7 days of observation, and levels of serum troponin did not change.[87]

Echocardiography is currently used routinely for screening potential donors for cardiac transplantation. Because of the often poor correlation between echocardiographic abnormalities and pathologic findings, physicians involved in the evaluation of donor candidates may need to develop more accurate techniques for identifying reversible myocardial dysfunction.[75,78]

Therefore, because recent pathologic studies have been inconsistent in documenting structural myocardial abnormalities, permanent myocardial damage likely contributes little to the hemodynamic profile. It is more probable that hypotension is caused by the collapse of vascular tone and an invariate heart rate.[37,38] Oscillations in heart rate are a product of parasympathetic and sympathetic stimuli to the heart, but the descending regulating connections from the brainstem become destroyed.[66]

Ultimately, the heart stops in brain death. In one recent study from Taiwan, despite full cardiovascular support, 97% of 73 patients who met the criteria for brain death developed asystole within 1 week.[42] The heart and the conduction system need continuous autonomic nervous system input.[27] When adrenergic input falls, a sudden decrease in contractility and decreases in coronary perfusion, myocardial ischemia, and cardiac arrhythmias occur in a downward spiral.[32] The terminal rhythms after disconnection from the ventilator are widening of the QRS complex, isolated atrial activity, slow junctional rhythm, sinus bradycardia, or ventricular tachycardia, but ECG activity may continue for 30 minutes or more after circulatory arrest.[49,61]

Pulmonary Function

Lungs may become damaged because of trauma, aspiration pneumonitis, and fat emboli.[6,59] Fiberoptic bronchoscopy may detect these abnormalities.[67] Only after these conditions have been excluded should the presence of pulmonary edema be considered. Sympathetic stimulation may lead to extreme degrees of pulmonary vasoconstriction. This results in pulmonary barotrauma and produces pulmonary capillary leakage of high-protein pulmonary fluid even after vascular pressures have returned to normal.[50,59,82] Acute left ventricular failure and a significant rise in left atrial pressure increase pulmonary artery pressure and cause a so-called blast injury. The mechanism of neurogenic pulmonary edema may be further elucidated by obtaining pleural fluid or analyzing pulmonary edema fluid. The protein in pulmonary edema fluid is compared with plasma protein, and ratios exceeding 0.7 suggest increased permeability. However, a large study found hydrostatic edema in 7 of 12 patients (ratio less than 0.7) with pulmonary edema. Hydrostatic pulmonary edema may be seen in cases of myocardial dysfunction,[85] but it can also be explained on the basis of profound venoconstriction due to an increase in epinephrine levels that may not be reflected in Swan-Ganz catheter measurements. This profound pulmonary venoconstriction disturbs the Starling forces in the lung, and even more fluid may be forced out when there is already increased permeability.

Considerable work has been published on the elucidation of a possible central nervous system effector site. Bilateral nucleus tractus solitarius (NTS) lesions produced a change in pulmonary vascular pressure and fluid influx independent of the systemic circulation.[83] Hypothalamic lesions may contribute, but through a complex regulating system that involves the NTS, the area postrema, and the ventrolateral medulla.

The radiologic features of pulmonary edema are typically a "whiteout snow-storm" pattern but may begin in the upper lobes due to recruitment of upper lobe vessels when the pulmonary vascular bed opens. Radiologic differentiation between cardiogenic and noncardiogenic pulmonary edema or aspiration pneumonitis is very difficult in brain death. Crystalloid fluid loading may further damage the lung and increase the alveolar-arterial gradient.[62] Clearance of alveolar liquid is mediated by epinephrine; therefore, beta-2 adrenergic agonist therapy (e.g., with isoproterenol or terbutaline) may theoretically accelerate reabsorption of alveolar fluid.[48,71] A recent experimental study in rats suggested that dopamine pretreatment could reduce reperfusion pulmonary edema.[35]

Lungs may become severely damaged from hypotension, and function may be impaired after reperfusion in a recipient.[90] Brief hypotension, such as in the apnea test, seems an unlikely component. A mean arterial blood pressure of 40 mm Hg sustained for at least 1 hour is probably needed to produce reperfusion lung injury. In our experience with over 250 consecutive patients with brain death, true neurogenic pulmonary edema after the diagnosis of brain death was uncommon, was easily managed with positive end-expiratory pressure (PEEP) and was fully reversible. In fact, if any patients had pulmonary dysfunction, it was from aspiration or direct trauma.

Kidney Function

Living-donor kidney grafts have a superb survival rate, because damage to the kidney is uncommon during procurement.[88] One study stated that 10% of cadaver grafts may be damaged before excision but seldom irreversibly. Often brief periods of hypotension are implicated.[34]

Dopamine may reduce allograft rejection,[77] not only through support of blood pressure but possibly also through more complex mechanisms that inhibit expression of adhesion molecules, which are required for leukocyte migration into the graft, to produce acute rejection. Plasma expanders, predominantly hydroxyethyl starch, may impair kidney function in recipients. Rapidly degradable solutions may cause less compromise of renal function.[17]

Liver Function

Very few experimental studies have evaluated liver function in brain-dead donors, but changes appear as early as 3 hours after the clinical determination of brain death.[89,100] Vacuolization in the vicinity of sinusoids and early disintegration of mitochondria and endoplasmic reticulum noted on electron microscopy, along with reduced bile production and stagnated leukocytes in sinusoids; endothelial cells, however, remain intact.[60]

Coagulopathy

Disseminated intravascular coagulation may occur at any time after a major destructive brain injury.[15] Multiple causes of this disorder may be put forward, and indeed, it is more common in polytrauma patients, who are at risk for fat emboli, and in women with complicated pregnancy causing embolization of amniotic fluid.

Penetrating traumatic head injury (e.g., gunshot wounds) may cause entry of brain tissue or its thromboplastin into capillaries and elicit a triggering mechanism for intravascular coagulation. Generally, however, the substantial amount of thromboplastin derived from brain necrosis readily causes fibrin deposition in the microcirculation, resulting in laboratory abnormalities such as reduced fibrinogen levels, prolonged partial thromboplastin time, and thrombocytopenia. Replacement of blood factors by means of fresh frozen plasma may not prevent microthrombi deposits in donor organs. The clinical relevance of microthrombi for graft function is unclear, but most studies appear to show no effect on liver, pancreas, and kidney graft function.[15,36]

Arterial Tone and Circulation

Hypotension can be caused by hypovolemia due to inadequate fluid resuscitation, use of osmotic agents, hyperglycemia-induced osmotic diuresis, cold diuresis, and sudden rewarming. Mostly loss of the sympathoexcitatory neurons in the rostroventrolateral medulla causes loss of vascular tone. These neurons also send glutaminergic (excitatory) tracts to the intermediolateral cell column in the spinal cord connecting to sympathetic ganglions and arteries. Loss of this output in sympathetic drive—together with loss of vagal output—will produce hypotension and an invariate heart rate. Vasopressors or inotropes (which may include vasopressin infusions) are often needed, but a sympathetic spinal overdrive may cause temporary blood pressure stabilization or even hypertension. The cause of hypertension after brain death is not clear but could be similar to early autonomic dysreflexia seen in acute spinal cord injury and perhaps from an early peripheral alpha-adrenoceptor hyperresponsiveness. Another possibility is that it represents a retained function of the most caudal medulla oblongata pressor areas. More typical is a gradual deterioration of blood pressure and increasing polyuria requiring progressively increasing doses of vasopressors or intropes. In our study of 92 patients we found that 70% of potential organ donors are rapidly hemodynamically unstable after brain death. The vast majority (78%) needed more than one agent at some point and many required 3 or 4 agents. The hemodynamic patterns we observed are shown in Figure 5-6.[31]

■ MEDICAL SUPPORTIVE CARE

Knowledge of organ injury associated with catastrophic injury leading to brain death assists in the preservation of organs destined for donation. Avoidance of injury remains the main objective, and this requires multiple intravenous drugs. The period of preservation often includes tests for suitability of organs, but the challenges rarely extend beyond the 36-hour period. Early evidence, however, suggested that delay in the declaration of brain death not only adds to the time of organ recovery but also may increase the risks to the transplantable organs, resulting in more complicated postoperative phases in the recipient.

Multiple reviews have been published on the best management of the organ donor, but the targets of supportive care have been arbitrarily defined. A distillation of common experiences is shown in Tables 5-7, 5-8 and 5-9.[8,29,39,73,74,76,79,96] The main objectives remain the maintenance of oxygenation and circulation, control of polyuria, and control of hyperglycemia. A recent evaluation of UNOS data involving 7 OPOs and 805 donors yielding 2685 organs for transplantation found that successful transplantation was related to reduced vasopressor usage (less than one agent and a low dose), maximizing oxygen (arterial PO_2 >80 mm Hg) and glucose control (<200 mg/dL). Thoracic organs appeared most vulnerable to changes in donor management.[26]

Principally, medical management of the organ donor consists of continuing care of the critically ill patient. Therefore, all aspects of intensive care are in play. However, life has ended and therapeutic options are merely supportive. The appropriate outcome is now a functioning organ in a recipient. The overriding principle is maintenance of normal or near-normal physiology. Therefore, several acute processes (i.e., pulmonary edema, hypovolemia) can and should be reversed. It is useful to present care of the organ donor in terms of multiple systems. (The evaluation and worksheets used by OPO coordinators are shown in Appendices.)

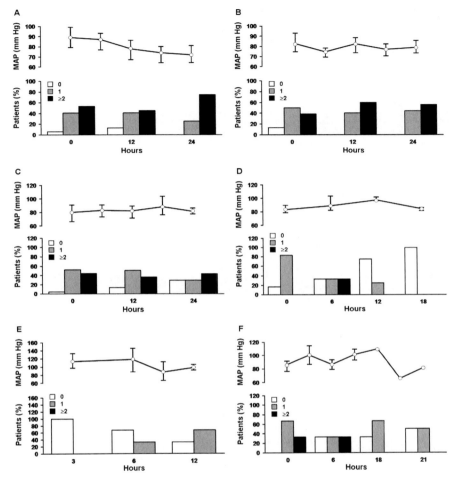

Figure 5-6 Patterns of Hemodynamic Instability after Brain Death Blood pressure patterns seen after brain death. Patterns A and B are more common. Line graph indicates mean arterial pressure (MAP) including 25th to 75th percentiles. Bars indicate number of vasopressors. A) Relentless hypotension despite increasing vasopressors. B) Stable blood pressure with increasing number or dose of vasopressors. C) Stable blood pressure with stable vasopressor requirement. D) Need for vasopressors followed by need for antihypertensives. E) Need for antihypertensives followed by need for vasopressors and F) Markedly labile blood pressure.

■ CARDIOVASCULAR MANAGEMENT

The main goal of cardiovascular management is adequate support of blood pressure and cardiac output. Many organ donors are stable with a combination of fluid resuscitation (mostly crystalloids such as 0.9% NaCl) and a combination of inotropes and vasopressors. Some protocols prefer norepinephrine; others prefer

TABLE 5-7 *Hormonal Resuscitation Therapy (HRT)*

Pre-medicate (in rapid succession)
1 amp 50% dextrose in water 2 grams solumedrol IV 20 units regular insulin IV 20 mcg levothyroxine (T4) IV
Levothyroxine (T4)
Start T4 IV 400 mcg/500 mL D5W infusion at 10 mcg/hour Goal T4 infusion at 50 mcg/hour Titrate to effect and wean off vasopressors

The pediatric doses are different and substantially reduced when weight is less than 35 kg.

Source: Adapted From Abdelnour and Rieke[1]

TABLE 5-8 *Avoidance of Injury to Transplantable Organs*

- Minimal volume strategy to limit extravascular lung water
- Preserve the PaO_2/FIO_2 gradient ≤300 mm Hg
- Give colloid solutions to maintain oxygenation and avoid pulmonary edema
- Give corticosteroids (15 mg/kg) to stabilize or reduce pulmonary edema
- Give packed red cells (Ht ≥30%)
- Avoid hypernatremia using hypotonic solutions
- Avoid acidosis (sodium bicarbonate at 50 mmol)
- Supplement electrolytes regularly (i.e., phosphate, magnesium, potassium)

TABLE 5-9 *Common Interventions during Procurement*

Maintenance of blood pressure
- Goal: SBP 90–160 mm Hg; MAP 70–90 mm Hg - Dopamine 3–5 mcg/kg/min (max 20 mcg/kg/min)* - Phenylephrine 40–60 mcg/min* - Vasopressin 1–2.5 units/h - Labetalol or esmolol (100 µg/kg) for incidental blood pressure surges - Hormonal therapy (see Table 5-7)
Maintenance of normoglycemia
- Goal: serum glucose 100–180 mg/dL - Titrate insulin infusion to effect
Maintenance of normonatremia
- Goal: serum sodium 135–145 mmol/L - Use a combination of IV 0.9% NaCl or 5% dextrose

* Low-dose strategy.

Abbreviations: MAP, mean arterial blood pressure; SBP, systolic blood pressure.

dopamine or dobutamine, alone or in combination with vasopressin. A satisfactory condition is achieved when the mean arterial blood pressure is >70 mm Hg, the heart rate is <100 beats per minute, and urine output is controlled, with production of <300 mL/h. Hemoglobin should be maintained at >7 g/dL using packet cells transfusion, if needed.

Vasopressin infusions are currently often used and stabilize the patient's hemodynamics well. Usually 0.5–2.5 units/h is sufficient. At high doses, vasopressin causes constriction of important arterial beds such as the coronary, renal, and splanchnic vasculature. Serum sodium values should be maintained (and checked three or four times a day) within 135–145 mol/L, and the vasopressin dose should be adjusted regularly to avoid overcorrection. Vasopressin (or desmopressin) has no adverse effect on graft function. Management of the hemodynamically unstable patient is discussed further in Chapter 6.

■ **RESPIRATORY MANAGEMENT**

Perhaps the more complicated part of management of the organ donor involves preservation of lung function. However, procurement of lungs is often limited by prior lung contusions or penetrating injury, pulmonary edema, aspiration pneumonitis, or pneumothorax requiring chest tubes. Nevertheless, if lungs are potentially procurable organs, adequate ventilator management and aggressive pulmonary toilet can be successful.[54]

The modern approach to ventilator management in critically ill patients also applies here. Ventilator management includes low tidal volume targets (6 mL/kg of ideal body weight), low PEEP (<7 cm H_2O) levels, a PaO_2/FIO_2 ratio of more than 300, and low plateau pressures (<30 cm H_2O). Oxygenation can be improved by a single dose of methylprednisolone (15 mg/kg IV). Bronchodilators may reduce mucous plugging, and albuterol nebulizers are used every 4 hours. Patients are provided with high oscillating vests to improve airway clearance, and turning and suctioning is performed every 2 hours. Bronchoalveolar lavage is typically performed, and the results will determine the suitability for transplantation (for that reason, lungs with a positive Gram stain or leukocytosis should likely not be used). In patients without transplantable lungs, the approach is simply to maintain oxygenation; other parameters become less crucial.

■ **ELECTROLYTE AND GLUCOSE MANAGEMENT**

Electrolytes are monitored every 2 hours and corrected. This may involve frequent supplementation of potassium, calcium chloride, magnesium sulfate, and potassium phosphate. Hypernatremia, hypokalemia, hypomagnesemia, and hypocalcemia are often a result of aggressive fluid resuscitation. Profound hypernatremia in the organ donor has been associated with posttransplantation renal dysfunction (acute tubular necrosis) and graft loss after liver transplantation. Glucose is managed using insulin protocols that aim at a glucose level of 100–180 mg/dL.[99] Large volumes of dextrose-containing fluids to treat diabetes insipidus are the main causes of prolonged hyperglycemia and should be avoided. Enteral feeding should continue until the organ donor is transferred to the operating room.

■ COAGULATION MANAGEMENT

Disseminated intravascular coagulation (DIC) is common after major traumatic brain injury and often after penetrating injury. Abnormalities in the prothrombin time (PT) and the partial thromboplastin time (PTT) can be corrected with vitamin K and fresh frozen plasma. Thrombocytopenia requires platelet transfusions, and a fibrinogen decrease can be treated with cryoprecipitate. When DIC occurs, transplantation may become seriously jeopardized and procurement may fail if the organ donor cannot be transferred to the operating room more quickly.

■ CONCLUSION

Procurement of organs and tissue after the clinical diagnosis of brain death is granted in more than 70% of requests. Procurement is, however, a major clinical undertaking requiring close monitoring and treatment by transplantation coordinators. There are many physiologic challenges to the organ donor. Overwhelming drive of the sympathetic nervous system may be detrimental to the heart and lungs. The initial major management concerns deal with hypotension (from collapse of arterial tone), an invariate heart rate (loss of autonomic control), and polyuria (diabetes insipidus). Hemodynamic status may also deteriorate from hypovolemia and hypotension. Hypotension may be initially reversible but progresses unrelentingly. Brain death leads to progressive deterioration of possible donor organs.

▪ **APPENDIX 1**

Example of Donor Management Orders Used by Organ Donor Coordinators

Source: LifeSource. Used with permission. This tool while not universal, incorporates the standard elements required by UNOS/OPTN and the Association of Organ Procurement Association (AOPO) Accreditation Standards.

Organ Donor Management Orders

1. Please copy ALL medical records since admission and give to LifeSource Donation Coordinator. If unable to copy while coordinator onsite, please fax to 651-917-5225 Attn: LifeSource Quality and Regulatory Coordinator as soon as possible. If questions please call LifeSource M-F at 651-603-7800 and ask for QA Coordinator.

2. Change all care and financial responsibilities to LifeSource.

3. Please discontinue all medications except for any vasopressor and antibiotic therapies currently in use.

4. Measure and document current height and weight.

5. Inform LifeSource Coordinator of the following:
   - CVP <4 or >6
   - SBP <100 or >150
   - DBP <50 or >90
   - Core temperature <96.0F or >100.5F
   - HR <60 or >120
   - Urine output <30 or >250cc/hr for 2 hours
   - SaO2 <96%

6. If SBP <100 and HR <90 Dopamine drip.-max 20mcg/kg/min. If SBP <100 and HR>90 then use Neosynephrine-max 200mcg/min. Titrate both medications to maintain SBP>100. Titrate all other Vasopressors off to keep SBP>100.

7. Place NG/OG tube. Low intermittent suction after placement.

8. Foley catheter with hourly urine output monitoring.

9. Triple lumen central IV access. CXR post placement confirming placement. PIV 2-#18 gauge (minimum 18 gauge).

10. Monitor and document CVP every 1hour.

11. Continuous arterial pressure monitoring. Monitor BP every 1hour and every 15 minutes with any instability or vasopressor medication adjustments.

12. Continuous cardiac monitoring, temperature and continuous SaO2 monitoring.

13. IV fluid therapy: **Input Total should be 100cc/hour-125cc/hour.**
    a. _____ at _____cc/hr.

14. Ventilatory settings:
    - Mode AC PCV
    - Rate _____ breaths/min. (PCO2 x rate/40). Goal PCO2 35-45.
    - AC TV 10cc/kg. If current setting <10cc/kg increase TV slowly.
    - IF PCV then adjust pressure settings to achieve TV of 10cc/kg and peak inspiratory pressure (PIP) <30.
    - FiO2 goal 40%. Adjust keeping SaO2 >95% and PaO2 >100.
    - PEEP 5cm
    - Consult RT for management assistance.

15. Zosyn 3.375 Grams IVPB every 6 hours.

16. Solumedrol 1gram every 12 hours or 15mg/kg if less than 70kg.

17. Albuterol/Atrovent nebulizers every 4 hours and every 2 hours PRN.

18. Consult LifeSource Donation Coordinator prior to giving Narcan 8mg IVP X 1.

19. Use Link Vest or CF vest if available for CPT. Turn and suction every 2 hours.

20. HOB >30 degrees except during CPT. During CPT Trendelenburg position (as patient tolerates) to facilitate secretions and suction after CPT cycle.

21. Levothyroxine (T4) protocol (wt. >35kg). K+ must be >3.5 prior to initiation. *LifeSource will provide T4 when able.*

    - Pre-medicate in rapid succession in order as follows:
      - 1 amp D50 IVP x1
      - 2 grams Solumedrol IVP x1 (If 1 gram already given as ordered above, give an additional 1 gram IVP)
      - 20 units regular insulin IVP X1
      - 20 mcg T4 IVP x1

22. T4 400mcg/500cc D5W -Start T4 IV drip at 10mcg/hour, max 50mcg/hour. Rate increases determined by LifeSource Donation Coordinator.

23. Follow ICU established K+, MG+ and phosphorous replacement protocols. If no established protocols consult with Donation Coordinator.

24. Follow ICU insulin drip management protocol. If no established protocol:
    - Regular insulin IV infusion
    - Glucose 80-120 goal
    - If >140-start drip at 2units/hour. Check glucose every 1hour with changes in drip. If glucose stable and no changes to drip in 2 hours may check

glucose every 2 hours. Increase regular insulin infusion by 1-2units/hour PRN keeping glucose <140 mg/dl. If glucose <80-discontinue infusion and check glucose in 1hour.

- If glucose increases >50mg/dl since previous check and increase in insulin drip-consult Donation Coordinator for intervention.

25. Artificial tears 2 drops both eyes every 4 hours.

LABS-all to be done STAT

26. ABO (blood typing) with subtype if able. Type and hold for 3 units PRBC's. If patient only has been typed once please repeat ABO testing for verification purposes with only 1 sub-typing needed.

27. Basic metabolic panel, Ionized Calcium, Mg, Phos, AST, ALT, GGT, T bili, D bili, alk phos, LDH, troponin I, CPK MB, amylase, lipase. **Repeat** BMP every 6 hours.

28. CBC w/diff, PT, PTT, INR stat. **Repeat** hemoglobin, hematocrit every 6 hours.

29. ABG now **and** every 4 hours all to be run STAT please.

30. UA/UC, blood cultures x2-(do not draw from invasive lines) timed 15" apart. Sputum Gram Stain and Culture. **Obtain all cultures prior to starting antibiotic therapy.**

31. PCXR every 4 hours with STAT interpretation. Indication-evaluate effusion vs. atelectasis.

32. Consult LifeSource Donation Coordinator on when to perform FIO2 challenge as follows: Increase FiO2 to 100% X30" then check ABG. Decrease FiO2 to 40% X30" and check ABG.

33. Consult Donation Coordinator for echocardiogram, 12 lead EKG, and bronchoscopy if applicable.

Signature:_____ Date:_____

■ **APPENDIX 2**

Evaluation and Management Forms Used by OPO Coordinators of LifeSource

Source: LifeSource. Used with permission. This tool while not universal, incorporates the standard elements required by UNOS/OPTN and the Association of Organ Procurement Association (AOPO) Accreditation Standards.

LifeSource
Organ & Tissue Donation

UNOS ID: _____ LifeSource #:_____

CONFIDENTIAL DONOR MANAGEMENT RECORD

Medical Record # _____   ☐ SCD   ☐ ECD   ☐ DCD

Coordinator(s) (First and Last Names) _____

DONOR INFORMATION

Donor Hospital _____   Hospital Unit _____   Provider # _____
City/State _____   Telephone # _____   Fax # _____
Date/Time Admission _____ / _____
Date/Time of Referral _____ / _____   Referring Person _____
Date/Time of LS Staff Arrival _____ / _____   Attending Physician _____

Donor Name_____   ☐ Brain Death   ☐ Cardiac Time of Death
SSN_____ DOB_____   Date/Time____/_____MD/DO_____
Address_____
City_____State_____ZIP_____   Date/Time____/_____MD/DO_____
Age_____ Sex _____ Race _____   Method(s) Used_____
Ht._____Wt._____BMI_____   ME/Coroner Case ☐ Yes ☐ No
   Permission for Donation ☐ Yes ☐ No Case # _____
HLA A___/___ B___/___ DR___/___   Restrictions _____
   Instructions_____
ABO _____ Rh _____ Sub _____   Name of ME/Coroner_____

Cause of Death (See Codes)_____   Date/Time of Contact _____/_____
Mechanism of Death (See Codes)_____   Autopsy ☐Yes ☐No   External Exam by ME prior to OR ☐Yes ☐No
Circumstances of Death (See Codes)_____   Autopsy Requested by Family? ☐ Yes ☐ No
Active Military ☐ Yes ☐ No ☐ Unknown   Funeral Home Name/Contact _____
☐ U.S. Born ☐ Not U.S. Born ☐ U.S. Citizen   Phone Number of Funeral Home _____
How long lived in U.S. _____years   Funeral Home Contacted Date/Time_____ / _____

CONSENT INFORMATION

Donor Designation? ☐ Yes ☐ No ☐ Unknown   Copy Attached ☐ Yes ☐ No
Next of Kin_____   **FUNERAL ARRANGEMENTS:**
Relationship_____   Viewing: ☐ Yes ☐ No ☐ Unknown
Address_____
   NOK Phone Number _____

Organ	Authorization Requested?	If not requested, write reason	Authorization Obtained?	If not, give reason
Kidney	☐ Yes ☐ No		☐ Yes ☐ No	
Liver	☐ Yes ☐ No		☐ Yes ☐ No	
Intestine	☐ Yes ☐ No		☐ Yes ☐ No	
Pancreas	☐ Yes ☐ No		☐ Yes ☐ No	
Heart	☐ Yes ☐ No		☐ Yes ☐ No	
Lung	☐ Yes ☐ No		☐ Yes ☐ No	
CV Tissue	☐ Yes ☐ No		☐ HV ☐ Saphenous ☐Femoral	
MS Tissue	☐ Yes ☐ No		☐ UE ☐ LE ☐ Skin ☐ Vert. Bodies	
Eye Tissue	☐ Yes ☐ No		☐ Corneas ☐ Sclera ☐ Whole eyes	

Authorization for Research ☐ Yes ☐ No ☐ Other _____
Any Limitations? _____

Authorization Obtained by _____   Date/Time_____ / _____

LifeSource
Organ & Tissue Donation

UNOS ID: _____ LifeSource #: _____

TISSUE INFORMATION

TISSUE INFORMATION

Tissue Agency Notified ☐ LifeSource ☐ Spirit of the North ☐ N/A

If Tissue recovered by LIFESOURCE (complete below):

Musculoskeletal (MTF-primary)
MTF   Screened ☐ Yes ☐ NA Name _____ Date/Time_____ Accepted Y/N, if no reason_____
LifeNet Screened ☐ Yes ☐ NA Name _____ Date/Time_____ Accepted Y/N, if no reason_____
Processor case # _____

Skin
MTF   Screened ☐ Yes ☐ NA Name _____ Date/Time_____ Accepted Y/N, if no reason_____
Processor case # _____

Vessel
Cryolife Screened ☐ Yes ☐ NA Name _____ Date/Time_____ Accepted Y/N, if no reason_____

Heart Valves (LifeNet-primary unless indicated on hospital cheat sheet)
LifeNet Screened ☐ Yes ☐ NA Name _____ Date/Time_____ Accepted Y/N, if no reason_____
Cryolife Screened ☐ Yes ☐ NA Name _____ Date/Time_____ Accepted Y/N, if no reason_____
Processor case # _____

EYE INFORMATION

☐ MLEB   ☐ NDLEB   ☐ SDLEB   ☐ WILEB   ☐ N/A
Name _____ Date/Time_____ / _____ Accepted Y/N, if no reason_____

Upon Completion of Case:

Funeral Home Notified? ☐ Yes ☐ Tissue/Eye Agency to call ☐ Other _____
By Whom? _____ Date / Time _____ / _____
Comments_____

ME/Coroner Notified? ☐ Yes ☐ NA ☐Tissue/Eye Agency to Call
By Whom? _____ Date / Time _____ / _____
Comments_____

UNOS Reference Codes

Cause of Death	Mechanism of Death		Circumstances of Death
Anoxia	Drowning	Gunshot Wound	Motor Vehicle Accident
Cerebrovascular/Stroke	Seizure	Stab	Alleged Suicide
Head Trauma	Drug Intoxication	Blunt Injury	Alleged Homicide
CNS Tumor	Asphyxiation	Sudden Infant Death	Alleged Child Abuse
Other	Cardiovascular	Intracranial Hemorrhage/Stroke	Non-Motor Vehicle Accident
	Electrical	Other	Other

LifeSource
Organ & Tissue Donation

UNOS ID: _____ LifeSource #: _____

ADMISSION COURSE/COMMENTS

Please identify any injuries, fractures, incisions, tattoos and, social indicators on the diagrams and describe below. Include any operative procedures or invasive lines/tubes.

☐ OR Procedures_____

_____

_____

☐ CPR/Downtime_____

Comments_____

_____

_____

1. Arterial Line
2. Central Line
3. Peripheral IV lines
4. Abrasions/Lacerations
5. Bruises/Hematomas
6. Fractures
7. Casts/splints/traction
8. Incisions/sutures
9. ICP monitor
10. Endotracheal tube
11. Foley Catheter

12. NG/OG
13. Chest tube
14. Tattoo (describe)
15. Piercing (describe)
16. Scars(surgical or trauma)
17. Non-therapeutic needle
      marks
18. Other (document)

LifeSource
Organ & Tissue Donation

UNOS ID: _____ LifeSource #: _____

INITIAL PHYSICAL ASSESSMENT

BODY IDENTIFIED BY ☐ Patient's Nurse ☐ Toe tag ☐ Wrist band ☐ Other_____

Person Identifying_____

Examination Performed By_____ Date / Time_____/_____

PHYSICAL EXAMINATION

EVIDENCE OF:				
Non-medical injection of drugs	☐ Yes ☐ No	Jaundice	☐ Yes ☐ No
Trauma to tissue retrieval sites	☐ Yes ☐ No	Infection	☐ Yes ☐ No
Genital lesions	☐ Yes ☐ No	Anal tears/perianal warts	☐ Yes ☐ No
Blue/purple spots	☐ Yes ☐ No	White spots in mouth	☐ Yes ☐ No
Enlarged lymph nodes	☐ Yes ☐ No	(comment below if unable to visualize oral cavity)	

PULMONARY

Tubes: ☐ Endotracheal Size_____mm Performed ☐ Prehospital ☐ Hospital
☐ Tracheostomy Size_____mm Performed ☐ Prehospital ☐ Hospital

Chest Tube ☐ Left Chest ☐ Right Chest Performed ☐ Prehospital ☐ Hospital
Drainage ☐ Yes_____ ☐ No

Breath Sounds ☐ Even ☐ Uneven ☐ Absent left/right ☐ Wheezes ☐ Clear
☐ Rales left/right ☐ Rhonchi left/right ☐ Decreased left/right

CARDIOVASCULAR

Lines: ☐ PA cath ☐ CVP ☐ Arterial line
Heart Rhythm ☐ Regular ☐ Irregular
Heart Tones ☐ Normal ☐ Murmur ☐ Rub
Periph. Pulses ☐ Present ☐ 1 2 3 4 ☐ Absent
Periph. Edema ☐ Present ☐ 1 2 3 4 ☐ Absent
Thoracic evaluation ☐ Chest trauma ☐ Intracardiac injections ☐ Other_____

INTEGUMENTARY

Color ☐ Pink ☐ Dusky ☐ Pale ☐ Other_____
Temperature ☐ Warm ☐ Cool Temp During Physical Exam: _____
Other ☐ Bruises ☐ Lacerations ☐ Track marks
☐ Piercings (professional or nonprofessional?) Describe:_____
☐ Tattoos (professional or nonprofessional?) Describe:_____

GASTROINTESTINAL

DPL ☐ Yes ☐ No ☐ Result_____
Tubes ☐ NG/OG ☐ Gastrostomy ☐ Surgical drains
Abdomen ☐ Incisions ☐ Surgical scars ☐ Other scars (describe below)
☐ Soft ☐ Firm ☐ Non-distended ☐ Distended
☐ + bowel sounds ☐ No bowel sounds

GENITOURINARY

Urine Volume ☐ <100 cc/hr ☐ 100 - 500 cc/hr ☐ >500 cc/hr ☐ Anuric
Appearance ☐ Clear ☐ Cloudy ☐ Hematuria

MUSCULOSKELETAL

Fractures ☐ Closed ☐ Compound/open ☐ Dressings/splint ☐ Traction ☐ None

---

Comments:

LifeSource
Organ & Tissue Donation

UNOS ID: _____ LifeSource #: _____

Lab Profile (Document any further labs on page 14)

Date												
Time												
Na+ (140-160)												
K+ (3.5-5.5)												
Cl- (96-115)												
CO$_2$												
BUN (<20)												
Creatinine (<1.5)												
GFR												
Glucose (65-150)												
Calcium (8.5-10.5)												
Phosphorous (1.8-2.6)												
Total Bili												
Direct/Conjugated Bili												
Indirect/Unconj. Bili												
SGOT(AST) (0-40)												
SGPT (ALT) (5-35)												
GGT (17-55)												
Albumin												
Total protein												
Mg												
Alk Phos (45-110)												
LDH (90-250)												
PT (11-15)												
PTT (24-36)												
INR												
Fibrinogen												
CPK/tot MB (0255/<5)												
Troponin												
Amylase (23-851)												
Lipase (0-80)												
HghA1c												
ETOH Level												
Toxicology Screening												
Pregnancy Screen												

Urinalysis (1 required w/in 24 hrs of XC) | **CBC/Differential**

Color			RBC							
Appearance			WBC							
pH			Hgb							
Spec. Grav.			Hct							
Protein			Plt							
Glucose			Segs							
Blood			Lymphs							
RBC			Bands							
WBC			Monos							
Epith			Eos							
Casts			Other							
Bacteria										

LifeSource
Organ & Tissue Donation

UNOS ID: _____ LifeSource #: _____

PRE-DONOR MANAGEMENT CULTURE RESULTS

Cultures	Date	Preliminary Result	Date	Final Results
Blood				
Blood				
Urine				
Sputum				
CSF				
Other_____				

Donor Management Cultures	Results	
Blood	Date/Time Drawn_____	☐ Report to Follow
Blood	Date/Time Drawn_____	☐ Report to Follow
Urine	Date/Time Drawn_____	☐ Report to Follow
Sputum	Date/Time Drawn_____	☐ Report to Follow

PRE-OPO (72 hours prior to Donor Management)

HEMODYNAMICS/TEMPERATURE								
From: Date								
Time								
To: Date								
Time								
Average BP								
Heart rate								
High BP								
Duration								
Low BP								
Duration								
CVP								
PA								
PAWP								
CO/CI								
Temp								
Drug/Dosage								
Drug/Dosage								
Drug/Dosage								
Drug/Dosage								

LifeSource
Organ & Tissue Donation

UNOS ID: _____ LifeSource #: _____

MEDICATIONS					
List all antibiotics during hospitalization, and **ALL medications administered 24 hours prior to Cross Clamp. These medications all need to be documented on the DDR in UNET.**					
Medication	Date/time started	Dosage	Peak dose	Duration	Date/time stopped

LifeSource
Organ & Tissue Donation

UNOS ID: _____   LifeSource #: _____

SEROLOGIES   *A non-hemodiluted sample is necessary for tissue/eye to proceed*

Specimen 1 Date/time drawn	Preinfusion ☐Yes ☐No Pretransfusion ☐Yes ☐No Hemodiluted ☐Yes ☐No	ANTI HIV I	ANTI HIV II	Anti-HTLV 1	Anti HTLV II	RPR-VDRL	Anti CMV	HbsAg	Anti-HBC	Anti-HCV	EBV	NAT I /II HCV/HIV
Specimen 2 Date/time drawn	Preinfusion ☐Yes ☐No Pretransfusion ☐Yes ☐No Hemodiluted ☐Yes ☐No	ANTI HIV I	ANTI HIV II	Anti-HTLV 1	Anti HTLV II	RPR-VDRL	Anti CMV	HbsAg	Anti-HBC	Anti-HCV	EBV	NAT I/ II HCV/HIV

Serology Codes: R .... REACTIVE   NR .... NON-REACTIVE   ND .... NOT DONE
                      U .... Unknown   C........... Cannot Disclose   I .... Indeterminate
Comments on reactive results (IgG/IgM, etc.)
_____

Serum Archive Specimen: Sent: ☐ Yes ☐ No   Draw Date _____   Time _____

Specimen Type:_____ Preinfusion: ☐ Yes ☐ No Pretransfusion: ☐ Yes ☐ No Hemodiluted: ☐ Yes ☐ No

Manufacturer Lot # _____   Expiration Date _____

Pre-OPO Intake (72 hours prior to Donor Management)						Pre-OPO Output (72 hours prior to Donor Management)			
Date (from/to)	Time (from/to)	Crystalloid	Colloid	Blood products	24° Total	Urine output/ hour average	Other output & Type	Total output	Lowest urine output per hour/ duration

BLOOD PRODUCT/COLLOID ADMINISTRATION SUMMARY SINCE ADMISSION				
Date	Time	Blood Product/Colloid Type	Unit #	Volume (ml)
		☐PRBCs ☐FFP ☐5%Albumin ☐25%Albumin ☐Cryo ☐Platelets ☐Other		
		☐PRBCs ☐FFP ☐5%Albumin ☐25%Albumin ☐Cryo ☐Platelets ☐Other		
		☐PRBCs ☐FFP ☐5%Albumin ☐25%Albumin ☐Cryo ☐Platelets ☐Other		
		☐PRBCs ☐FFP ☐5%Albumin ☐25%Albumin ☐Cryo ☐Platelets ☐Other		
		☐PRBCs ☐FFP ☐5%Albumin ☐25%Albumin ☐Cryo ☐Platelets ☐Other		
		☐PRBCs ☐FFP ☐5%Albumin ☐25%Albumin ☐Cryo ☐Platelets ☐Other		

LifeSource
Organ & Tissue Donation

UNOS ID: _____ LifeSource #: _____

CARDIAC DATA

EKG   ☐ Normal   ☐ Abnormal

Date / Time _____ / _____   Consulting Physician_____
Interpretation:_____
_____
_____

☐ **2-D ECHO** ☐ **TRANS–ESOPHAGEAL ECHO**   ☐ Not Performed/Reason_____
See Echo Report ☐
Date / Time_____ / _____   Consulting Physician_____
Interpretation:_____
_____
_____
_____

CVP_____	EF_____	BP _____	HR_____	Cardiac rhythm_____
CO_____	CI_____	PAWP_____	SF_____	PA pressure_____

Pressors   ☐ Yes   ☐ No

During echo: ☐ Dopamine   Dosage_____
☐ Neosynephrine   Dosage_____
☐ Levophed   Dosage_____
☐ T4   Dosage_____
☐ Other_____Dosage_____

ANGIOGRAPHY

Date / Time_____ / _____Consulting Physician_____
Interpretation_____
_____
_____

DEFIBRILLATION ☐ Yes ☐ No

Duration_____
Date/time: _____ / _____

CHEST COMPRESSIONS   ☐ Yes ☐ No

Duration _____
Date/time: _____ / _____

EPISODES OF ARRHYTHMIA

Date/Time	Rhythm	Duration	Treatment

LifeSource
Organ & Tissue Donation

UNOS ID: _____ LifeSource #: _____

PULMONARY DATA

CXR
Date/ Time _____**Read By** _____ Change from previous CXR? ☐ Yes ☐ No

Interpretation_____

CXR
Date/ Time _____**Read By** _____ Change from previous CXR? ☐ Yes ☐ No

Interpretation_____

CXR
Date/ Time _____**Read By** _____ Change from previous CXR? ☐ Yes ☐ No

Interpretation_____

CXR
Date/ Time _____**Read By** _____ Change from previous CXR? ☐ Yes ☐ No

Interpretation_____

CXR
Date/ Time _____**Read By** _____ Change from previous CXR? ☐ Yes ☐ No

Interpretation_____

Chest CT Results_____

BRONCHOSCOPY   **See Bronchoscopy Report** ☐
Date / Time_____/_____   Consultant_____
Interpretation_____
_____
_____

Sputum Gram Stain Date/Time_____/_____Result _____
_____

1. Length of Right Lung_____
2. Length of Left Lung_____
3. Aortic Knob Width_____
4. Diaphragm Width_____
5. Dist. RCPA to LCPA_____
6. Chest Circ.@ Nipple Line_____
7. Total Lung Capacity_____
8. Vital Capacity_____

Males
$TLC = (0.094 \times Ht.\ cm) - (0.015 \times Age\ in\ Yrs.) - 9.167$
$VC = (0.064 \times Ht.\ cm) - (0.031 \times Age\ in\ Yrs.) - 5.335$
Females
$TLC = (0.079 \times Ht.\ cm) - (0.008 \times Age\ in\ Yrs.) - 7.49$
$VC = (0.052 \times Ht.\ cm) - (0.018 \times Age\ in\ Yrs.) - 4.36$
(1 inch = 2.54 cms)

ARTERIAL BLOOD GASES

DATE/TIME	pH	pCO_2	pO_2	HCO_3/BE	O_2Sat	FiO_2	Mode	Rate	TV	PEEP	PiP

LifeSource
Organ & Tissue Donation

UNOS ID: _____ LifeSource #: _____

INTRAOPERATIVE MANAGEMENT

Enter OR ....Date_____ Time_____ ☐ Central Time
Incision ....Date_____ Time_____
Clamp ....Date_____ Time_____ ☐ Mountain Time
Exit OR ....Date_____ Time_____
Average BP_____ Low BP_____ Duration_____ High BP_____ Duration_____
Average HR_____ Low HR_____ Duration_____ High HR _____ Duration _____
Average urine output_____ Last hour urine output_____ Total urine output in OR_____
See attached DCD flowsheet? ☐ Yes ☐ No
Anesthesia Guidelines provided to MDA/CRNA? ☐ Yes ☐ No

MEDICATIONS

☐Heparin Dosage/Time _____/_____   ☐ Vasodilators ☐ Nipride Dosage_____
☐Thorazine Dosage/Time _____/_____   ☐ Other_____ Dosage_____
☐ Mannitol Dosage/Time _____/_____   ☐ Vasopressors ☐ Dopamine Dosage_____
☐ Lasix Dosage/Time _____/_____   ☐ Neosynephrine Dosage_____
☐ Solumedrol Dosage/Time _____/_____   ☐ Levophed Dosage_____
☐ T4 Dosage/Time _____/_____   ☐ Other Dosage_____
☐ Other_____ Dosage/Time _____/_____   ☐ Blood products type/volume_____/_____
☐ Decadron Dosage/Time _____/_____   ☐ Blood products type/volume_____/_____
☐ PGE 1 Dosage/Time _____/_____   ☐ Crystalloids type/volume_____/_____

RECOVERY TEAM NAMES (PRINT)

Heart	Heart/Lung	Right Lung	Left Lung

Liver	Kidneys	Pancreas	Intestine

Abdominal and chest cavities visually inspected for contraindications to donation by_____
Comments/Labs_____
_____
_____

Donation Coordinator_____ Surgical Recovery Coordinator _____

ME form completed and faxed to ME office?   ☐ Yes ☐ No ☐ NA

Verification of Accuracy Form Completed?   Date / Time_____/_____

Preservation Solution Additives:
No Additives added to HTK or SPS-1 or Celsior or Kidney Perfusate Solution (KPS)
For MNUM per 1liter bag Perfadex: 4cc THAM/60 mg CACL/125ugm PGE1 in NaCl
For MNUM per 1 liter bag Cardioplegia: D5W 1000cc/32mEq KCL/26mEqNaHCO3/15,000mgMannitol
For MNSM per 2800cc bag Perfadex: 9.24 mls THAM

LifeSource
Organ & Tissue Donation

UNOS ID: _____ LifeSource #: _____

RENAL DATA

☐ Warm Ischemic Time   ☐ Yes ☐ No   Duration_____

Insitu Flush   ☐Yes ☐No Flush Solution_____ Volume_____ Flush Characteristics ☐1+ ☐2+ ☐3+ ☐4+

Storage Solution_____ Backtable Flush ☐ Yes ☐ No Volume_____ Sent en bloc ☐ Yes ☐ No

Typing Materials   ☐ Nodes   ☐ Spleen   ☐ Blood Clot

Recovering Surgeon _____ Assistant Surgeon_____

Left kidney	Left	Renal anatomy	Right	Right kidney
HardSoft	☐Yes ☐No	**Aortic plaque**	☐Yes ☐No	Hard Soft
Hard Soft	☐Yes ☐No	**Arterial plaque**	☐Yes ☐No	Hard Soft
	☐Yes ☐No	**Infarcted area(s)**	☐Yes ☐No	
	☐Yes ☐No	**Capsule tears(s)**	☐Yes ☐No	
	☐Yes ☐No	**Subcapsular hematoma(s)**	☐Yes ☐No	
	☐Yes ☐No	**Cysts/Discoloration**	☐Yes ☐No	
	☐Yes ☐No	**Pumped**	☐Yes ☐No	
	☐Yes ☐No	**Biopsy**	☐Yes ☐No	

Left Kidney Anatomy

☐Not recovered/reason _____

Length _____cm   Width _____cm

Arteries # _____   Aortic cuff ☐Yes ☐No

Are multiple arteries on a common cuff? ☐Yes ☐No

Length _____cm_____cm_____cm

Diameter _____mm_____mm_____mm

Distance apart _____mm _____mm

Veins #_____Full vena cava ☐Yes ☐ No

Length _____cm_____cm_____cm

Diameter _____mm_____mm_____mm

Distance apart _____cm _____cm

Ureter single/double/triple

Length _____cm_____cm_____cm

Abnormalities ☐Yes ☐No

Surgical Damage ☐Yes ☐No

Comments_____

_____

_____

See Biopsy Form ☐

Biopsy Results_____

_____

_____

Right Kidney Anatomy

☐Not recovered/reason_____

Length _____cm   Width _____cm

Arteries # _____   Aortic cuff ☐Yes ☐No

Are multiple arteries on a common cuff? ☐Yes ☐No

Length _____cm_____cm_____cm

Diameter _____mm_____mm_____mm

Distance apart _____mm _____mm

Veins #_____Full vena cava ☐Yes ☐ No

Length _____cm_____cm_____cm

Diameter _____mm_____mm_____mm

Distance apart _____cm _____cm

Ureter single/double/triple

Length _____cm_____cm_____cm

Abnormalities ☐Yes ☐No

Surgical Damage ☐Yes ☐No

Comments_____

_____

_____

See Biopsy Form ☐

Biopsy Results_____

_____

_____

Kidney Score _____	**Kidney Pumped** ☐ Yes ☐ No	Kidney Score _____	**Kidney Pumped** ☐ Yes ☐ No
Grade _____	If yes, renal perfusion record attached	Grade _____	If yes, renal perfusion record attached

LifeSource
Organ & Tissue Donation

UNOS ID: _____　LifeSource #: _____

HEART DATA

☐ Heart for Valves　☐ Research Program_____　☐ Not Recovered/Reason _____
Flush Time _____ Flush Solution _____Volume_____ Storage Solution _____
For Valves: Storage Solution Manufacturer _____ Lot _____ Expiration Date _____
　　　　　　Shipping Container Lot _____ Batch # _____
Anatomical Abnormality ☐ Yes　☐ No　Comments_____
Surgical Damage　　　　☐ Yes　☐No　Comments_____
Evidence/CV disease?　☐ Yes　☐No　Comments_____
Recovery Surgeon_____　　Transplant Program_____

LUNG DATA

☐ Transplanted　☐ Research Program_____　☐ Not Recovered/Reason _____
Flush Time _____ Flush Solution _____ Volume _____ Storage Solution_____
Lung Recovered　☐ Right　☐ Left　☐ Heart/Lung　☐ Double Lung
Intraoperative Bronchoscopy Results_____
Anatomical Abnormality ☐ Yes　☐ No　Comments_____
Surgical Damage　　　　☐ Yes　☐ No　Comments_____
Recovery Surgeon_____　　　Transplant Program_____

PANCREAS DATA

☐ Transplanted　☐Islet cells　☐ Research Program_____ ☐ Not Recovered/Reason_____
Aortic flush　　　Start Time_____ Solution_____ Volume_____ Char 1 2 3 4
Whole ☐ Yes ☐ No　Celiac ☐ Yes ☐ No　Spleen Attached ☐Yes ☐ No　Portal Vein ☐ Yes ☐ No
Anatomical Abnormality　☐ Yes　☐ No　　Comments_____
Surgical Damage　　　　　☐ Yes　☐ No　　Comments_____
Vessels Sent　　　　　　　☐ Yes　☐ No　　Comments_____
Duodenal Flush　　　　　　☐ Yes　☐ No ☐ LS solution: 25 mg Fungizone, 1 gm Ancef, 50mg Gentamicin all in 500 cc NaCl
Recovery Surgeon_____　　　Transplant Program_____

LIVER DATA

☐ Transplanted　☐ Research Program_____　☐ Not Recovered/Reason_____
Aortic Flush　　　Start Time_____　Solution_____　Volume_____ Char 1 2 3 4
Portal Flush　　　Start Time_____　Solution_____　Volume_____ Char 1 2 3 4
Anatomical Abnormality　　　☐ Yes　☐ No Comments_____
Surgical Damage　　　　　　　☐ Yes　☐ No Comments_____
Hematoma　　　　　　　　　　☐ Yes　☐ No Comments_____
Vessels Sent　　　　　　　　　☐ Yes　☐ No Comments_____
Gall Bladder Incised　　　　　☐ Yes　☐ No Comments_____
Replaced Hepatic　　☐ No　　☐ Right ☐ Left Comments_____
Biopsy　　　　　　　　　　　☐ Yes　☐ No Result (include % fat)
Biopsy Per Mayo protocol　　☐ Yes　☐ No _____

Recovery Surgeon_____　　　Transplant Program_____

INTESTINE DATA

☐ Transplanted　☐ Research Program_____　☐ Not Recovered/Reason_____
Flush_____　　Start Time_____　Solution_____　Volume_____ Char 1 2 3 4
Anatomical Abnormality ☐ Yes　☐ No　Comments_____
Surgical Damage　　　　☐ Yes　☐ No　Comments_____
Bowel Prep　　　　　　☐ Yes　☐ No
Recovery Surgeon_____　　　Transplant Program_____

UNOS #: Date: / / Admit Weight: Todays Weight: Previous Day Fluid Balance:

Time

Systolic BP V
Diastolic BP ∧
Pulse •

250 240 230 220 210 200 190 180 170 160 150 140 130 120 110 100 90 80 70 60 50 40 30 20 10 0

Hemodynamics
- Temperature/SaO2
- RA/CVP
- PAS/PAD
- LA/PAW
- CO/CI

Infusions
- Dopamine Mcg/Kg/Min
- Dopamine ml/hr
- Pitressin u/hr
- Pitressin ml/hr
- T4 Mcq/hr
- T4 ml/hr
- Glucose
- Insulin units/hr
- Insulin ml/hr

Colloid
- Albumin
- Blood

Output
- Urine

LifeSource
Organ & Tissue Donation

UNOS ID:_____ LifeSource #: _____

ORGAN/TISSUE SCREENING WORKSHEET

Organ	Center	Person Contacted	Response
Heart	MNAN		
	MNMC		
	MNUM		
Lungs	MNSM		
	MNUM		
Liver	MNMC		
	MNUM		
Pancreas	MNMC		
	MNUM		
	NDSL		
	SDMK		
Kidney	MNAN		
	MNHC		
	MNMC		
	MNUM		
	NDMC		
	NDSL		
	SDMK		
	SDSV		
Intestine	MNUM		

Tissue	Center	Person Contacted	Response
Tissue	LifeSource		
	Spirit of the North		
	Other		
Eye	MNLEB		
	NDLEB		
	SDLEB		
Valves	LifeNet		
	Cryolife		

Research	Program	Person Contacted	Response
	IIAM		
	NDRI		

LifeSource
Organ & Tissue Donation

UNOS ID:_____ LifeSource #: _____

DONOR HOSPITAL PERSONNEL

Department	First Name	Last Name	Credentials
ICU			
HUC/Secretary			
Respiratory Therapy			
Cardiology/Angiography Techs			
Chaplaincy			
PHYSICIANS			
Neurology			
Intensivists/Attending Other MDs			
Cardiology			
OPERATING ROOM			
Nurses/Scrub Techs			
Anesthesiology/CRNAs			
ME/MEI			
Other			

■ REFERENCES

1. Abdelnour T, Rieke S. Relationship of hormonal resuscitation therapy and central venous pressure on increasing organs for transplant. *J Heart Lung Transplant* 2009;28:480–485.
2. ACRE Trial Collaborators. Effect of "collaborative requesting" on consent rate for organ donation: randomized controlled trial (ACRE trial). *BMJ* 2009;339:b3911.
3. Adrie C, Monchi M, Fulgencio J-P, et al. Immune status and apoptosis activation during brain death. *Shock* 2010;33:353–362.
4. Alghanim SA. Knowledge and attitudes toward organ donation: a community-based study comparing rural and urban populations. *Saudi J Kidney Dis Transplant* 2010;21:23–30.
5. Atkinson JL. The neglected prehospital phase of head injury: apnea and catecholamine surge. *Mayo Clin Proc* 2000;75:37–47.
6. Avlonitis VS, Fisher AJ, Kirby JA, et al. Pulmonary transplantation: the role of brain death in donor lung injury. *Transplantation* 2003;75:1928–1933.
7. Barklin A. Systemic inflammation in the brain-dead organ donor. *Acta Anaesthesiol Scand* 2009;53:425–435.
8. Botha P, Rostron AJ, Fisher AJ, et al. Current strategies in donor selection and management. *Semin Thoracic Surg* 2008;20:143–151.
9. Boucek MM, Mathis CM, Kanakriyeh MS, et al. Donor shortage: use of the dysfunctional donor heart. *J Heart Lung Transplant* 1993;12:S186–S190.
10. Brown CV, Foulkrod KH, Dworaczyk S, et al. Barriers to obtaining family consent for potential organ donors. *J Trauma* 2010;68:447–451.
11. Bruinsma GJ, Nederhoff MG, Geertman HJ, et al. Acute increase of myocardial workload, hemodynamic instability, and myocardial histological changes induced by brain death in the cat. *J Surg Res* 1997;68:7–15.
12. Cantin B, Kwok BWK, Chan MCY, et al. The impact of brain death on survival after heart transplantation: time is of the essence. *Transplantation* 2003;76:1275–1279.
13. Carey ME, Sarna GS, Farrell JB, et al. Experimental missile wound to the brain. *J Neurosurg* 1989;71:754–764.
14. Carlos TM, Clark RS, Franicola-Higgins D, et al. Expression of endothelial adhesion molecules and recruitment of neutrophils after traumatic brain injury in rats. *J Leukoc Biol* 1997;61:279–285.
15. Cheng SS, Pinson CW, Lopez RR, et al. Effect of donor-disseminated intravascular coagulation in liver transplantation. *Arch Surg* 1991;126:1292–1296.
16. Christmas AB, Mallico EJ, Burris GW, et al. A paradigm shift in the approach to families for organ donation: honoring patients' wishes versus request for permission in patients with Department of Motor Vehicles donor designations. *J Trauma* 2008;65:1507–1509.
17. Cittanova ML, LeBlanc I, Legendre C, et al. Effect of hydroxyethyl starch in brain-dead kidney donors on renal function in kidney-transplant recipients. *Lancet* 1995;348:1620–1622.
18. Connor RC. Heart damage associated with intracranial lesions. *BMJ* 1968;3:29–31.
19. Cooper DK, Basker M. Physiologic changes following brain death. *Transplant Proc* 1999;31:1001–1002.
20. Dae MW, O'Connell JW, Botvinick EH, et al. Scintigraphic assessment of regional cardiac adrenergic innervation. *Circulation* 1989;79:634–644.
21. de Groot YJ, Jansen NE, Bakker J, Kuiper MA, et al. Imminent brain death: point of departure for potential heart beating organ donor recognition. *Intensive Care Med* 2010;36:1488–1494.
22. de Groot YJ, Jansen NE, Bakker J, et al. Donor conversion rates depend on assessment tools of the potential organ donor. *Intensive Care Med* 2011, in press.

23. Dimopoulou I, Tsagarakis S, Anthi A, et al. High prevalence of decreased cortisol reserve in brain-dead potential organ donors. *Crit Care Med* 2003;31:1113–1117.
24. Doshi R, Neil-Dwyer G. A clinicopathological study of patients following a subarachnoid hemorrhage. *J Neurosurg* 1980;52:295–301.
25. Dujardin KS. McCully RB, Wijdicks EFM, et al. Myocardial dysfunction associated with brain death: clinical, echocardiographic, and pathologic features. *J Heart Lung Transplant* 2001;20:350–357.
26. Franklin GA, Santos AP, Smith JW, et al. Optimization of donor management goals yields increased organ use. *Am Surg* 2010;76:587–594.
27. Freitas J, Puig J, Rocha AP, et al. Heart rate variability in brain death. *Clin Auton Res* 1996;6:141–146.
28. Frontera JA. How I manage the adult potential organ donor: donation after cardiac death (part 2). *Neurocrit Care* 2010;12:111–116.
29. Frontera JA, Kalb T. How I manage the adult potential organ donor: donation after neurological death (part 1). *Neurocrit Care* 2010;12:103–110.
30. Fugate JE, Stadler M, Rabinstein AA, Wijdicks EFM. Variability in after Cardiac Death protocols: a national survey.*Transplantation.* 2011;91:386–389.
31. Fugate JE, Rabinstein AA,Wijdicks EFM. Blood pressure patterns after brain death. Submitted for publication
32. Goldstein B, Toweill D, Lai S, et al. Uncoupling of the autonomic and cardiovascular systems in acute brain injury. *Am J Physiol* 1998;275:R1287–R1292.
33. Gramm HJ, Meinhold H, Bickel U, et al. Acute endocrine failure after brain death? *Transplantation* 1992;54:851–857.
34. Halloran PF, Aprile MA, Farewell V, et al. Early function as the principal correlate of graft survival. A multivariate analysis of 200 cadaveric renal transplants treated with a protocol incorporating anti-lymphocyte globulin and cyclosporine. *Transplantation* 1988;46:223–228.
35. Hanusch C, Nowak K, Torlitz P, et al. Donor dopamine treatment limits pulmonary edema and inflammation in lung allografts subjected to prolonged hypothermia. *Transplantation* 2008;85:1449–1455.
36. Hefty TR, Cotterell LW, Fraser SC, et al. Disseminated intravascular coagulation in cadaveric organ donors. Incidence and effect on renal transplantation. *Transplantation* 1993;55:442–443.
37. Herijgers P, Borgers M, Flameng W. The effect of brain death on cardiovascular function in rats. Part I. Is the heart damaged? *Cardiovasc Res* 1998;38:98–106.
38. Herijgers P, Flameng W. The effect of brain death on cardiovascular function in rats. Part II. The cause of the *in vivo* hemodynamic changes. *Cardiovasc Res* 1998;38:107–115.
39. Herijgers P, Flameng WJ. Graft protection in organ transplantation. *Best Pract Res Clin Anesthesiol* 2008;22:225–239.
40. Howlett TA, Keogh AM, Perry L, et al. Anterior and posterior pituitary function in brain-stem-dead donors. A possible role for hormonal replacement therapy. *Transplantation* 1989;47:828–834.
41. Huang RC, Fishman JA. Screening of deceased organ donors: no easy answers. *Transplantation* 2011;91:146–149.
42. Hung TP, Chen ST. Prognosis of deeply comatose patients on ventilators. *J Neurol Neurosurg Psychiatry* 1995;58:75–80.
43. Karch SB, Billingham ME. Myocardial contraction bands revisited. *Hum Pathol* 1986;17:9–13.
44. Kashap R, Ryan C, Sharma R, et al. Liver grafts from donors with central nervous system tumors: a single center perspective. *Liver Transpl* 2009;15:1204–1208.
45. Kirsch M, Farhat F, Garnier JP, et al. Acute brain death abolishes the cardioprotective effects of ischemic preconditioning in the rabbit. *Transplantation* 2000;69:2013–2019.

46. Kono T, Morita H, Kuroiwa T, et al. Left ventricular wall abnormalities in patients with subarachnoid hemorrhage: neurogenic stunned myocardium. *J Am Coll Cardiol* 1994;24:636–640.

47. Kotsch K, Ulrich F, Reutzel-Selke A, et al. Methylprednisolone therapy in deceased donors reduces inflammation in the donor liver and improves outcomes after liver transplantation. *Ann Surg* 2008;248:1042–1050.

48. Lane SM, Maender KC, Awender NE, et al. Adrenal epinephrine increases alveolar liquid clearance in a canine model of neurogenic pulmonary edema. *Am J Respir Crit Care Med* 1998;158:760–768.

49. Logigian EL, Ropper AH. Terminal electrocardiographic changes in brain-dead patients. *Neurology* 1985;35:915–918.

50. Maron MB, Holcomb PH, Dawson CA, et al. Edema development and recovery in neurogenic pulmonary edema. *J Appl Physiol* 1994;77:1155–1163.

51. Masson F, Thicoipe M, Gin H, et al. The endocrine pancreas in brain-dead donors. A prospective study in 25 patients. *Transplantation* 1993;56:363–367.

52. Mayer SA, LiMandri G, Sherman D, et al. Electrocardiographic markers of abnormal left ventricular wall motion in acute subarachnoid hemorrhage. *J Neurosurg* 1995;83: 889–896.

53. McCormick WF, Halmi NS. The hypophysis in patients with coma depasse ("respirator brain"). *Am J Clin Pathol* 1970;54:374–383.

54. McElhinney DB, Khan JH, Babcock WD, et al. Thoracic organ donor characteristics associated with successful lung procurement. *Clin Transplant* 2001;15:68–71.

55. Nicolas-Robin A, Barouk JD, Amour J, et al. Hydrocortisone supplementation enhances hemodynamic stability in brain-dead patients. *Anesthesiology* 2010;112:1204–1210.

56. Novitzky D, Cooper DK, Morrell D, et al. Change from aerobic to anaerobic metabolism after brain death and reversal following triiodothyronine therapy. *Transplantation* 1988;45:32–36.

57. Novitzky D, Cooper DK, Reichart B. Hemodynamic and metabolic responses to hormonal therapy in brain-dead potential organ donors. *Transplantation* 1987;43: 852–854.

58. Novitzky D, Cooper DKC, Rosendale JD, et al. Hormonal therapy of the brain-dead organ donor: experimental and clinical studies. *Transplantation* 2006;82: 1396–1401.

59. Novitzky D, Wicomb WN, Rose AG, et al. Pathophysiology of pulmonary edema following experimental brain death in the chacma baboon. *Ann Thorac Surg* 1987;43: 288–294.

60. Okamoto S, Corso CO, Kondo T, et al. Changes in hepatic microcirculation and histomorphology in brain-dead organ donors: an experimental study in rats. *Eur J Surg* 1999;165:759–766.

61. Ouaknine G. Bedside procedures in the diagnosis of brain death. *Resuscitation* 1975;4:159–177.

62. Pennefather SH, Bullock RE, Dark JH. The effect of fluid therapy on alveolar arterial oxygen gradient in brain-dead organ donors. *Transplantation* 1993;56:1418–1422.

63. Pollick C, Cujec B, Parker S, et al. Left ventricular wall motion abnormalities in subarachnoid hemorrhage: an echocardiographic study. *J Am Coll Cardiol* 1988;12: 600–605.

64. Power BM, Van Heerden PV. The physiological changes associated with brain death-current concepts and implications for treatment of the brain dead organ donor. *Anaesth Intensive Care* 1995;23:26–36.

65. Randell TT, Hockerstedt KA. Triiodothyronine treatment in brain-dead multiorgan donors—a controlled study. *Transplantation* 1992;54:736–738.

66. Rapenne T, Moreau D, Lenfant F, et al. Could heart rate variability analysis become an early predictor of imminent brain death? A pilot study. *Anesth Analg* 2000;91: 329–336.

67. Riou B, Guesde R, Jacquens Y, et al. Fiberoptic bronchoscopy in brain-dead organ donors. *Am J Respir Crit Card Med* 1994;150:558–560.
68. Rithalia A, McDaid C, Suekarran S, et al. A systemic review of presumed consent systems for deceased organ donation. *Health Technol Assess* 2009;13:1–95.
69. Rosendale JD, Kauffman HM, McBride MA, et al. Hormonal resuscitation yields more transplanted hearts, with improved early function. *Transplantation* 2003;75:1336–1341.
70. Rosner MJ, Newsome HH, Becker DP. Mechanical brain injury: the sympathoadrenal response. *J Neurosurg* 1984;61:76–86.
71. Sakuma T, Folkesson HG, Suzuki S, et al. Beta-adrenergic agonist stimulated alveolar fluid clearance in ex vivo human and rate lungs. *Am J Respir Crit Care Med* 1997;155:506–512.
72. Salim A, Martin M, Brown C, et al. Using thyroid hormone in brain-dead donors to maximize the number of organs available for transplantation. *Clin Transplant* 2007;21:405–409.
73. Salim A, Martin M, Brown C, et al. The effect of a protocol of aggressive donor management: implications for the national organ donor shortage. *J Trauma* 2006;61:429–435.
74. Salim A, Velmahos GC, Brown C, et al. Aggressive organ donor management significantly increases the number of organs available for transplantation. *J Trauma* 2005;58:991–994.
75. Satur CM, Doyle D, Darracott-Cankovic S, et al. Can technetium-99m pyrophosphate be used to quantify myocardial injury in donor hearts? *Ann Thorac Surg* 1999;68:2225–2230.
76. Scheinkestel CD, Tuxen DV, Cooper DJ, et al. Medical management of the (potential) organ donor. *Anaesth Intensive Care* 1995;23:51–59.
77. Schnuelle P, Lorenz D, Mueller A, et al. Donor catecholamine use reduces acute allograft rejection and improves graft survival after cadaveric renal transplantation. *Kidney Int* 1999;56:738–746.
78. Seiler C, Laske A, Gallino A, et al. Echocardiographic evaluation of left ventricular wall motion before and after heart transplantation. *J Heart Lung Transplant* 1992;11:867–874.
79. Shah VR. Aggressive management of multiorgan donor. *Transplant Proc* 2008;40:1087–1090.
80. Siminoff LA, Mercer MB, Graham G, et al. The reasons families donate organs for transplantation: implications for policy and practice. *J Trauma* 2007;62:969–978.
81. Siminoff LA, Traino HM, Gordon N. Determinants of family consent to tissue donation. *J Trauma* 2010;69:956–963.
82. Simon RP. Neurogenic pulmonary edema. *Neurol Clin* 1993;11:309–323.
83. Sirois BC, Sears SF, Marhefka S. Do new drivers equal new donors? An examination of factors influencing organ donation attitudes and behaviors in adolescents. *J Behav Med* 2005;28:201–212.
84. Skrabal CA, Thompson LO, Potapov EV, et al. Organ-specific regulation of pro-inflammatory molecules in heart, lung, and kidney following brain death. *J Surg Res* 2005;123:118–125.
85. Smith WS, Matthay MA. Evidence for a hydrostatic mechanism in human neurogenic pulmonary edema. *Chest* 1997;111:1326–1333.
86. Sullivan HG, Martinez J, Becker DP, et al. Fluid-percussion model of mechanical brain injury in the cat. *J Neurosurg* 1976;45:520–534.
87. Taniguchi S, Kitamura S, Kawachi K, et al. Effects of hormonal supplements on the maintenance of cardiac function in potential donor patients after cerebral death. *Eur J Cardiothorac Surg* 1992;6:96–101.
88. Terasaki PI, Cecka JM, Gjerson DW, et al. High survival rates of kidney transplants from spousal and living unrelated donors. *N Engl J Med* 1995;333:333–336.

89. Totsuka E, Fung JJ, Ishii T, et al. Influence of donor condition on postoperative graft survival and function in human liver transplantation. *Transplant Proc* 2000;32: 322–326.
90. Van Gelder F, Manyalich M, Conta AN, et al. 2009 International donation and transplantation activity. IROD aT Preliminary data. *Organs, Tissues, Cells* 2010;13:5–8.
91. Venkateswaran RV, Steeds RP, Quinn DW, et al. The hemodynamic effects of adjunctive hormone therapy in potential heart donors: a prospective randomized double-blind factorially designed controlled trial. *Eur Heart J* 2009;30:1771–1780.
92. von Pohle WR. Obtaining organ donation: who should ask? *Heart Lung* 1996;25: 304–309.
93. Walker AE, Kollros JJ, Case TJ. Physiological basis of concussion. *J Neurosurg* 1944;1: 103–116.
94. Weiss S, Kotsch K, Francuski M, et al. Brain death activates donor organs and is associated with a worse I/R injury after liver transplantation. *Am J Transplant* 2007;7:1584–1593.
95. Wijdicks EFM. *The Comatose Patient.* Oxford University Press; New York, NY 2008.
96. Wood KE, Becker BN, McCartney JG, et al. Care of the potential organ donor. *N Engl J Med* 2004;351:2730–2739.
97. Wood KE, Coursin DB. Intensivists and organ donor management. *Curr Opin Anaesthesiol* 2007;20:97–99.
98. Yee AH, Rabinstein AA, Thapa P, et al. Factors influencing time to death after withdrawal of life support in neurocritical care patients. *Neurology* 2010;74: 1380–1385.
99. Yoshida H, Hiraide A, Yoshioka T, et al. Transient suppression of pancreatic endocrine function in patients following brain death. *Clin Transplant* 1996;10:28–33.
100. Zhu C, Li J, Zhang G, et al. Brain death disrupts structure and function of pig liver. *Transplant Proc* 2010;42:733–736.

6   Clinical Problems in Brain Death

■ CONTENTS

1. The Qualification of the Examiner 150
2. Clinical Mimics 155
3. Acid-Base Disturbances 158
4. Electrolyte Abnormalities 160
5. Acute Intoxications 162
6. Reliability of Ancillary Tests 165
7. Ancillary Tests and Confounders 168
8. Primary Brainstem Lesion 171
9. Uncertainty About Interpreting Spinal Reflexes 174
10. Ventilator Autocycling 177
11. Chronic CO_2 Retention and the Apnea Test 179
12. Terminating the Apnea Test 181
13. Breathing During the Apnea Test 184
14. Cardiopulmonary Resuscitation and Brain Death 187

15. Extracorporeal Membrane Oxygenation (ECMO) and Brain Death 190
16. Anencephaly and Brain Death 193
17. Shaken Baby Syndrome and Brain Death 196
18. Maternal Brain Death 200
19. Legal Challenges in Brain Death 204
20. Family Opposition to Accepting Brain Death 209
21. Sperm and Oocyte Retrieval in Brain Death 211
22. Organ Donation and the Hemodynamically Unstable Donor 214
23. Organ Donation in Prisoners 218
24. Organ Donation, Consent, and Costs 220
25. Organ Donation and Directing the Gift 222

There are clear guiding principles in the determination of brain death and subsequent discussion about organ donation. In most situations, brain death is straightforward to diagnose, consent is obtained for organ donation and—for the endlessly waiting recipients—all goes well. But questions can arise and occasionally we encounter problems. For some physicians these queries are mostly a consequence of unfamiliarity with the process, uncertainty about explaining discrepancies during clinical testing, problems with interpreting ancillary tests, and less than full understanding of procurement and transplantation logistics. For others, carrying the apnea test to completion creates unease and some troubleshooting.

Advances in medical practice have also changed the way physicians approach catastrophic neurologic illness. Not long ago, physicians did not have to be concerned about the effects of therapeutic hypothermia after cardiopulmonary resuscitation or the complexities of extracorporeal membrane oxygenation, but now the consequences of these therapeutic interventions need to be considered. The number of available ancillary tests also has increased over the years (MR imaging, CT angiogram) creating difficulties with its interpretation when the validity of the tests is insufficiently known. The diagnosis of brain death also may generate moral dilemmas.

This chapter seeks to address common clinical problems in practice.

Clinical Problem

1

The Qualification of the Examiner

■ THE COMMON CLINICAL QUESTIONS

How can we define physician competence? Are physicians in all specialties allowed to determine brain death? How many physicians are required?

■ THE FACTS

There are no studies of the accuracy and performance skills of physicians performing a brain death examination. No formal audits of intensivists, emergency physicians, neurosurgeons, or neurologists have been performed recently, but there is no reason to suggest incompetence. In our experience with hundreds of brain death determinations performed by neurologists and neurosurgeons, trauma surgeons, and medical intensivists, grossly incomplete examinations were nonexistent.[6] Some imperfections can always be found and physicians are not infallible. Whether published cases may have been wrongly assessed is difficult to know for sure, but incomplete descriptions of brain death determinations in the non-neurology literature are quite common (Chapters 2 and 4 and clinical problem 18). Errors can be made with failure to recognize potential mimics or with the interpretation of the neurologic examination, but the more common problem is an incomplete examination by an inexperienced physician. The most commonly 'forgotten' parts of the examination involve oculovestibular responses, the cough reflex, and the apnea test. It is even possible that organ transplantation agencies or families are approached for donation before the examination is completed. Expectedly, this will result in major distrust of the physician if the examination later fails to show brain death.

The Uniform Determination of Death Act (UDDA) states that "A determination of death must be made in accordance with accepted medical standards." The UDDA implies that the examiner should meet certain qualifications and have professional personal experience, but it does not further define a standard. Several position papers have specifically addressed the examiner.[1,3,4,6] The American Academy of Neurology (AAN) 2010 guideline states, "Legally, all physicians are allowed to determine brain death in most U.S. states. Neurologists, neurosurgeons, and intensive care specialists may have specialized expertise. It seems reasonable to require that all physicians making a determination of brain death be intimately familiar with brain death criteria."[6] The Society of Critical Care Medicine and American Academy of Pediatrics Task Force states that "qualified clinicians include: pediatric intensivists and neonatologists, pediatric neurologists and neurosurgeons, pediatric trauma surgeons, and pediatric anesthesiologists with critical care training" and adds that "adult specialists should have appropriate neurologic and critical care training to diagnose brain death when caring for the pediatric patient from birth to 18 years of age."[3] However, such limitations on the specialty type will put some specialists at a disadvantage and will create problems of availability in smaller community hospitals. For that reason, the AAN guideline did not further restrict the specialty.[3]

There is notable variation in hospital guidelines from highly ranked medical institutions in the U.S. A neurologist or neurosurgeon is required to be involved in less than half of the guidelines in a recent survey.[1] In one-third of the guidelines, the attending physician is required to be involved (Figure 6-1). One survey noted that in more than two-thirds of the hospital practice guidelines, multiple examinations were required; almost half of the hospital practice guidelines specifically stipulated two different examiners.[1] Several U.S. states and hospital protocols require two physicians to assess the patient independently.

Lack of availability of neurologists may be a problem, and not all neurologists are comfortable doing a brain death examination (neurologists may take a hospital service only a few times a year). Having designated neurologists or neurointensivists in a hospital may lead to a gradual shift toward those with the most experience.[5]

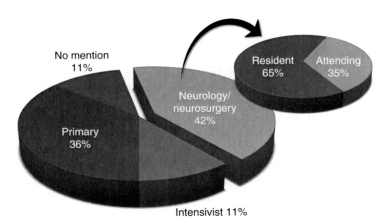

Figure 6-1 Review of 38 hospital practice guidelines for the determination of brain death. Institutions varied widely regarding who could perform brain death determination. Options included an intensivist, the patient's primary attending physician, a neurologist or neurosurgeon, or no stipulation. A neurologist or neurosurgeon is required to be involved in only 42% of guidelines, and of these, only 35% require an attending neurologist or neurosurgeon to be involved. Data from Greer et al.[1] Used with permission from *Neurology.*

The "better to be safe than sorry" argument has been used to justify two inde-pendent examinations. However, it assumes that one physician is more likely to err than two physicians. This has not been demonstrated, and in my experience, near misses always involve two physicians making the same judgment error (i.e., under-estimation of sedative effects). With multiple physicians, there may be a feeling of false security, and as a result of reduced attentiveness, knowing that another physi-cian has already examined the patient, errors may result.

Some hospital protocols demand two examinations with a certain time interval between them. In New York State, a 6-hour interval was recommended, but in actuality it became two to three times longer (Figure 6-2). Moreover, 12% of the organ donors developed a terminal cardiac arrest during this unnecessarily prolonged waiting period and were lost to procurement.[2]

The central message is that a comprehensive clinical evaluation of brain death is diagnostically accurate when done by skillful specialists, preferably in the neu-rosciences, who likely better appreciate the potential confounders. This may include a sufficient observation period before starting the examination, but one careful clinical neurologic examination should suffice. Clinical determination of brain death is by no means simple. Competency involves proficiency with a neu-rologic examination, skill in performing an apnea test, interpretation of ancillary tests, and experience in leading a family conference.

So, who does qualify? A separate team or service would be ideal and would minimize errors and even facilitate communication with organ donation agen-cies. Intensive care neurologists and neurosurgeons are eminently qualified, but anesthesiologists and medical or surgical intensivists should be considered if they have maintained their clinical skills. Intensivists are quite comfortable with the determination of brain death but often prefer a specialist in the neurosciences to make a definitive assessment. In some instances, in an unusual display of physi-cian collaboration, the intensivist will perform the apnea test after the neurolo-gist has documented irreversible coma and absent brainstem reflexes. Not having residents or fellows in neurology and neurosurgery perform such an examination is understandable unless it is performed under the close supervision of an attend-ing physician. By law, physician assistants and registered nurses are allowed to determine brain death in some U.S. states under the supervision of a medical doctor, but whether this practice is prevalent is not known. Both physician assis-tants and nursing staff are often closely involved in support of the family.

Physicians who have been attending and caring for the patient should be allowed to determine brain death, and although one could imagine a possible conflict of interest, it is very implausible. This is different in donation after cardiac death (DCD) protocols. Removing oneself from a DCD protocol is common practice, with the attending physician deciding to withdraw support separately from another physician involved with the DCD protocol in the operating room.

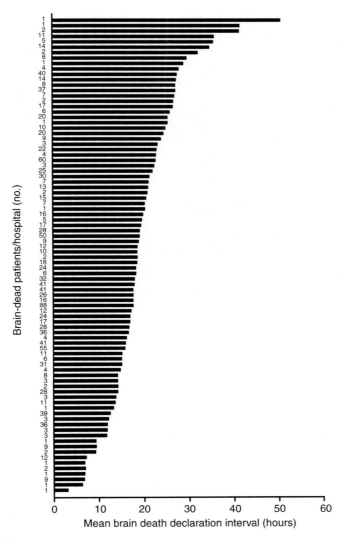

Figure 6-2 The mean brain death declaration interval is defined as the time in hours between the first and second clinical brain death examinations. Data were obtained for all hospitals serviced by the New York Organ Donor Network (NYODN) from June 1, 2007, to December 31, 2009, including 88 hospitals with at least one brain-dead patient more than 1 year of age for whom the brain death interval was less than 96 hours. The overall brain death interval for 1311 patients was: mean, 19.2 hours; median, 18.5 hours; range 3 to 50 hours. (Data from Lustbader et al.[2] Used with permission from *Neurology*.)

Development of special certificates, as in resuscitation medicine, may need consideration, but how specific training will be organized is not known. How to test competence has not been defined, and how to administer certification is not known. Brain death is an uncommon outcome of acute catastrophic neurologic disease. Most hospitals with multiple intensive care units (ICUs), even in densely populated areas in the United States, determine brain death at most 30 times a year, and it requires a small group of physicians to gain sufficient expertise in brain death determination. The truth of the matter is that most physicians have not performed more than a handful of such examinations.

■ REFERENCES

1. Greer DM, Varelas PN, Haque S, et al. Variability of brain death determination guidelines in leading U.S. neurologic institutions. *Neurology* 2008;70:284–289.
2. Lustbader D, O'Hara D, Wijdicks EFM, et al. Second brain death examination may negatively affect organ donation. *Neurology* 2011;76:119–124.
3. Nakagawa TA, Ashwal S, Mathur M, et al. Guidelines for the determination of brain death in infants and children: an update of the (1987) task force recommendations. *Crit Care Med.* 2011 in press.
4. Uniform Determination of Death Act, 12 uniform laws annotated 589 (West 1993 and West supp 1997).
5. Wijdicks EFM, Rabinstein AA, Manno EM, et al. Pronouncing brain death: contemporary practice and safety of the apnea test. *Neurology* 2008;71:1240–1244.
6. Wijdicks EFM, Varelas P, Gronseth GS, et al. Evidence-based guideline update: determining brain death in adults: report of the quality standards subcommittee of the American Academy of Neurology. *Neurology* 2010;74:1911–1918.

Clinical Problem
2

Clinical Mimics

■ **THE COMMON CLINICAL QUESTIONS**

Are there any neurologic or medical conditions that can mimic brain death? What are the warning signs?

■ **THE FACTS**

There are no reports in peer-reviewed medical journals of conditions mimicking brain death that have described a complete brain death examination.

Several studies have claimed that brain death can be mimicked by fulminant Guillain-Barré syndrome,[1,5,6,11,12,14] baclofen overdose,[10] barbiturate overdose,[8,16] and delayed vecuronium clearance.[7] Most commonly, Guillain-Barré syndrome with absent brainstem reflexes have been described, but in all cases, respiratory drive was not adequately assessed (and likely present) and vasopressors were not required. Loss of most brainstem reflexes for 2 months was described in one instance.[6] (In some of these patients there was an uncomfortable feeling with the attending physician, leading to tests such as magnetic resonance imaging (MRI) and electroencephalography (EEG) and they showed normal findings.)

Several clinical signs should warn against a premature assessment for brain death. Table 6-1 summarizes these warning signs.

TABLE 6-1 *Serious Warning Signs that Should Defer Brain Death Examination*

• Normal CT scan
• Unsupported blood pressure (no need for vasopressors)
• Absent diabetes insipidus
• Marked heart rate variations
• Fever and shock
• Marked metabolic acidosis
• Hypothermia <32°C (more often accidental and reversible)
• Marked miosis (heroin or organophosphate intoxication)
• Myoclonus (lithium, SSRIs)
• Rigidity (SSRI, haloperidol)
• Profuse sweating (organophosphates)
• Abnormal laboratory values (acidosis, liver function tests, renal function tests)
• Traces in drug screens

Abbreviations: CT, computed tomography; SSRI, selective serotonin reuptake inhibitor.

Any major intoxication with a sedative agent may mimic brain death, but in the vast majority of cases, pupil responses remain intact. Even a high dose of pheno-barbital will not mute the pupillary reflexes. In our experience with several cases of high-dose barbiturate infusion resulting in an isoelectric EEG, the patients continued to trigger the ventilator and, in some instances, could even be placed on continuous positive airway pressure (CPAP).

Another major mimicking condition is hypothermia. Hypothermia is a manifestation of brain death (poikilothermia), but temperatures are rarely below 32°C. Moreover, Osborn (camel hump) waves are not seen on the electrocardiogram (ECG) and, if present, often point to a far more severe accidental form of hypothermia.

Severe hypothermia is defined as a core temperature of 35°C or less. The degrees of hypothermia have been arbitrarily categorized. Hypothermia results in progressive loss of neurologic function and brainstem reflexes.[3] Exceptions exist; a confused patient with a core temperature of 24°C has been reported, emphasizing a potentially poor correlation of the degree of hypothermia with the level of consciousness.[9]

Hypothermia (usually mild) may occur in a setting of acute neurologic illness in which the patient is no longer protected against the ambient temperature, in a setting of an endocrine crisis such as hypoglycemic coma, or coma from hypothyroidism. It is very important to exclude coingestion of drugs. Opioids such as heroin, barbiturates, benzodiazepines, phenothiazines, tricyclic antidepressants, and lithium may all cause significant hypothermia when a patient is exposed to a cold environment.

Patients with hypothermia are vasoconstricted, may not shiver when their core temperature is below 30°C, and may exhibit a profoundly cold axilla ("cold as marble"). Tachycardia with conversion to bradycardia will occur at a core temperature of 28°C, together with Osborne waves, but this configuration may be absent in up to 20% of patients and is not specific for hypothermia. Pupillary dilatation and sluggish light responses occur at core temperatures between 32°C and 28°C, and other brainstem reflexes disappear below 28°C.[2]

Management of hypothermia invariably involves aggressive resuscitation.[13,15] One study from Bern, Switzerland, in 32 young, hypothermic (less than 28°C) patients with circulatory arrest (mostly due to mountaineering accidents) found no neurologic deficits in 15 resuscitated survivors.[17] Therefore, there is no baseline hypothermia below which resuscitation is definitively unsuccessful. Successful resuscitation with good cognition after 9 hours of resuscitative efforts has recently been reported in a patient with a temperature of 13.7°C.[4] The critical significance of these reports is that an expeditious response is needed, no matter how severe the presenting findings are.[2]

Initial management of a mildly hypothermic patient is gentle handling (repeated painful stimuli to assess motor response or grimacing may facilitate the development of cardiac arrhythmias), oxygenation, and crystalloid resuscitation. In most instances, with a core temperature above 32°C, rewarming with heating blankets suffices. Extracorporeal rewarming using a cardiopulmonary bypass circuit is indicated when no perfusing cardiac rhythm is present.

■ REFERENCES

1. Bakshi N, Maselli RA, Gospe SM Jr, et al. Fulminant demyelinating neuropathy mimicking cerebral death. *Muscle Nerve* 1997;20:1595–1597.
2. Boyd J, Brugger H, Shuster M. Prognostic factors in avalanche resuscitation: a systematic review. *Resuscitation* 2010;81:645–652.
3. Fischbeck KH, Simon RP. Neurological manifestations of accidental hypothermia. *Ann Neurol* 1981;10:384–387.
4. Gilbert M, Busund R, Skagseth A, et al. Resuscitation from accidental hypothermia of 13.7 degrees C with circulatory arrest. *Lancet* 2000;355:375–376.
5. Hassan T, Mumford C. Guillain-Barré syndrome mistaken for brain stem death. *Postgrad Med J* 1991;67:280–281.
6. Joshi MC, Azim A, Gupta GL, et al. Guillain-Barré syndrome with absent brainstem reflexes: a report of two cases. *Anaesth Intensive Care* 2008;36:867–869.
7. Kainuma M, Miyake T, Kanno T. Extremely prolonged vecuronium clearance in a brain death case. *Anesthesiology* 2001;95:1023–1024.
8. Kirshbaum RJ, Carollo VJ. Reversible isoelectric EEG in barbiturate coma. *JAMA* 1970;212:1215.
9. Lloyd EL. Accidental hypothermia. *Resuscitation* 1996;32:111–124.
10. Ostermann ME, Young B, Sibbald WJ, et al. Coma mimicking brain death following baclofen overdose. *Intensive Care Med* 2000;26:1144–1146.
11. Rajdev SK, Sarma D, Singh R, et al. Guillain-Barré syndrome mimicking cerebral death. *Indian J Crit Care Med* 2003;7:50–52.
12. Rigamonti A, Basso F, Stanzani L, et al. Guillain-Barré syndrome mimicking brain death. *J Peripher Nerv Syst* 2009;14:316–319.
13. Silfvast T, Petilla V. Outcome from severe accidental hypothermia in southern Finland: a 10 year review. *Resuscitation* 2003;59:285–290.
14. Stojkovic T, Verdin M, Hurtevent JF, et al. Guillain-Barré syndrome resembling brainstem death in a patient with brain injury. *J Neurol* 2001;248:430–432.
15. Vassal T, Benoit-Gonin B, Carrat F, et al. Severe accidental hypothermia treated in an ICU: prognosis and outcome. *Chest* 2001;120:1998–2003.
16. Wakamoto H, Nakamura Y, Ebihara T, et al. Reversible coma associated with prolonged high-dose phenobarbital therapy in bilateral Sturge-Weber syndrome. *J Child Neurol* 2009;24:1547–1551.
17. Walpoth BH, Walpoth-Aslan BN, Mattle HP, et al. Outcome of survivors of accidental deep hypothermia and circulatory arrest treated with extracorporeal blood warming. *N Engl J Med* 1997;337:1500–1505.

Clinical Problem
3

Acid-Base Disturbances

■ THE COMMON CLINICAL QUESTIONS

How should an acid-base disturbance be interpreted, and how does it confound the neurologic examination?

■ THE FACTS

Acid-base disturbances are expected in patients who have become brain dead, but most of these changes are inconsequential. A typical aberration is a respiratory alkalosis as a result of induced hyperventilation in an attempt to reduce intracranial pressure. Usually, respiratory alkalosis is corrected before a brain death examination is performed by simply reducing minute ventilation on the mechanical ventilator.

A more complex issue involves a patient with metabolic or respiratory acidosis. Metabolic acidosis may occur in comatose patients after cardiopulmonary resuscitation, in those with recurrent seizures causing lactate acidosis, and in those who are comatose in an evolving severe sepsis syndrome. Most importantly, an acid-base disturbance should point to a possible drug intoxication, particularly if the patient is first seen in the emergency department.[3–11] Metabolic acidosis can be associated with ingestion of ethanol, methanol, ethylene glycol, salicylates, and cocaine, among other drugs. The acidosis may be due to uncoupled oxidative phosphorylation (salicylates), seizures (cocaine), or anaerobic glycolysis (cyanide).[2] Opioids, ethanol, and barbiturates can cause respiratory acidosis. Pure metabolic or respiratory alkalosis is seldom a direct manifestation of poisoning. These profound changes point to a certain type of intoxification, and generally, the determination of brain death should be deferred in the presence of acidosis or alkalosis. These derangements may in fact indicate a possible reversible medical illness.[1,11] A guide in identifying the toxin is presented in Table 6-2.

Correction of the acid-base disturbance is warranted. Sodium bicarbonate is needed to correct severe acidemia (pH <7.20). A continuous infusion of sodium bicarbonate usually at about 8 mmol/L per 12 hours may suffice. Treatment can then be directed to correction of the underlying trigger.[5]

TABLE 6-2 *Drug-Induced Acid-Base Abnormalities*

Metabolic Acidosis
Acetaminophen
Ethanol, methanol, ethylene glycol
Salicylates
Cyanide
Cocaine
Strychnine
Papaverine
Toluene
Respiratory Acidosis
Opiates
Ethanol, methanol, ethylene glycol
Barbiturates
Anesthetics

Metabolic alkalosis is quite common after the diagnosis of brain death and is a direct result of intravascular depletion from diabetes insipidus. The abnormality is noted at the time of the diagnosis of brain death or even before and may be more apparent with insufficient management. Metabolic alkalosis may also be a result of giving multiple doses of osmotic diuretics in an attempt to lower the intracranial pressure. The treatment is fluid resuscitation with isotonic saline and potassium replacement.

■ **REFERENCES**

1. Androgue HJ, Madias NE. Management of the life-threatening acid-base disorders, first of two parts. *N Engl J Med* 1998;338:26–34.
2. Coentrão L, Moura D. Acute Cyanide poisoning among jewelry and textile industry workers. *Am J Emerg Med* 2010; 29:78–81.
3. Flanagan RJ. The poisoned patient: the role of the laboratory. *Br J Biomed Sci* 1995;52: 202–213.
4. Flohenbaum N, Mokhlesi B, Corbridge T. Toxicology in the critically ill patient. *Clin Chest Med* 2003;24:689–711.
5. Nelson L, Lewin NA, Howland MA, et al, eds, *Goldfrank's Toxicologic Emergencies.* 9th ed. New York: McGraw–Hill Professional; 2010.
6. Ngo AS, Anthony CR, Samuel M, et al. Should a benzodiazepine antagonist be used in unconscious patients presenting to the emergency department? *Resuscitation* 2007;74: 27–27.
7. Roberts DM, Buckley NA. Pharmacokinetic considerations in clinical toxicology: clinical applications. *Clin Pharmacokinet* 2007;46:897–939.
8. Shannon MW, Borron SW, Burns M. *Haddad and Winchester's Clinical Management of Poisoning and Drug Overdose.* 4th ed. New York: U.S. Elsevier Health Sciences; 2007.
9. Thundiyil JG, Stober J, Besbelli N, et al. Acute pesticide poisoning: a proposed classification tool. *Bull World Health Organ* 2008;86:205–209.
10. Timmer R, Sands J. Lithium intoxication. *J Am Soc Nephrol* 1999;10:666–674.
11. Wijdicks EFM. *Neurologic Complication of Critical Illness.* 3rd ed. New York: Oxford University Press; 2009.

Clinical Problem 4

Electrolyte Abnormalities

■ THE COMMON CLINICAL QUESTIONS

What level of hypernatremia is acceptable in brain death? When do electrolyte abnormalities warrant correction?

■ THE FACTS

A recent study found a high incidence of hyperosmolality (68%) together with hyperglycemia (75%), hypophosphatemia (72%), and hypokalemia (70%). However, these values were noted during procurement and not at the time of brain death declaration.[3] Hypernatremia was associated with high lactate levels suggesting hypoperfusion—induced tissue ischemia.[3]

Of all electrolyte abnormalities, hypernatremia is most common and is often considered a possible confounder. As expected, hypernatremia in brain death is typically caused by net water loss and central diabetes insipidus.[2,7] Hypernatremia may also preexist before the diagnosis is made and may be due to multiple doses of mannitol 20% or hypertonic (10%, 23%) saline, both of which can cause significant osmotic diuresis. Unreplaced water loss in mannitol causes hypernatremia. Sodium overload is the cause of hypernatremia when using hypertonic solutions. In one study, hypernatremia from osmotic agent use was the most commonly identifiable cause.[2]

Some degree of hypernatremia occurs long after brain death determination and during procurement, and is a consequence of the difficulty of matching urinary output with fluid intake.[4] Once the diagnosis of brain death is made and established, maintenance of normal sodium values is important because prolonged hypernatremia—and basically dehydration—has been associated with poor organ function in recipients.

The level at which the clinical examination could be confounded by hypernatremia is generally defined at 160 mmol/L or more.[1] However, plasma osmolality may be better correlated with the level of consciousness than an absolute value of hypernatremia. Plasma osmolality above 350 mosm/L will result in progressive drowsiness in other situations.[1,8] As in many other electrolyte disorders, the rapid development of hypernatremia is more important than the absolute value.

TABLE 6-3 *Laboratory Values Requiring Correction before Brain Death Examination*

Derangement	Serum
Hyponatremia	<110 mmol/L
Hypernatremia	>160 mmol/L
Hypercalcemia	>12 mg/dL
Hypoglycemia	<70 mg/dL
Hyperglycemia	>300 mg/dL

Although severe hypernatremia may be considered a possible confounder in brain death more generally, in other series of hospital-acquired hypernatremia, it is associated with marked hypotension and eventually cardiac arrest.[5,6] At the time of brain death examination, plasma sodium should likely be less than 160 mmol/L and should be corrected if higher values are present. Treatment usually consists only of correction of the water deficit using D5W. The rate of correction can be calculated using the Adrogue–Madias formula (see also www.medcalc.com).

Other electrolyte abnormalities pertain to glucose derangements. Both hyperglycemia and hypoglycemia are major confounders, and any major deviation from the norm is obviously unacceptable. Severe hyperglycemia can be associated with ketoacidosis. A diabetic nonketotic hyperosmolar state can increase the glucose serum level to over 600 mg/dL.[8] Another most complicated situation involves patients who have been overdosed with hypoglycemic drugs. The brain injury may be permanent after glucose has been corrected, and little may be found on the initial computed tomography (CT) scan.

In daily practice, a simple set of electrolytes will be available, and the values should be repeated before any formal evaluation is made to determine brain death. The major electrolyte abnormalities that require correction—with estimated cutoffs—are shown in Table 6-3.

■ REFERENCES

1. Adrogue HY, Madias NE. Hypernatremia. *N Engl J Med* 2000;342:1493–1499.
2. Aiyagari V, Deibert E, Diringer MN. Hypernatremia in the neurologic intensive care unit: how high is too high? *J Crit Care* 2006;21:163–172.
3. Dominguez-Roldan JM, Jimenez-Gonzalez PI, Garcia-Alfaro C, Hernandez-Hanzanas F, Fernandez-Hinojosa E, Bellido-Sanchez R. Electrolyte disorders, hyperosmolar states, and lactic acidosis in brain dead patients. *Transplant Pro* 2005;37:1987–1989.
4. Grigoras I, Blaj M, Chelarescu O, Craus C, Florin G. Functional improvement between brain death declaration and organ harvesting. *Transplant Proc* 2010;42:147–149.
5. Holley AD, Green S, Davoren P. Extreme hypernatremia: a case report and brief review. *Crit Care Resusc* 2007;9:55–58.
6. Morris-Jones PH, Houston IB, Evans RC. Prognosis of the neurological complications of acute hypernatremia. *Lancet* 1967;2:1385–1389.
7. Powner DJ, Boccalandro C, Alp MS, Vollmer DG. Endocrine failure after traumatic brain injury in adults. *Neurocrit Care* 2006;5:61–70.
8. Wijdicks EFM. Neurologic complications of critical illness. Oxford University Press 2009.

Acute Intoxications

■ **THE COMMON CLINICAL QUESTIONS**

How can we exclude the effect of alcohol? Which drugs are included in drug screens? Are serum levels of suspected drugs useful?

■ **THE FACTS**

The most common confounding intoxication is alcohol. The clinical manifestations of drunkenness depend on whether the patient was a naive drinker. Common clinical scenarios involve patients in motor vehicle accidents while driving under the influence of alcohol. In any patient, it may take 24 hours after considerable alcohol consumption to metabolize it, and the decrease in concentration should be monitored using blood ethanol concentrations. Generally, blood ethanol levels cause respiratory depression and hypothermia with levels above 0.2%. Severe binge drinking may be associated with much higher values and often results in ketoacidosis. In some instances, traumatic head injury is associated with ingestion of both alcohol and illegal drugs, and the neurologic examination will be very unreliable. A blood ethanol concentration of 0.08% determines the inability to drive, and that level can be used as a target value to exclude any effects of alcohol.

Unfortunately, detailed clinical neurologic findings in intoxicated patients are mostly absent in published cases, and often only pupillary responses are reported. When an intoxication is considered, the pupil response to light remains an important distinguishing feature and can be elicited in many cases. A magnifying glass may be needed to appreciate pupillary contraction to light. Mydriasis (8 or 9 mm) or midposition pupils (6 or 7 mm) can be seen after toxic exposure to antihistamines, tricyclic antidepressants, amphetamines, cocaine, phenylephrine, and other sympathicomimetics. Miosis (1–2 mm) points to any of the anticholinesterase agents, organophosphates, opioids (heroine), pilocarpine, and barbiturates. Naturally, toxins, poisons, sedative drugs, and many other agents may cause coma when patients are exposed to large quantities, but only a few pharmaceutical agents produce a clinical syndrome frighteningly similar to that of brain death from structural injury.[1,2] Barbiturates and tricyclic antidepressants are best known, but in many instances, some brainstem reflexes remain intact and that will make the distinction easy.

Toxins may also induce a structural lesion as a result of anoxia (carbon monoxide), inhibition of phosphorylation (carbon disulfide, cyanide, and hydrogen sulfide), or direct structural neuronal destruction (manganese, 1-methyl-4-phenyl-1,2,3,6-tetrahydropyridine [MPTP]). In these patients the injury is structural, and the effect of the toxin is brief and devastating. Brain death examination can usually proceed in these unusual instances.

A much more complex problem is the presence of metabolites or traces of circulating pharmaceutical agents in drug screens, and whether they can even be considered confounders in the first place in the clinical determination of brain death. Even though a drug has been identified, a critical threshold is often not known. Traces of benzodiazepines and opioids may be linked to a prior intubation procedure and may not be relevant.

Although drug screens may be helpful, quantitative measurements take time. The toxicology assays in serum and urine usually available in the emergency department are shown in Table 6-4 and 6-5.[3-6] A quantitative assay is useful only if there is a specific therapy.

Certain toxins are not detectable by emergency toxicity screens. Examples include cyanide, lithium, isoniazid, antibiotics (too polar), aromatic and halogenated hydrocarbon solvents, hydrogen sulfide and nitrogen dioxide (too volatile), and fentanyl, LSD, ergot alkaloids, and digoxin (the volume of distribution is large and the concentration is too low).

It is plain and simple: brain death determination cannot and should not proceed when there is evidence of drug or alcohol ingestion. Use of antiepileptic drugs by patients with prior epilepsy can be allowed and should only confound the neurologic examination if toxicity is suspected. When the degree of intoxication is not

TABLE 6-4   *Stat Quantitative Serum Toxicology Assays Available in an Emergency Department*[a]

Acetaminophen
Lithium
Salicylate
Carboxyhemoglobin and methemoglobin
Theophylline
Valproic acid
Carbamazepine
Digoxin
Phenobarbital (if urine barbiturates are positive)
Iron
Transferrin
Methyl alcohol[b]
Ethylene glycol[b]

[a] May be available within an hour.

[b] More realistic time for these assays is 2–4 h.

Source: From Wu et al.[6] with permission of the publisher.

164 ■ BRAIN DEATH

TABLE 6-5 *Stat Qualitative Urine Toxicology Assays Available in an Emergency Department*

Cocaine
Opiates
Barbiturates
Amphetamines
Propoxyphene
Phencyclidine
Tricyclic antidepressants

Source: From Wu et al.[6] with permission of the publisher.

known, flumazenil or naloxone administration cannot be assumed to be a sufficient antidote. Some patients may have ingested benzodiazepines with very long half-lives (i.e., clonazepam or diazepam), and the reversal effect—if anything is observed—may be short-lived. Charcoal hemoperfusion can be considered in patients with toxic levels of barbiturates, but a considerable time of observation still is needed until the plasma levels decline to subtherapeutic and "acceptable" levels (pentobarbital less than 5 mcg/mL and phenobarbital less than 40 mcg/mL).

In most cases, elimination is five times the drug's half-life, and this will need to be calculated to ensure the absence of confounding sedation (Chapter 2).

■ REFERENCES

1. Barry JD. Diagnosis and management of the poisoned child. *Pediatr Ann* 2005;34: 937–946.
2. Pitetti RD, Whitman E, Zaylor A. Accidental and nonaccidental poisonings as a cause of apparent life-threatening events in infants. *Pediatrics* 2008;122:e359–e362.
3. Thomas SH, Watson ID. Laboratory analyses for poisoned patients. *Ann Clin Biochem* 2002;39:327.
4. Rentsch KM. Laboratory diagnostics in acute poisoning: critical overview. *Clin Chem Lab. Med* 2010;48:1381–1387.
5. Watson ID. Laboratory support for the poisoned patient. *Ther Drug Monit* 1998;20: 490–497.
6. Wu AHB, McKay C, Broussard LA, et al. National Academy of Clinical Biochemistry laboratory medicine practice guidelines: recommendations for the use of laboratory tests to support poisoned patients who present to the emergency department. *Clin Chem* 2003;49:357–379.

Clinical Problem
6

Reliability of Ancillary Tests

■ THE COMMON CLINICAL QUESTIONS

What is the validity of current ancillary laboratory tests? How do these tests compare with each other?

■ THE FACTS

The determination of brain death is based on a comprehensive clinical assessment. Ancillary tests are helpful when they do what they are supposed to do: confirm the clinical diagnosis of brain death. Besides their use as a diagnostic safeguard, the most common indication for ancillary tests for adults with suspected brain death is failure to complete the apnea test. In the United States, ancillary laboratory testing is not mandatory for adults or children. In most other countries, a comprehensive evaluation with a single neurologic examination is adequate (Chapter 1). However, in 40% of 80 recently surveyed nations, an ancillary test was legally required.[15] Requirements to perform an ancillary test vary commonly within a continent. For example, laboratory tests are legally required in approximately half of the countries of the European Union.[15]

These tests can be divided into those that test the electrical function of the brain and those that test cerebral blood flow. If ancillary tests are used to confirm the clinical examination, the tests should be identical in reliability. Thus, an isoelectric EEG with the appropriate recording settings and no response with any form of stimulation or a cerebral blood flow study with absent intracranial blood flow, should always coincide with absence of all brainstem reflexes and apnea, and no patient should improve. This is however not the reality, and persistent blood flow and EEG activity has been found in patients who meet the clinical criteria. Furthermore, lack of improvement has only been proven with a clinical examination—not with laboratory tests (i.e., there are multiple examples in the literature of patients with isoelectric EEGs who improved clinically).

An ancillary test can be labeled false positive or false negative when two tests are compared with each other and one test is used as a reference test.[7,10,18] However, a false-positive result can also mean that the ancillary test suggests brain death but the patient does not meet the clinical criteria.[16] False-positive ancillary tests

TABLE 6-6 *Selected Studies with Discrepancies (False Positives)*

Authors	N	Comparison	False Positive, N
Hassler et al.[9]	33	CA vs *TCD*	1
Newell et al.[13]	12	Clinical vs *TCD*	1
Flowers and Patel[6]	24	Clinical vs *TCD*	3
Reid et al,[17]	11	Clinical vs *Nuclear brain scan*	3
Yatim et al.[19]	17	Nuclear brain scan vs *CA*	1
Zurynski et al.[20]*	107	CA vs *TCD*	1
Nebra et al.[12]†	25	TCD vs *Nuclear brain scan*	1
Dosemeci et al.[4]	28	Clinical vs *TCD*	1
Berenguer et al.[1]	25	CTA vs *Nuclear brain scan*	3

Abbreviations: CA, cerebral angiogram; CTA, computed tomography angiogram; TCD, transcranial doppler ultrasound.

* In nine cases there were absent middle cerebral artery signals with normal basilar artery signals.

† Mainly comparison of flow in the posterior fossa.

  Italic indicates a false-positive study.

Source: From Wijdicks EFM. The case against confirmatory tests for determining brain death in adults. *Neurology* 2010;75:77–83. Used with permission from *Neurology*.

are seen with transcranial Doppler, nuclear scan, and CT angiogram (Table 6-6).[7] With transcranial Doppler ultrasound, there may be absent anterior circulation signals while the posterior circulation signals are present.

Far more common are false-negative results when the patient has met the clinical criteria for brain death but the ancillary test shows flow or brain activity on the EEG (Table 6-7).[8] As expected, brain blood flow is a direct consequence of the degree of intracranial pressure. Very high intracranial pressures will not allow blood to pierce through the dura, and brain flow stops at that level. Therefore, when there is no increase in intracranial pressure, such as early after asphyxia or after cardiopulmonary resuscitation, cerebral blood flow may be easily demonstrated while the patient meets all of the clinical criteria for brain death. There is a possibility that patients may appear brain dead on one laboratory

TABLE 6-7 *Selected Studies with Discrepancies (False Negatives)*

Authors	N	Studies	False Negative, N
Petty et al.[14]	23	Clinical vs *TCD*	2
Flowers and Patel[6]	219	Clinical vs *Nuclear brain scan*	6
Munari et al.[11]	20	Clinical vs *Nuclear brain scan*	1
de Freitas and André,[3]	270	Clinical vs *TCD*	47
Quesnel et al.[16]	21	Clinical vs *CTA*	10
Combes et al.[2]	30	Clinical vs *CTA*	13
Escudero et al.[5]	27	Clinical vs *CTA*	2

Abbreviation: CTA, computed tomography angiography; TCD, transcranial Doppler ultrasound.

Italic indicates a false-negative study.

Source: From Wijdicks EFM. The case against confirmatory tests for determining brain death in adults. *Neurology* 2010;75:77–83. Used with permission from *Neurology*.

test (EEG) but not on another (TCD). In countries that require mandatory confirmatory tests, delay in final diagnosis can be substantial and it may take days until the discrepancy between tests is resolved. Regrettably there is too much emphasis on these imperfect tests.

■ REFERENCES

1. Berenguer CM, Davis FE, Howington JU. Brain death confirmation: comparison of computed tomography with nuclear medicine perfusion scan. *J Trauma* 2010;68: 553–559.
2. Combes J-C, Chomel A, Ricolfi F, et al. Reliability of computed tomographic angiography in the diagnosis of brain death. *Transplant Proc* 2007;39:16–20.
3. de Freitas GR, Andre C. Sensitivity of transcranial Doppler for confirming brain death: a prospective study of 270 cases. *Acta Neurol Scand* 2006;113:426–432.
4. Dosemeci L, Dora B, Yilmaz M, et al. Utility of transcranial Doppler ultrasonography for confirmatory diagnosis of brain death: two sides of the coin. *Transplantation* 2004;77:71–75.
5. Escudero D, Otero J, Marques L, et al. Diagnosing brain death by CT perfusion and multislice CT angiography. *Neurocrit Care* 2009;11:261–271.
6. Flowers WM Jr, Patel BR. Radionuclide angiography as a confirmatory test for brain death: a review of 229 studies in 219 patients. *South Med J* 1997;90:1091–1096.
7. Greer DM, Strozyk D, Schwamm LH. False positive CT angiography in brain death. *Neurocrit Care* 2009;11:272–275.
8. Hansen AVE, Lavin PJM, Moody EB, et al. False-negative cerebral radionuclide flow study, in brain death, caused by a ventricular drain. *Clin Nucl Med* 1993;18:502–505.
9. Hassler W, Steinmetz H, Gawlowski J. Transcranial Doppler ultrasonography in raised intracranial pressure and in intracranial circulatory arrest. *J Neurosurg* 1988;68: 745–751.
10. Lampl Y, Gilad R, Eshcel Y, et al. Diagnosing brain death using the transcranial Doppler with a transorbital approach. *Arch Neurol* 2002;59:58–60.
11. Munari M, Zucchetta P, Carollo C, et al. Confirmatory tests in the diagnosis of brain death: comparison between SPECT and contrast angiography. *Crit Care Med* 2005;33:2068–2073.
12. Nebra AC, Virgos B, Santos S, et al. Clinical diagnosis of brain death and transcranial Doppler, looking for middle cerebral arteries and intracranial vertebral arteries: agreement with scintigraphic techniques. *Rev Neurol* 2001;33:916–920.
13. Newell DW, Grady MS, Sirotta P, et al. Evaluation of brain death using transcranial Doppler. *Neurosurgery* 1989;24:509–513.
14. Petty GW, Mohr JP, Pedley TA, et al. The role of transcranial Doppler in confirming brain death. Sensitivity, specificity, and suggestions for performance and interpretation. *Neurology* 1990;40:300–303.
15. Powers AD, Graeber MC, Smith RR. Transcranial Doppler ultrasonography in the determination of brain death. *Neurosurgery* 1989;24:884–889.
16. Quesnel C, Fulgencio J-P, Adrie C, et al. Limitations of computed tomographic angiography in the diagnosis of brain death. *Intensive Care Med* 2007;33:2129–2135.
17. Reid RH, Gulenchyn KY, Ballinger JR. Clinical use of technetium-99m HM-PAO for determination of brain death. *J Nucl Med* 1989;30:1621–1626.
18. Wieler H, Marohl K, Kaiser KP, et al. Tc-99m HMPAO cerebral scintigraphy: a reliable noninvasive method for determination of brain death. *Clin Nucl Med* 1993;18:104–109.
19. Yatim A, Mercatello A, Coronel B, et al. 99mTc-HMPAO cerebral scintigraphy in the diagnosis of brain death. *Transplant Proc* 1991; 23:2491.
20. Zurynski Y, Dorsch N, Pearson I, et al. Transcranial Doppler ultrasound in brain death: experience in 140 patients. *Neurol Res* 1991;13:248–252.

Clinical Problem
7

Ancillary Tests and Confounders

■ THE COMMON CLINICAL QUESTIONS

Can an ancillary test be used in patients with confounders? Isn't the absence of cerebral blood flow to the brain sufficient to make the diagnosis of brain death?

■ THE FACTS

Staying on the same subject as in clinical problem 6, a frequently asked question is what to do with a patient in pentobarbital coma with high intracranial pressures. Patients may "look" brain dead and may have very high intracranial pressures that do not respond to any osmotic agents, and cerebral blood flow studies show no uptake of a tracer or contrast entering the dura. In practice, there may be a push to come to closure. The only issue that prevents a final decision is a lingering confounding barbiturate. Waiting for its clearance is sometimes not acceptable to a grieving family, and physicians are asked to withdraw support or to proceed with organ donation.

If confounders are identified, the neurologic examination is most often confounded by recent administration of drugs, alcohol or as a result of severe penetrating craniofacial injury. An ancillary test is often considered in these situations.[2,4,5,7] Because EEGs are also confounded by sedation, a cerebral flow study is the preferred test. The ancillary test is now elevated to become a diagnostic test.

Some studies have actually reported on the use of cerebral flow studies because EEGs would not be reliable in "sedated" patients.[3,6,8] One study from Barcelona suggested the use of a transcranial Doppler or nuclear scan to "speed up" the diagnosis of brain death in patients with recent administration of barbiturates, benzodiazepines, or opiates.[5] One study suggested the use of CT perfusion to circumvent the confounding effect of barbiturates.[2] Another study reported nuclear scanning in patients in barbiturate coma for the treatment of increased intracranial hypertension.[3] In this study of 22 patients with high doses of barbiturates, brain death was suspected. Monitoring of intracranial pressure revealed that with a major rise in pressure, pupils became fixed and dilated and intracranial uptake of the isotope tracer was absent. When cerebral perfusion pressure was normal, the isotope was visualized in the brain.

One recent study also found 28% of patients with confounders and clinical suspicion of brain death had intracranial blood flow.[7]

Another study likely also involving patients with lingering sedatives compared cerebral angiogram with CT angiogram and found agreement in only 9 of the 24 comparisons.[1] CT angiogram often showed intracranial flow where cerebral angiogram showed none and vice versa.

One can only conclude that cerebral blood flow studies in "sedated patients suspected of brain death" often show intracranial flow, but it depends on the flow study used. No flow on one study may mean flow on another. Cerebral blood flow, in sedated patients, may still depend on intracranial pressure.

These challenging clinical scenarios are all too common. Strictly speaking, only in the absence of confounders and after a full neurologic examination can the patient be declared brain dead or even considered for a donation protocol. One could also argue that antidotes (flumazenil or naloxone) would be insufficient to absolutely ensure that the effects of benzodiazepines or opioids have been reversed. The problem here is what constitutes an adequate dose for reversal of pharmacologic intoxication.

To proceed with withdrawal of support or organ procurement would then be in a patient without a reliable neurologic examination and without a reliable assessment of the prognosis. None of these ancillary studies can replace this examination, and none give conclusive answers.[10,11] One should be concerned about using any surrogate technical test to definitively determine brain death. Patients with high ICPs may have residual breathing drive. Massively increased ICP does not

TABLE 6-8 *Pitfalls of Confirmatory Tests*

Cerebral angiogram

- Image variability with injection of arch or selective arteries
- Image variability with injection or/and push technique
- No guidelines for interpretation

Transcranial Doppler ultrasound

- Technical difficulties and skill dependent
- Normal in brain death with no increased intracranial pressure

EEG

- Artifacts in intensive care settings
- Information from mostly cortex only

Evoked potentials

- Absent in patients without brain death

CT angiogram

- Interpretation difficulties
- Retained blood flow in 20% of cases
- Possibility to miss slow flow states because of rapid acquisition of images

Nuclear brain scan

- Interpretation difficulties
- Requires experience

Adapted from Wijdicks. Used with permission of *Neurology*.[10]

always correspond with absent intracranial bloodflow (cerebral perfusion pressure is a better guide, see Chapter 2). To further illustrate that in one study a median ICP of 102 mm Hg was associated with intracranial opacification on selective 4 vessel cerebral angiogram.[8] Using a cerebral blood flow test to diagnose brain death in a patient with a major confounder is bound to cause errors. No one would want to experience reappearance of clinical signs in patients with confounded clinical examination and a false positive test blood flow test. There are simply too many pitfalls with ancillary tests (Table 6-8). All these major problems, however, can be avoided if treating physicians do not use long-acting drugs in patients who are imminently brain dead. Barbiturates to treat increased ICP likely should be replaced with more modern approaches such a hypothermia and decompressive craniectomy.

■ REFERENCES

1. Bohatyrewicz R, Sawicki M, Walecka A, Computed Tomographic Angiography and Perfusion in the Diagnosis of Brain Death. *Transplant Proc* 2010 42, 3941–3946.
2. Braun M, Ducrocq X, Huot J-C, et al. Intravenous angiography in brain death: report of 140 patients. *Neuroradiology* 1997;39:400–405.
3. Facco E, Zuchetta P, Munari M, et al. 99m TC–HMPAO SPECT in the diagnosis of brain death. *Intensive Care Med* 1998;24:911–917.
4. Goodman JM, Heck LJ, Moore BD Confirmation of brain death with portable isotope angiography: a review of 204 consecutive cases. *Neurosurgery* 1985;16:492–497.
5. López-Navidad A, Caballero F, Domingo P, et al. Early diagnosis of brain death in patients treated with central nervous system depressant drugs. *Transplantation* 2000;70:131–135.
6. Nau R, Prange HW, Klingelhofer J, et al. Results of four technical investigations in fifty clinically brain dead patients. *Intensive Care Med* 1992;18:82–88.
7. Qureshi AI, Kirmani JF, Xavier AR, et al. Computed tomographic angiography for the diagnosis of brain death. *Neurology* 2004;62:652–653.
8. Savard M, Turgeon AF, Gariépy JL. Selective 4 Vessels Angiography in Brain Death: A Retrospective Study. *Can J Neurol Sci* 2010;37:492–497.
9. Wijdicks EFM. Brain death worldwide: accepted fact but no global consensus in diagnostic criteria. *Neurology* 2002;58:1367–1372.
10. Wijdicks EFM. The case against confirmatory tests for determining brain death in adults. *Neurology* 2010;75:77–83.
11. Young GB, Shemie SD, Doig CJ, et al. Brief review: the role of ancillary tests in the neurological determination of death. *Can J Anaesth* 2006;53:620–627.

Clinical Problem 8

Primary Brainstem Lesion

■ THE COMMON CLINICAL QUESTIONS

Could a primary brainstem lesion result in brain death? What other tests are necessary to diagnose brain death?

■ THE FACTS

Acute catastrophic injury may be confined to the brainstem. In most instances this is a destructive pontine hemorrhage, an acute basilar artery embolus, or a head injury that involves primarily the brainstem.[1,3-5] Gunshot wounds, especially when the barrel of the gun has been placed inside the mouth, can destroy the brainstem preferentially. Brainstem compression from a large cerebellar hemorrhage is also a common clinical condition. The brain hemispheres remain initially untouched unless acute hydrocephalus—from obstruction at the fourth ventricle or aqueduct— increases the intracranial pressure and impedes intracranial flow.

A few detailed comments are warranted. First, a primary brainstem lesion or a lesion that compresses the brainstem, such as in a cerebellar hemorrhage, usually does not produce complete loss of brain function. In most instances there is sparing of the medulla oblongata, which is detected by the presence of a breathing drive that may have to be demonstrated with a formal apnea test.[9] Often blood pressures do not need to be pharmacologically supported. These patients despite loss of upper brainstem reflexes may eventually be supported long term. This clinical condition is technically different from brain death, not only because breathing is preserved but also because there is autonomic regulation of cardiac function and maintenance of vascular tone. Such a case is shown in Figure 6-3.[7]

Second, a destructive primary brainstem lesion is as irreversible as a lesion that involves the hemispheres and brainstem; therefore, it is unnecessary to perform an ancillary test. These tests often show preserved blood flow when the intracranial pressure has not increased to extreme values, and EEG may show nonreactive alpha or spindle coma patterns.[6]

The AAN guideline does not differentiate between a primary brainstem lesion and a lesion of the hemisphere and brainstem, and simply states that the clinical examination should be sufficient.[8] Coma, absent brainstem reflexes, and confirmed

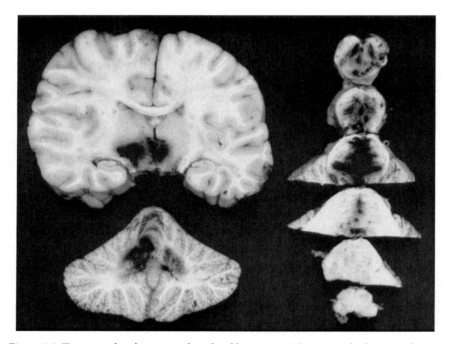

Figure 6-3 Traumatic head injury and epidural hematoma. The patient had a normal breathing drive and cough responses, but all pontomesencephalic reflexes remained absent. After 1 week of full support and no clinical change, the family decided to withdraw support. Neuropathologic examination showed thalamic, cerebellar, and upper brainstem lesions but sparing of the medulla. From Wijdicks et al.[7] with permission of the publisher. *See* Figure 6-3 in the color insert.

apnea in a predominant brainstem lesion is not reversible—not even after emergent decompressive surgery—and no brainstem reflex will return.[8] Brainstem reflexes may return if only some are absent, but not when all are lost.

Some institutions have extended their observation time to 24 hours; others have extended it even longer until an ancillary test shows no intracranial flow or a flat EEG. The German Brain Death Guidelines require 72 hours of observation and a confirmatory test for lesions of the posterior fossa but not when the lesions are supratentorial.[2]

The most important responsibility for physicians is to perform a complete examination in patients with a primary lesion in the brainstem. More often than not, physicians will find that patients with a primary brainstem lesion or a compressed brainstem from a cerebellar lesion do not fulfill all the criteria for brain death and may even benefit from aggressive intervention (ventriculostomy or suboccipital craniotomy).

■ REFERENCES

1. Britt RH, Herrick MK, Mason RT, et al. Traumatic lesions of pontomedullary junction. *Neurosurgery* 1980;6:623–631.
2. Dritte Fortschreibung 1997 mit Erganzungen gemaβ Transplantationsgesez (TPG). Richtlinien zur Feststellung des Hirntodes. *Deutsches Arzteblatt* 1998;95, Heft 30.
3. Firsching R, Woischneck D, Klein S, et al. Brainstem lesions after head injury. *Neurol Res* 2002;24:145–146.
4. Kosteljanetz M, Ohrstrom JK, Skjodt S, et al. Clinical brain death with preserved cerebral arterial circulation. *Acta Neurol Scand* 1988;78:418–421.
5. Ogata J, Imakita M, Yutani C, et al. Primary brainstem death: a clinico-pathological study. *JNNP* 1988;51:646–650.
6. Rodin E, Tahir S, Austin D, et al. Brainstem death. *Clin Electroencephalogr* 1985;16: 63–71.
7. Wijdicks EFM, Atkinson JL, Okazaki H. Isolated medulla oblongata function after severe traumatic brain injury. *J Neurol Neurosurg Psychiatry* 2001;70:127–129.
8. Wijdicks EFM, Varelas P, Gronseth GS, et al. Evidence-based guideline update: determining brain death in adults: report of the quality standards subcommittee of the American Academy of Neurology. *Neurology* 2010;74:1911–1918.
9. Woischneck D, Kappa T, Heissler HE, et al. Respiratory function after lesions in medulla oblongata. *Neurol Res* 2009;31:1019–1022.

Clinical Problem
9

Uncertainty About Interpreting Spinal Reflexes

■ THE COMMON CLINICAL QUESTIONS

What are common spinally generated reflexes and movements? How can these observations be distinguished from preserved brain function?

■ THE FACTS

Patients meeting the criteria of brain death are motionless. However, body movements after death have occasionally been observed during the apnea test, during preparation for transport, at the time of abdominal incision for organ retrieval, and in the morgue itself.[1,2,5,6,7,17] A prospective study of 38 patients with brain death, mostly young adults, found a surprisingly high frequency of spinal-generated movements (39%), but also included a triple flexion response and minor twitches such as facial myokymias, and finger jerks.[19-22] In our experience, these movements are very rare, with only a few patients in our series demonstrating finger flexion or arm lifting. A provoked triple flexion response is more common and may remain for hours up to the time of transfer to the operating room.

The early papers on brain death contained descriptions of body movements brought on by any type of stimulation—triple flexion of the legs, adduction or abduction of the arm to the stimulated area, and head rotation. These movements have puzzled the unprepared, and have concerned family members. Evidence that the movements represent only spinal activity is the consistent clinical documentation of brain death, often with confirmation by an isoelectric EEG or the absence of intracranial flow. In general, they do not even remotely resemble voluntary movements or decerebrate or decorticate rigidity, and similar movements have been demonstrated experimentally in isolated spinal cord preparations. The most impressive body movement is a brief attempt of the body to sit up to 40 to 60 degrees, but generally not in a full sitting position. Arms may raise independently of each other but legs seldom move. Rhythmic flexion of the hip and knee mimicking stepping has occurred with progressive brainstem destruction, but it often disappears in brain death. These are all very slow movements, lasting for 10 to 20 seconds, and some are barely noticeable or even reproducible.

TABLE 6-9 *Movements and Reflexes in Brain Death*

Head and neck
Neck-abdominal muscle contraction
Neck-hip flexion
Neck-arm flexion
Shoulder protrusion
Head turning to one side
Upper extremity
Flexion-withdrawal reflex
Unilateral extension-pronation
Isolated finger jerks; finger pinch-finger flexion
Flexion elevation of arms
Trunk
Asymmetric opisthotonic posturing of trunk
Flexion of trunk, causing partial sitting movement
Abdominal twitches
Lower extremity
Plantar flexion of toes after percussion
Triple flexion response

Adapted from references 9–16 and 24–26.

There has been quite a bit of fascination in the literature with these spinal reflexes, but some published responses, however, are dubious.[23] The most commonly reported reflexes and movements are shown in Table 6-9.[9-16,24-26]

These movements have been named *Lazarus signs*, referring to the biblical person said to have been raised by Jesus, but the term is disrespectful to the patient and family and should be avoided in conversation.[8,18] It may be seen more often in the final stages of circulatory collapse in a markedly hypoxemic, cyanotic, apneic patient after withdrawal of support. Some of this spinal activity may be triggered by the ventilator, synchronous with pulmonary insufflation, and disappears after disconnection of the ventilator.[20]

Other manifestations include the undulating toe sign (snapping the big toe leads to an undulating movement of the toes resembling those of a sea anemone); a persistent Babinski response; any tendon, abdominal, or cremaster reflex; flushing; shivering; sweating; and myoclonic twitching in limb muscles.

The pathophysiology is a polysynaptic, polysegmental reflex from the spinal cord and may be stimulated in patients who are markedly polysegmental hypoxemic. Prolonged apnea tests causing acidosis and hypoxemia have traditionally been associated with spontaneous spinal cord reflexes. However, a noxious stimulus or one simple touch may produce these complex movements, and they may occur after forceful flexion of the neck or rotation of the body.

■ REFERENCES

1. Araullo ML, Frank JI, Goldenberg FD, et al. Transient bilateral finger tremor after brain death. *Neurology* 2007;68:E22.
2. Bohatyrewicz R, Walecka A, Bohatyrewicz A, et al. Unusual movements, "spontaneous" breathing, and unclear cerebral vessels sonography in a brain-dead patient: a case report. *Transplant Proc* 2007;39:2707–2708.
3. Bolger C, Bojanic S, Phillips J, et al. Ocular microtremor in brain stem death. *Neurosurgery* 1999;44:1201–1206.
4. Conci F, Procaccio F, Arosio M, et al. Viscero-somatic and viscera-visceral reflexes in brain death. *J Neurol Neurosurg Psychiatry* 1986;49:695–698.
5. de Freitas GR, Lima MA, Andre C. Complex spinal reflexes during transcranial Doppler ultrasound examination for the confirmation of brain death. *Acta Neurol Scand* 2003;108:170–173.
6. Dosemeci L, Cengiz M, Yilmaz M, et al. Frequency of spinal reflex movements in brain-dead patients. *Transplant Proc* 2004;36:17–19.
7. Han SG, Kim GM, Lee KH, et al. Reflex movements in patients with brain death: a prospective study in a tertiary medical center. *J Korean Med Sci* 2006;21:588–590.
8. Heytens L, Verlooy J, Gheuens J, et al. Lazarus sign and extensor posturing in a brain-dead patient. Case report. *J Neurosurg* 1989;7:449–451.
9. Jain S, DeGeorgia JS. Brain death–associated reflexes and automatisms. *Neurocrit Care* 2005;3:122–126.
10. Jordan JE, Dyess E, Cliett J. Unusual spontaneous movements in brain-dead patients. *Neurology* 1985;35:1082.
11. Jung KY, Hann SG, Lee KH, et al. Repetitive leg movements mimicking periodic leg movement during sleep in a brain-dead patient. *Eur J Neurol* 2006;13:e3–e4.
12. Kuwagata Y, Sugimoto H, Yoshioka T, et al. Hemodynamic response with passive neck flexion in brain death. *Neurosurgery* 1991;29:239–241.
13. Lang CJ, Sittl H, Erbguth F. Autonomous stump movements in brain death. *Eur Neurol* 1997;37:249.
14. Marti-Fabregas J, Lopez-Navidad A, Caballero F, et al. Decerebrate-like posturing with mechanical ventilation in brain death. *Neurology* 2000;54:224–227.
15. McNair NL, Meador KJ. The undulating toe flexion sign in brain death. *Mov Disord* 1992;7:345–347.
16. Poulton TJ. Spontaneous movements in brain-death patients. *JAMA* 1986;225:2028.
17. Rodrigues W, Vyas H. Movements in brain death. *Eur J Neurol* 2001;8:209–213.
18. Ropper AH. Unusual spontaneous movements in brain-dead patients. *Neurology* 1984;34:1089–1092.
19. Saposnik G, Basile VS, Young GB. Movements in brain death: a systematic review. *Can J Neurol Sci* 2009;36:154–160.
20. Saposnik G, Bueri JA, Maurino J, et al. Spontaneous and reflex movements in brain death. *Neurology* 2000;54:221–223.
21. Saposnik G, Maurino J, Saizar R. Facial myokymia in brain death. *Eur J Neurol* 2001;8:227–230.
22. Saposnik G, Maurino J, Saizar R, et al. Undulating toe movements in brain death. *Eur J Neurol* 2004;11:723–727.
23. Shulgman D, Parulekar M, Elston JS, et al. Abnormal pupillary activity in a brainstem-dead patient. *Br J Anaesth* 2001;86:717–720.
24. Spittler JF, Wortmann D, von During M, et al. Phenomenological diversity of spinal reflexes in brain death. *Eur J Neurol* 2000;7:315–321.
25. Turmel A, Roux A, Bojanowski MW. Spinal man after declaration of brain death. *Neurosurgery* 1991;28:298–301.
26. Zubkov AY, Wijdicks EFM. Plantar flexion and flexion synergy in brain death. *Neurology* 2008;70:e74.

Clinical Problem 10

Ventilator Autocycling

■ THE COMMON CLINICAL QUESTIONS

How can a patient's breathing drive be differentiated from ventilator autocycling? What predisposes to this phenomenon?

■ THE FACTS

Most alarming to the ICU staff is when a brain dead patient suddenly appears to trigger the ventilator. The patient appears to be breathing over a set frequency and the ventilator may even indicate a good tidal volume. This phenomenon may indicate ventilator autocycling.[1,4,5–10]

This false triggering may be more common than is generally appreciated, and we have observed ventilatory autocycling in at least 10% of our brain death examinations.[9] In a pressure-triggered ventilator setting, a drop in airway pressure from an inspiratory effort by the patient triggers the ventilator to provide a breath. In a flow-triggered setting, gas flows continuously within the ventilator circuit (flow-by). The patient's effort to obtain a breath is much less, making a flow-triggered mode more often a preferred setting. However, the flow-triggered mode is very susceptible to noise. The ventilator then senses a change in flow in the circuit and provides a mechanical breath. Autotriggering of the ventilator may occur from leaks in the circuit or flow fluctuations from condensed water in the circuit.[4,5] Leaks in the endotracheal tube or ventilator tubing or simply the presence of chest tubes are common triggers.[8] These changes usually trigger if sensitivity is set at a low level and decreasing the trigger sensitivity level will cause these breaths to disappear. Changing to pressure triggering is the most simple solution, but with added pressure support and low pressure sensitivity setting ventilator autocycling may still occur.[8] Ventilator auto-cycling may also be due to precardiac movements.[1,6] It is a result of a decrease in airway pressure synchronous with the cardiac heartbeat and, therefore, changing from a flow-triggered setting on the ventilator to a pressure setting may not always solve the problem. An algorithm to troubleshoot this phenomenon is shown in Figure 6-4. Not uncommonly, another apnea test with disconnection from the ventilator may be needed to differentiate between two possibilities. Some physicians have proceeded with an ancillary test, only to find that the test is not compatible with circulatory arrest in the brain causing more confusion than resolution.[2,3]

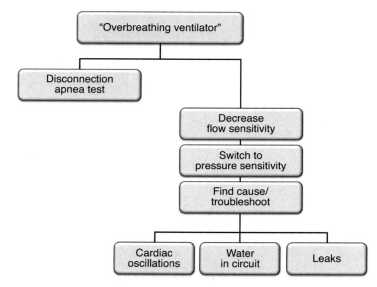

Figure 6-4 Algorithm to check for causes of ventilator autocycling.

There is real concern that some patients with a "retained breathing drive" are excluded from formal testing, or worse, that a prolonged waiting time for the respiratory drive to disappear may lead to premature cardiac arrest in a potential organ donor or to a switch to a DCD protocol preventing donation of the heart and lungs.[7]

■ REFERENCES

1. Arbour R. Cardiogenic oscillation and ventilator autotriggering in brain-dead patients: a case series. *Am J Crit Care* 2009;18:496:488–495.
2. Bertagna F, Barozzi O, Puta E, et al. Residual brain viability, evaluated by 99mTc-ECD, SPECT, in patients with suspected brain death and with confounding clinical factors. *Nuclear Med Commun* 2009;30:815–821.
3. Bohatyrewicz R, Walecka A, Bohatyrewicz A, et al. Unusual movements, "spontaneous" breathing, and unclear cerebral vessels sonography in a brain-dead patient: a case report. *Transplant Proc* 2007;39:2707–2708.
4. Harboe S, Hjalmarsson S, Søreide E. Autocycling and increase in intrinsic positive end-expiratory pressure during mechanical ventilation. *Acta Anaesthesiol Scand* 2001;45:1295–1297.
5. Hill LL, Pearl RG. Flow triggering, pressure triggering, and autotriggering during mechanical ventilation. *Crit Care Med* 2000;28:579–581.
6. Imanaka H, Nishimura M, Takeuchi M, et al. Autotriggering caused by cardiogenic oscillation during flow triggered mechanical ventilation. *Crit Care Med* 2000;28:579–581.
7. McGee W, Mailloux P. Ventilator autocycling and delayed recognition of brain death. *Neurocrit Care* 2011; in press.
8. Schwab RJ, Schnader JS. Ventilator autocycling due to an endotracheal tube cuff leak. *Chest* 1991;100:1172–1173.
9. Wijdicks EFM, Manno EM, Holets SR. Ventilator self-cycling may falsely suggest patient effort during brain death determination. *Neurology* 2005;65:774.
10. Williatts SM, Drummond G. Brainstem death and ventilator trigger settings. *Anaesthesia* 2005;55:676–677.

Chronic CO$_2$ Retention and the Apnea Test

■ THE COMMON CLINICAL QUESTIONS

Can the apnea test be reliably performed in a patient with chronic hypercapnia? Is there a target arterial PCO$_2$? How do we recognize chronic hypercapnia?

■ THE FACTS

The centrally guided respiratory drive is determined by a certain threshold and sensitivity.[1] The chemoreceptor areas are located anterior and laterally in the medulla.[3-5] A quick chemoresponse is present under normal conditions and also in normocapnic patients with chronic obstructive pulmonary disease (COPD).[10] An increase in arterial PCO$_2$ results in a decrease in cerebrospinal fluid (CSF) pH, but within hours, the CSF pH normalizes due to changes in CSF bicarbonate level. Normally, the rise in arterial PCO$_2$ occurs within minutes, followed by an increase in respiratory depth and rate. In a catastrophic neurologic illness leading to brain death, abnormal function of the respiratory centers causes apnea (assuming no abnormality in neuromuscular transmission and intact respiratory mechanics). Carbon dioxide (CO$_2$) responsiveness in brain death patients has been a matter of debate. The debate centered largely on the level of the arterial PCO$_2$ that would result in maximal stimulation of the respiratory centers (Chapter 2).

In hypercapnic COPD patients (also known as *CO$_2$ retainers*) respiratory sensitivity to CO$_2$ is decreased,[2] but when severe airway disease is present, sensitivity is low, arterial PCO$_2$ rises, and patients become dependent on a hypoxemic stimulus.[6-8] Thus, hyperoxygenation during the oxygen-diffusion apnea test will already result in a reduction of this response. Most of the responses rise hyperbolically. Figure 6-5 shows that the threshold level in hypoxemic patients is between 40 and 50 mm Hg arterial PCO$_2$; and in normoxemic or hyperoxemic patients, end tidal PCO$_2$ might be slightly higher, in the 50 mm Hg range.[9] In chronic hypercapnia, however, evidence has suggested not only that the threshold is increased in chronically hypercapnic patients but also that the response may be muted. It is therefore impossible to set a target in chronically hypercapnic patients.

Apart from morbid obesity or long-standing COPD, chronic hypercapnia is typically recognized by a baseline blood gas that shows a marked increase in

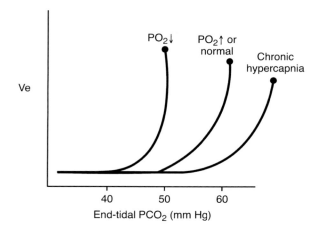

Figure 6-5 Expected ventilatory responses to hypoxemia in normal conditions and in patients with CO_2 retention. PCO_2, partial pressure of carbon dioxide; PO_2, partial pressure of oxygen; Ve, Ventilation.

bicarbonate and an arterial PCO_2 usually between 50 and 70 mm Hg. When these conditions are present, an apnea test with a CO_2 challenge cannot be reliably performed. In our experience, patients with chronic hypercapnia who have become brain dead are actually rare. It is possible that patients with chronic hypercapnia are less often struck by a neurologic illness that leads to brain death. Perhaps hypoxic-ischemic encephalopathy occurs more often in these patients, with cortical injury sparing the brainstem.

■ **REFERENCES**

1. Ainslie PN, Duffin J. Integration of cerebrovascular CO_2 reactivity and chemoreflex control of breathing: mechanisms of regulation, measurement, and interpretation. *Am J Physiol Regul Integr Comp Physiol* 2009;295:R1473–R1495.
2. Duffin J. The chemoreflex control of breathing and its measurement. *Can J Anaesth* 1990;37:933–942.
3. Duffin J. The role of the central chemoreceptors: a modeling perspective. *Respir Physiol Neurbiol* 2010;173:230–243.
4. Duffin J, McAvoy GF. The peripheral-chemoreceptor threshold to carbon dioxide in man. *J Physiol* 1988;406:15–26.
5. Guyenet PG, Stornetta RL, Abbott SB, et al. Central CO_2-chemoreception and integrated neural mechanisms of cardiovascular and respiratory control. *J Appl Physiol* 2010;108:995–1002.
6. Kepron W, Cherniack RM. The ventilatory response to hypercapnia and to hypoxemia in chronic obstructive lung disease. *Am Rev Respir Dis* 1973;108:843–850.
7. Khodadadeh B, Safwan Badr M, Mateika JH. The ventilatory response to carbon dioxide and sustained hypoxia is enhanced after episodic hypoxia in OSA patients. *Respir Physiol Neurobiol* 2006;150:122–134.
8. O'Donnell TV, Hood LJ. Decreased chemoreceptor sensitivity and chronic obstructive lung disease. *J R Coll Physicians Lond* 1971;6:53–63.
9. Ogoh S, Ainslie PN, Miyamoto T. Onset responses of ventilation and cerebral blood flow to hypercapnia in humans: rest and exercise. *J Appl Physiol* 2009;106:880–886.
10. Scano G, Spinelli A, Duranti R, et al. Carbon dioxide responsiveness in COPD patients with and without chronic hypercapnia. *Eur Respir J* 1995;8:78–85.

Clinical Problem
12

Terminating the Apnea Test

■ THE COMMON CLINICAL QUESTIONS

When should the apnea test be discontinued? What factors predispose to stopping the apnea test?

■ THE FACTS

Concerns about the safety of the apnea test have remained. Some ICU experiences have shown complications in more than two-thirds of patients[1,3,5,10] but not others.[4,11,12] Premature discontinuation of the apnea test may be related to the method used, susceptability of the patient, and mostly pretest cardiovascular and respiratory status. All clinically used apnea tests induce hypercapnia, resulting in concomitant respiratory acidosis.[2,6-9,12]

The most commonly identified factors that anticipate a possible problematic apnea test are shown in Table 6-10. Pretest hypoxemia was a major risk factor in two studies, and in one study the risk remained despite administration of 100% oxygen.[4,13] However, preoxygenation—providing an oxygen reservoir and removing alveolar nitrogen—resulted in safe completion of most of our apnea tests. Another study showed that pretest acidemia may predispose to hypotension, but the prevalence of premature discontinuation of the apnea test remains low (<5%).[14]

TABLE 6-10 *Factors Associated with Aborting the Apnea Test*

- Insufficient preoxygenation
- T-piece oxygen administration
- High intratracheal flow of oxygen (>10 L/min)
- High A-a gradient (>300)
- Hypotension (systolic blood pressure <90 mm Hg)
- Mild acidosis (arterial pH < 7.30)
- Chest tubes for pneumothorax
- Polytrauma
- Younger age

How acidosis could cause worsening of hypotension is not exactly known. (A transesophageal echocardiogram during the apnea test—with an end pH around 7.0—did not show any evidence of left ventricular dysfunction.[3]) The apnea test may remain a very tricky procedure in young patients after polytrauma and with chest tubes in place. These patients, in an unstable hemodynamic condition from polytrauma, may have lost all brain function, but the apnea test is virtually impossible to perform.

Apnea tests are rarely discontinued as a result of a sudden development of pneumothorax. High oxygen flows (>10 L/min) or large insufflation catheters may cause trapping of gas moreover insertion of a catheter with sharp endings, may damage the bronchial wall (for details on the insufflation catheter, see Chapter 2).

A major concern is when the apnea test is performed without adequate preparation and clinical assessment of the potential risks. Patients should be normovolemic, normotensive, and normocapnic, and preoxygenation should have resulted in a PaO_2 of at least 200 mm Hg. Ventilator requirements should be evaluated, and in particular adequate oxygenation with low PEEP (5 cm H_2O) requirement should be demonstrated. The apnea test is rarely aborted when these preconditions are met.

The apnea test is usually terminated due to failure to maintain adequate oxygenation and blood pressure after disconnection of the ventilator. Usually the first minutes of the apnea test will make it clear whether the test can be continued. Oxygen desaturation generally occurs rather quickly after disconnection of the ventilator, leading to a decrease of the pulse oximeter reading to below 85%. The apnea test is also aborted if systolic blood pressure decreases to less than 90 mm Hg. However, hypotension may be brief and may respond well to a bolus of 100 mcg of intravenous phenylephrine. In some patients, the apnea test can be completed after a single dose of phenylephrine because the observation time is short. The decision to abort the apnea test should not be postponed if the response to phenylephrine is incomplete or marginal (e.g., systolic blood pressure remains below 90 mm Hg). Systolic blood pressure may irreversibly decrease quickly, resulting in cardiac asystole.

Cardiac arrest following the sudden appearance of hypotension is very uncommon, with no such instance in the recent Mayo Clinic series. Cardiovascular collapse occurs if the apnea test is not terminated in time and a rapidly developing hypoxemia or hypotension is underappreciated by the physician.

Another trial of apnea testing can be considered, but this time using a T-piece, a CPAP valve of 10 cm H_2O, and 100% oxygen at a rate of 12 L/min. There is some evidence that this technique may better secure oxygenation.[11] Problems with oxygenation may remain difficult to overcome. These patients probably cannot be declared brain dead and, therefore, could become candidates for a DCD protocol after the decision to withdraw support has been made.

■ **REFERENCES**

1. Combes JC, Nicolas F, Cros N, et al. Severe pulmonary arterial hypertension during the apnea test for brain death. *Transplant Proc* 1996;28:375.

2. Dominguez R, Barrera C, Murillo CF, et al. Clinical factors in influencing the increment of blood carbon dioxide during the apnea test for the diagnosis of brain death. *Transplant Proc* 1999;31:2599–2600.
3. Ebata T, Watanabe Y, Amaha K, et al. Hemodynamic changes during the apnea test for diagnosis of brain death. *Can J Anesth* 1991;38:438–440.
4. Goudreau JL, Wijdicks EFM, Emery SF. Complications during the determination of brain death: predisposing factors. *Neurology* 2000;55:1045–1048.
5. Jeret JS, Benjamin JL. Risk of hypotension during apnea testing. *Arch Neurol* 1994;51: 595–599.
6. Lang CJG, Heckman JG. Apnea testing for the diagnosis of brain death. *Acta Neurol Scand* 2005;112:358–369.
7. Outwater KM, Rockolf MA. Apnea testing to confirm brain death in children. *Crit Care Med* 1984;12:357–358.
8. Perel A, Berger M, Cortev S. The use of continuous flow oxygen and PEEP during apnea in the diagnosis of brain death. *Int Care Med* 1983;9:25–27.
9. Pitts LH, Kaktis J, Caronna, et al. Brain death, apneic diffusion, oxygenation and organ transplantation. *J Trauma* 1978;18:180–183.
10. Sasponik G, Rizzo G, Vega A, et al. Problems associated with apnea test in the diagnosis of brain death. *Neurol India* 2004;52:342–345.
11. Simon L, Martin RL, Pierre CN, et al. Efficacy of a T-piece system and a continuous positive airway pressure system for apnea testing in the diagnosis of brain death. *Crit Care Med* 2006;34:2213–2216.
12. Wijdicks EFM, Rabinstein AA, Manno EM, et al. Pronouncing brain death: contemporary practice and safety of the apnea test. *Neurology* 2008;71:1240–1241.
13. Wu XL, Fang G, Li L, et al. Complications associated with the apnea test in the determination of the brain death. *Chin Med J* 2008;121:1169–1177.
14. Yee AH, Mandrekar J, Rabinstein AA, et al. Predictors of apnea test failure during brain death determination. *Neurocrit Care* 2010;12:352–355.

Clinical Problem 13

Breathing During the Apnea Test

■ **THE COMMON CLINICAL QUESTIONS**

How often has breathing been observed during apnea testing? What is the best course of action when breathing occurs?

■ **THE FACTS**

Preserved breathing drive is generally present in a comatose patient with a major catastrophic neurologic injury. Even in patients suspected of brain death, if the patient is examined more closely, traces of a cough reflex may be elicited as a sign that brainstem function is still present. Conversely, breathing during the apnea test when all other brainstem reflexes and a motor response are absent is very uncommon. If the apnea test is performed in patients with absent brainstem reflexes and also if the blood pressure is supported with vasopressors or inotropes, it is unlikely that the test will document an effective breathing drive.

Breathing during the apnea test may occur at different time intervals from the start of the test and at different arterial PCO_2 values. In our recent study of 228 consecutive patients, the apnea test was performed only after all other brainstem reflexes were absent. Disconnection from the ventilator documented a normal breathing drive in two patients, but repeat apnea testing 12 hours and 3 days later resulted in a positive test (since this study was published, two more patients have been observed).[9]

There are several important observations to note. First, breathing may be a single gasp, an irregular or regular breathing pattern. A single agonal gasp may occur unexpectedly and is usually brief, with little chest and abdomen expansion. Such a trace of breathing may be difficult to ascertain with confidence and should prompt a repeat of the entire procedure. Several inspiratory gasps may be observed with clear chest excursions, and in some patients a fairly regular breathing pattern may appear that suggests good tidal volumes (the volume of inspiratory breaths may be measured later by the ventilator after reconnection).

Second, breathing may occur immediately after disconnection or several minutes into the apnea test. Breathing effort is dependent on the arterial PCO_2

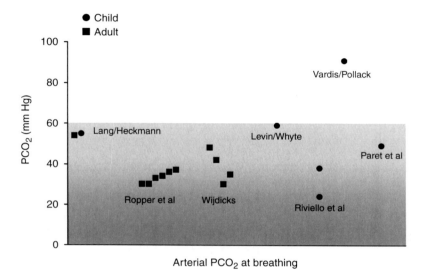

Figure 6-6 Summary of patients tested for brain death and those who started to breath during apnea testing.

value and most often starts in the 30–55 mm Hg range.[5-8] A breathing effort may therefore not appear if the arterial PCO_2 value is below 30 mm Hg, and in some patients, more than 10 minutes may be needed to achieve a 20 mm Hg increase or the target value of 60 mm Hg. Simple disconnection from the ventilator for 5 to 10 minutes is not sufficient to document lack of ventilatory drive. Arterial blood gas determinations are needed to prove an actual arterial PCO_2 increase.

There have been some reports of spontaneous respiration in children and neonates but also breathing at high arterial PCO_2 thresholds.[5,7,8] A few case reports in neonates and children documenting arterial breathing at PCO_2 values of 67, 69, 91, and 112 mm Hg were published in the past, but not recently; therefore, the reliability of these observations is questionable.[2] None of these exceptional cases has resulted in reconsideration of the apnea test procedure or a change in the arterial PCO_2 threshold.[2] The recently reported thresholds are shown in Figure 6-6.

Third, disconnection from the ventilator is absolutely essential to exclude ventilator auto cycling or any ventilator influence in the assessment of apnea.

Once breathing has been established, decisions will have to be made. In most instances, the ventilatory drive is reexamined within 24 hours of the first apnea test. Families may not want to wait and decide to withdraw support. Some of them also do not want to proceed with a DCD protocol and simply want to end the state of extremity they are in. Careful discussion of the potential benefits of organ donation may be needed at this point, and help convince the family to wait a little longer.

Once the apnea test is positive (no breathing effort), breathing does not return in adults. Two reports in children have documented "return of respiration." One dubious report describes a 3-month-old Japanese infant who met all the criteria for brain death after cardiopulmonary arrest associated with hypoglycemia including two apnea tests ($PaCO_2$ of 69 and 62 mm Hg, respectively) and a flat EEG. The child was supported—the Japanese physicians were legally unable to declare the infant brain dead—and a month later, the child developed irregular (2–3/min) respirations with low (40–50 mL) tidal volumes at an arterial PCO_2 of 30 mm Hg.[4] A cerebral angiogram was normal, and an autopsy showed largely cortical necrosis. A second case has been reported of return of "hiccups" in a 10-month-old infant 15 hours after documentation of brain death. In this case, prior use of barbiturates was a confounder, and may have muted the respiratory drive initially.[1]

■ REFERENCES

1. Joffe AR, Kolski H, Duff J, et al. A 10-month-old infant with reversible findings of brain death. *Pediatr Neurol* 2009;41:378–382.
2. Lang CJG, Heckmann JG. Apnea testing for the diagnosis of brain death. *Acta Neurol Scand* 2005;112:358–369.
3. Levin SD, Whyte RK. Brain death sans frontières. *N Engl J Med* 1988;318:852–853.
4. Okamoto K, Sugimoto T. Return of spontaneous respiration in an infant who fulfilled current criteria to determine brain death. *Pediatrics* 1995;96:518–520.
5. Paret G, Barzilay Z. Apnea testing in suspected brain dead children—physiologic and mathematical modeling. *Intensive Care Med.* 1995;21:247–252.
6. Ropper AH, Kennedy SK, Russell L. Apnea testing in the diagnosis of brain death. *J Neurosurg* 1981;55:942–946.
7. Riviello JJ, Sapin JI, Brown LW, et al. Hypoxemia and hemodynamic changes during the hypercarbia stimulation test. *Pediatr Neurol* 1988;4:213–218.
8. Vardis R, Pollack MM. Increased apnea threshold in a pediatric patient with suspected brain death. *Crit Care Med* 1998;26:1917–1919.
9. Wijdicks EFM, Rabinstein AA, Manno EM, et al. Pronouncing brain death: contemporary practice and safety of the apnea test. *Neurology* 2008;71:1240–1244.

Clinical Problem 14

Cardiopulmonary Resuscitation and Brain Death

■ **THE COMMON CLINICAL QUESTIONS**

How much does therapeutic hypothermia confound the neurologic examination? Are there different guidelines with the diagnosis of brain death after cardiopulmonary resuscitation (CPR)?

■ **THE FACTS**

Anoxic-ischemic injury irreversibly damages the cortical layers, but a more significant injury may have involved the brainstem.[6] Brain death is a possible outcome after CPR and is due to development of cerebral edema or is present at onset. In our recent prospective series of comatose patients following CPR, only 8 of 192 (4%) patients met the criteria for brain death.[9] Even in patients with fixed pupils on admission, only one in three met the criteria for brain death later. In some patients with fixed pupils, brain death was suspected, but the examination could not be completed due to the presence of confounders (cardiogenic shock or profound liver dysfunction and drug administration).[9] Another study found brain death more frequently after CPR and in about one in six patients.[1] Patients who meet the clinical criteria for brain death immediately after resumption of circulation typically have had either prolonged resuscitation for asystole or resuscitation for exsanguination from major trauma.

Therapeutic hypothermia has become a common treatment of comatose patients following CPR.[2-4,16-18] It is estimated to be initiated in approximately 60–70% of the patients who are then also entered into a protocol that may involve sedatives and neuromuscular junction blockers.[7] Most cooling protocols use short-acting benzodiazepines or propofol but may also include fentanyl. Neuromuscular blockade to prevent shivering usually is achieved with atracurium or vecuronium. The clinical benefit of therapeutic hypothermia has resulted in its increased practice in coronary care units. A Cochrane systemic review identified four randomized, controlled trials and documented an improved outcome with cooling protocols varying from 12 to 72 hours.[2]

However, patients who fulfill the criteria for brain death after CPR more often are hemodynamically unstable, and many of them die from irreversible cardiac shock before brain death can be determined. The clinical examination of brain death may be difficult to complete due to persistent hypotension and use of multiple vasopressors. The apnea test may also be compromised due to the development of significant pulmonary edema from cardiac failure.

The major issue in protocols of therapeutic hypothermia is the use of drugs providing analgesia and anesthesia. Many protocols use midazolam, but the metabolism of this drug is markedly changed after hypothermia in patients. This happens not only in patients with associated hepatic dysfunction and renal dysfunction that may have occurred during CPR, but also as a result of reduced clearance caused by hypothermia.

There is evidence that hypothermia may lead to a fivefold increase in midazolam plasma concentration; this increase can be explained by depressed CYP3A4 and CYP3A5 activity. A recent study found that midazolam clearance was reduced 11% for each 1°C decrease in core temperature from 36.5°C.[11]

Midazolam is administered in varying doses, and the residual effect is dependent on the initial dose. A high dose (more than 5 mg/h) will make brain death determination virtually impossible. Alternative drugs, such as propofol, may also be problematic, and plasma concentrations may increase up to 30% in patients with hypothermia due to intracompartmental clearance.[14]

Fentanyl is used in many protocols, and depending on the dose (usually starting at 25 mcg/kg/h), the metabolism and clearance of fentanyl is markedly decreased up to four times.[8] Neuromuscular blocking drugs such as vecuronium, pancuronium, and rocuronium all produce active metabolites in the setting of hypothermia, and rocuronium metabolism is prolonged in patients who have hepatic dysfunction.[5,10,15]

Additional clearance of anticonvulsant drugs can be markedly impaired during hypothermia.[13] If phenytoin has been used to treat seizures, elimination is markedly different and both free and total serum levels should be monitored. Recent studies have found up to 180% increase in serum levels with a temperature of 34°C.[12] The decreased elimination was due not to a change in plasma protein binding but to decreased P450 metabolism.[19] The changes in clearance rate of several drugs are shown in Table 6-11.

How to interpret these changes in clearance is downright problematic. Therapeutic hypothermia in a patient with an infusion of fentanyl or midazolam—certainly both—will seriously confound neurologic examination. Better tissue perfusion following rewarming resulting in drug redistribution may further increase drug levels. Ischemic liver injury may also contribute. Even in the best circumstances, physicians may have to conclude that a brain death examination

TABLE 6-11 *Estimates in Clearance Change in Drugs Used in Therapeutic Hypothermia after Cardiopulmonary Resuscitation*

Midazolam	11% per 1°C decrease
Remifentanil	6% per 1°C decrease
Vecuronium	11% per 1°C decrease
Fentanyl	6% per 1°C decrease
Propofol	8% per 1°C decrease

Source: Data from Tortorici et al.[19]

is unreliable. Donation through DCD protocol could, nevertheless, proceed. Factors that may preclude organ donation are prolonged resuscitation efforts resulting in worsening liver function tests (bedside liver biopsy may be performed) or severe acute tubular necrosis.

■ REFERENCES

1. Adrie C, Haouache H, Saleh M, et al. An underrecognized source of organ donors: patients with brain death after successfully resuscitated cardiac arrest. *Intensive Care Med* 2008;34:132–137.
2. Arrich J, Holzer M, Herkner H, et al. Hypothermia for neuroprotection in adults after cardiopulmonary resuscitation. *Cochrane Database Syst Rev* 2009;4:CD004128.
3. Bernard SA, Gray TW, Buist MD, et al. Treatment of comatose survivors of out-of-hospital cardiac arrest with induced hypothermia. *N Engl J Med* 2002;346:557–563.
4. Broccard A. Therapeutic hypothermia for anoxic brain injury following cardiac arrest: a "cool" transition toward cardiopulmonary cerebral resuscitation. *Crit Care Med* 2006;34:2008–2009.
5. Caldwell JE, Heier T, Wright PM, et al. Temperature-dependent pharmacokinetics and pharmacodynamics of vecuronium. *Anesthesiology* 2000;92:84–93.
6. Callans DJ. Out-of-hospital cardiac arrest—the solution is shocking. *N Engl J Med* 2004;351:632–634.
7. Chamorro C, Borrallo JM, Romera MA, et al. Anesthesia and analgesia protocol during therapeutic hypothermia after cardiac arrest: a systematic review. *Anesth Analg* 2010;110:1328–1335.
8. Fritz HG, Holzmayr M, Walter B, et al. The effect of mild hypothermia on plasma fentanyl concentration and biotransformation in juvenile pigs. *Anesth Analg* 2005;100:996–1002.
9. Fugate JE, Wijdicks EFM, Mandrekar J, et al. Predictors of neurologic outcome in hypothermia after cardiac arrest. *Ann Neurol* 2010;68:907–914.
10. Heier T, Clough D, Wright PM, et al. The influence of mild hypothermia on the pharmacokinetics and time course of action of neostigmine in anesthetized volunteers. *Anesthesiology* 2002;97:90–95.
11. Hostler D, Zhou J, Tortorici MA, et al. Mild hypothermia alters midazolam pharmacokinetics in normal health volunteers. *Drug Metab Disposition* 2010;38:781–788.
12. Iida Y, Nishi S, Asada A. Effect of mild therapeutic hypothermia on phenytoin pharmacokinetics. *The Drug Monit* 2001;23:192–197.
13. Kadar D, Tang BK, Conn AW. The fate of phenobarbitone in children in hypothermia and at normal body temperature. *Can Anaesth Soc J* 1982;29:16–23.
14. Leslie K, Sessler DI, Bjorksten AR, et al. Mild hypothermia alters propofol pharmacokinetics and increases the duration of action of atracurium. *Anesth Analg* 1995;80:1007–1014.
15. Michelsen LG, Holford NH, Lu W, et al. The pharmacokinetics of remifentanil in patients undergoing coronary artery bypass grafting with cardiopulmonary bypass. *Anesth Analg* 2001;93:1100–1105.
16. Nolan JP, Morley PT, Vanden Hoek TL, et al. International Liaison Committee on Resuscitation. Therapeutic hypothermia after cardiac arrest: an advisory statement by the advanced lift support task force of the International Liaison Committee on Resuscitation. *Circulation* 2003;108:118–121.
17. Polderman KH, Herold I. Therapeutic hypothermia and controlled normothermia in the intensive care unit: practical considerations, side effects, and cooling methods. *Crit Care Med* 2009;37:1101–1120.
18. Sessler DI. Complications and treatment of mild hypothermia. *Anesthesiology* 2001;95:531–543.
19. Tortorici MA, Kochanek PM, Poloyac SM. Effects of hypothermia on drug disposition, metabolism, and response: a focus of hypothermia-mediated alterations on the cytochrome P450 enzyme system. *Crit Care Med* 2007;35:2196–2204.

Clinical Problem
15

Extracorporeal Membrane Oxygenation (ECMO) and Brain Death

■ THE COMMON CLINICAL QUESTIONS

What is the role of ECMO in an unstable brain death donor? How can we safely perform an apnea test in a patient on ECMO?

■ THE FACTS

Extracorporeal membrane oxygenation is an uncommon treatment modality and has been offered to limited numbers of patients in multiple settings. In large referral centers, only 50 to 60 adult patients were treated with ECMO over nearly a decade.[6,12] Extracorporeal membrane oxygenation provides extracirculatory support to adult patients and children in cardiac or respiratory failure who would otherwise be expected to die.[1-5,9] Intensive care with ECMO allows select patients to regain sustainable organ function and survive. Extracorporeal membrane oxygenation is not routinely used in adults, but it has been found to improve survival in some patients who undergo cardiopulmonary resuscitation (E-CPR) or experience other forms of severe cardiopulmonary injury. In 2009, the national Extracorporeal Life Support Organization registry reported on 295 adults treated with E-CPR.[2] In this large series, brain death occurred in 28% of patients.[2]

Extracorporeal membrane oxygenation has been extensively studied in infants. In the pediatric population, the most common cause of death on ECMO is intracranial hemorrhage rather than cardiopulmonary failure.[3,7] This raises concern that adult patients on ECMO are similarly at risk of death from neurologic injury; this could be related both to the precipitating event that led to ECMO and to ECMO therapy itself.[10]

In our experience with neurologic complications in ECMO, several patients lost their brainstem reflexes. Typically, such patients can be assessed using the standard criteria and assessments, but challenges in evaluation may include multiorgan failure, marked metabolic acidosis, and difficulty in performing an apnea test.

One way to resolve the difficulty with the apnea test is to blend in CO_2 through the circuit while measuring arterial blood gases. The patient is maintained on an anesthesia bag with a PEEP valve, and end-tidal CO_2 can be monitored to detect

TABLE 6-12 *Apnea Test in a Patient on ECMO*

- Place patient on CPAP through the anesthesia bag
- Maintain the necessary cardiac output through the ECMO circuit
- Provide the necessary oxygen concentration through the blender on the circuit at the lowest sweep flow possible (>90% oxygen saturation on pulse oximetry)
- Obtain a baseline arterial blood gas determination
- Blend in CO_2 incrementally from a baseline $PaCO_2$ of 40 mm Hg
- Measure arterial blood gas at 4-minute intervals and until a $PaCO_2$ of 60 mm Hg is reached (monitor with $ETCO_2$ device)

Abbreviations: CO_2, carbon dioxide; ECMO, extracorporeal membrane oxygenation; $ETCO_2$, end-tidal carbon dioxide; $PaCO_2$, arterial pressure of carbon dioxide.

breathing by the patient (Table 6-12). An alternative option is the use of an ancillary laboratory test. Cerebral blood flow studies require transport of the patient outside the ICU, which is virtually impossible. Moreover, in patients with diffuse anoxic-ischemic injury, these studies usually show persistent flow (cerebral edema may not have caused sufficiently increased intracranial pressure). An EEG may be easier to perform, but isoelectric EEGs may be associated with residual brainstem function and artifacts may be substantial.

Extracorporeal membrane oxygenation has also been used in patients who are markedly unstable following brain death examination. Despite receiving vasopressors, thyroid hormone, and vasopressin, some patients have systolic blood pressures barely reaching 60 mm Hg. This can rapidly lead to loss of organs. If there is a strong impetus for organ donation, and usually there is, ECMO can be successful in maintaining an adequate hemodynamic status. The mean arterial blood pressure can be maintained with ECMO support, even following cessation of cardiac activity. The Wisconsin solution can then be infused through the ECMO circuit, and kidneys can be placed on pulsatile pump perfusion. Extracorporeal membrane oxygenation has been employed less frequently to maintain organ function in DCD protocols, but there is growing interest. In these situations, ECMO is inserted through arterial and venous catheters before circulatory arrest, and maintaining the flow of oxygenated blood to the organs will reduce ischemia time.[8,11]

■ REFERENCES

1. Amigoni A, Pettenazzo A, Biban P, et al. Neurologic outcome in children after extracorporeal membrane oxygenation: prognostic value of diagnostic tests. *Pediatr Neurol* 2005;32:173–179.
2. Cardarelli MG, Young AJ, Griffith B. Use of extracorporeal membrane oxygenation for adults in cardiac arrest (E-CPR): a meta-analysis of observational studies. *ASAIO J* 2009;55:581–586.
3. Cilley RE, Zwischenger JB, Andrews AF, et al. Intracranial hemorrhage during extracorporeal membrane oxygenation in neonates. *Pediatrics* 1986;78:699–704.
4. Glass P, Miller M, Short B. Morbidity of survivors of extracorporeal membrane oxygenation: neurodevelopmental outcome at 1 year of age. *Pediatrics* 1989;83:72–78.

5. Huang S, Wu E, Chen Y, et al. Extracorporeal membrane oxygenation rescue for cardio-pulmonary resuscitation in pediatric patients. *Crit Care Med* 2008;36:1607–1613.

6. Lan C, Tsai P, Chen Y, et al. Prognostic factors for adult patients receiving extracorporeal membrane oxygenation as mechanical circulatory support—a 14-year experience at a medical center. *Artificial Organs* 2010;32:E59–E64.

7. Lidegran MK, Mosskin M, Ringertz HG, et al. Cranial CT for diagnosis of intracranial complications in adult and pediatric patients during ECMO: clinical benefits in diagnosis and treatment. *Acad Radiol* 2007;14:62–71.

8. Magliocca JF, Magee JC, Rowe SA, et al. Extracorporeal support for organ donation after cardiac death effectively expands the donor pool. *J Trauma Injury Infect Crit Care* 2005;58:1095–1102.

9. Massetti M, Tasle M, Le Page O, et al. Back from irreversibility: extracorporeal life support for prolonged cardiac arrest. *Ann Thorac Surg* 2005;79:178–184.

10. Risnes I, Wagner K, Nome T, et al. Cerebral outcome in adult patients treated with extracorporeal membrane oxygenation. *Ann Thorac Surg* 2006;81:1401–1407.

11. Rudich SM, Arenas JD, Magee JC, et al. Extracorporeal support of the nonheart-beating organ donor. *Transplantation* 2002;73:158–159.

12. Thiagarajan RR, Brogan TV, Scheuer MA, et al. Extracorporeal membrane oxygenation to support cardiopulmonary resuscitation in adults. *Ann Thorac Surg* 2009;87: 778–785.

Anencephaly and Brain Death

■ THE COMMON CLINICAL QUESTIONS

Can brain death be diagnosed in a neonate with anencephaly? Should anencephalics be intubated just for organ donation alone?

■ THE FACTS

Anencephaly is a rare neural tube closure defect.[5] The appearance of an anencephalic neonate is characteristic, with absence of the cranial vault and eye protrusion from shallow orbits. The brain consists of a poorly differentiated mass, but with recognizable glia, ependyma, and even choroid plexus.[8] There are different types of anencephaly, with some infants demonstrating a rudimentary brainstem and more or less absent midbrain and pons (Figure 6-7). In others, better differentiation of the upper brainstem can be found. The medulla oblongata may be well preserved.

Clinical examination is variable and is not necessarily dependent on the degree of preservation of the brainstem. One landmark study with detailed clinical findings at birth identified spontaneous movements; startle movements; suck, root, and gag responses; and also measurable pupillary, corneal, and oculocephalic reflexes.[2] In this study, only two patients were declared brain dead. Both infants were declared brain dead on the day of birth, but positive corneal, suck, and gag responses were present initially. Autopsy in one of the two brain-dead anencephalic neonates showed acute and chronic hemorrhage in the pons. Most remarkable, autopsy in these anencephalic infants showed poorly differentiated brainstem neuronal tissue but apparently sufficiently organized to produce reflex arcs. The neuropathology varied from rare primitive neuronal tissue to a few scattered neurons in the medulla and an absent pons to a near-normal-appearing brainstem.[2]

Anencephaly is often diagnosed prenatally, and most parents decide on elective pregnancy termination.[6] If the pregnancy continues, delivery may result in death in 35% of the cases, with mostly stillbirth or neonatal survival time of a few hours.[11]

Although the intervention is futile, neonates with anencephaly may be intubated following delivery at the request of the parents. (The hospital is required to

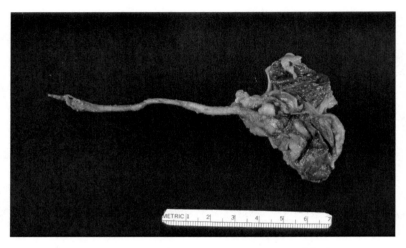

Figure 6-7 Gross macroscopic view showing some preservation of the brainstem structures but amorf cerebrum. *See* Figure 6-7 in the color insert.

treat an anencephalic infant if the parents insist.) These neonates may progress to loss of all brainstem function, but it is unknown if the parents would then accept brain death or even organ donation.

There are little data on the practice of determining brain death in anencephalic infants. Diagnosis of brain death in an anencephalic infant is similar to that in any other neonate; however, examination can be difficult to perform, and an observation period of to 24 to 48 hours has been recommended.[1-4,6,9] Long-term support of the anencephalic neonate is also on record. ("Baby K" in the United States is best known; her parents demanded that the physician keep her on a ventilator. When the physician tried to obtain a court order to withdraw support, the judge decided that aggressive care was warranted under the Americans with Disabilities Act, and Baby K lived for more than 2 years.[7,14])

A controversy started in the United States when the parents of an anencephalic infant ("Baby Theresa") asked a Florida court for permission to donate her organs.[12,13,15,16] The Florida Supreme Court, however, decided against organ donation because the baby did not meet the brain death criteria (there was intact brainstem function, and the child was breathing on her own).[14] Moreover, disabilities and right-to-life advocates created an outcry after the Council on Ethical and Judicial Affairs of the American Medical Association stated that anencephalic infants could be organ donors while still alive. However, the Council later rescinded the statement and reported that live-born anencephalic infants who do not meet the brain death criteria cannot be considered for organ donation.

Others have argued that anencephalic infants will die quickly, a considerable number of organs—about 1000 annually—will be lost, and an exception should be made concerning these unconscious neonates without a brain.[15,16] However, several organizations believe that such an exception may result in poor public policy, a slippery slope, and, ultimately, distrust.

Recently, the International Federation of Gynecology and Obstetrics published the statement that "the principal protection of the vulnerable newborn may apply in that an anencephalic infant may need protection against being treated only as a mean to another advantage."[10]

The discussion on anencephalic neonates is complicated. Strictly speaking, these infants have a functioning brainstem, but in some cases barely so, with little recognizable structure on neuropathology examination and the truth lies somewhere in between. If DCD protocols are in place in the hospital where the neonate is born, organ donation may still proceed after withdrawal of support, but the logistics and emotions may be very difficult to handle and there is no published experience.

■ REFERENCES

1. American Medical Association Council on Ethical and Judicial Affairs. The use of anencephalic neonates as organ donors. *JAMA* 1995;273:1614–1618.
2. Ashwal S, Peabody JL, Schneider S, et al. Anencephaly: clinical determination of brain death and neuropathologic studies. *Pediatr Neurol* 1990;6:233–239.
3. Bard JS. The diagnosis is anencephaly and the parents ask about organ donation: now what? A guide for hospital council and ethics committees. *West N Engl Law Rev* 1999;21:49–95.
4. Botkin JR. Anencephalic infants as organ donors. *Pediatrics* 1988;82:250–256.
5. Cameron M, Moran P. Prenatal screening and diagnosis of neural tube defects. *Prenat Diagn* 2009;29:402–411.
6. Cranford RE. Anencephalic infants as organ donors. *Transplant Proc* 1992;24: 2218–2220.
7. Doczy LC, Trieger R, Gedik A. Anencephaly and right to life. *Lancet* 1993;342: 1558–1559.
8. *Greenfield's Neuropathology*. 6th ed. Love S, Louis DN, Ellison DW, eds.London: Hodder Arnold; 2008.
9. Harrison MR. Organ procurement for children: the anencephalic fetus as donor. *Lancet* 1986;132:1383–1386.
10. Milliez J. FIGO Committee for the Ethical Aspects of Human Reproduction and Women's Health. Anencephaly and organ transplantation. *Int J Gynecol Obstet* 2008;102:99.
11. Obeidi N, Russell N, Higgins JR, et al. The natural history of anencephaly. *Prenat Diagn* 2010;30:357–360.
12. Paris JJ, Signorello G. The use of anencephalic organ donors: lesson of Baby Theresa. *Ann Clin Ethics Rep* 1992;6:3–6.
13. Reagan JE. Ethics consultation: anencephaly and organ donation. *J Law Med Ethics* 1995;23:402–403.
14. Stumpf DA, Cranford RE, Elias S, et al. The infant with anencephaly. The Medical Task Force on anencephaly. *N Engl J Med* 1990;322:669–674.
15. Truog RD, Fletcher JC. Brain death and the anencephalic newborn. *Bioethics* 1990;4: 199–215.
16. Walters J, Shawl S, Masek T. Anencephaly: where do we now stand? *Semin Neurol* 1997;17:249–255.

Clinical Problem 17

Shaken Baby Syndrome and Brain Death

■ THE COMMON CLINICAL QUESTIONS

What are the indicators of neurologic injury from child abuse? What are the neuroimaging features in shaken baby syndrome?

■ THE FACTS

The term *shaken baby syndrome* has many synonyms (*shaken impact syndrome, battered baby, nonaccidental head injury*).[2,18,20] Shaken baby syndrome is typically observed in children less than 3 years of age, with a peak incidence in the first year.[5,25] A history of child abuse and foul play is commonly inconsistent or incomplete.[24]

It may be prevalent, with one study in children with subdural hematomas suggesting that more than half had abusive injury.[10] A prospective epidemiologic study in pediatric units in Scotland found a high annual incidence of 24.6 per 100,000 children younger than 1 year.[8] In the United States, it is common in urban regions and during fall and winter months. Risk factors for shaken baby syndrome are younger parents, low socioeconomic status, child disability, and premature birth. Fathers, boyfriends, and female babysitters most often cause the injuries; less commonly, the mother of the child is implicated.[9,14] Although the clinical features are well delineated, the syndrome is still shrouded in controversy and hyperbolized in legal proceedings.[3,4,6,7,11-13,22]

Brain death is a consequence of sustained increased intracranial pressure that usually appears in close proximity to the injury. The clinical examination of a brain-dead infant after abuse is similar to that in any other infant. In some countries, cerebral flow studies are performed to document absent flow, but with increasing intracranial pressure, the fontanelles bulge and may allow considerable pressure.[23] On examination, the infant is comatose, is commonly mildly to moderately anemic, and may display signs of severe disseminated intravascular coagulation. Pancreatic traumatic damage may be seen, with high amylase levels, and liver injury may also be present.[17] Femur, humerus, and rib fractures (i.e., of different ages and bilateral) and superficial bruises should be actively sought (Figure 6-8). Other fracture locations that are suspicious are scapula, spinous process, and sternum, but the metaphyseal

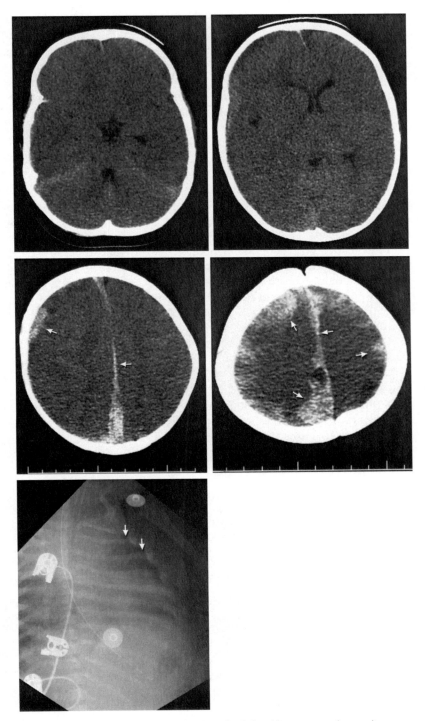

Figure 6-8 Both subarachnoid hemorrhage and subdural hematomas (arrows) are seen on CT scans of a child with shaken baby syndrome. Multiple rib fractures are noted on the chest x-ray (arrows).

fracture of the distal tibia and fibula (toddler's fracture) is a high-specificity indicator in a child not walking.[1,21] A fairly common finding is bilateral retinal hemorrhage (60%), which should be specifically sought. The presence of retinal hemorrhages together with retinal folds or detachments, which can be seen only after expert evaluation by an ophthalmologist, is much more suggestive of the diagnosis.[15,16] In children with increased intracranial pressure a rhythmic pulse of the fontanelle is often found and transmits the systolic wave of the cerebrospinal fluid.

The CT scan may detect skull fractures (on bone windows) that could be multiple and cross suture lines. The CT scan typically detects a subarachnoid hemorrhage and subdural hematomas or diffuse brain edema indistinguishable from the patterns seen in anoxic-ischemic injury.[19] The CT scan may also include petechial or punctate hemorrhages along the gyral surfaces and the inferior surface of the frontal and temporal poles (Figure 6-8). The brain is hypodense, with loss of white matter–gray matter differentiation but with sparing of the basal ganglia and posterior fossa structures. Intentional injury is more likely when the CT scan shows subdural hematoma over the convexity or in the interhemispheric fissure. The presence of layers of subdural hematomas of different ages is very suggestive of nonaccidental traumatic brain injury. The age of the subdural hematoma may be difficult to estimate, and an MRI could be more useful in this determination.[19] Contrecoup lesions are perhaps more common and are a reflection of acceleration/deceleration force.

The coroner will perform an autopsy. Eventually, pathologic examination is an important adjunct in confirming the clinical diagnosis. However, the interpretation of injury is complex, and a meticulous autopsy is usually performed by experts in this field. Courts have often questioned shaking as a major impact. Relevant studies have recently been published.[11,24]

■ REFERENCES

1. Adamsbaum C, Méjean N, Merzoug V, et al. How to explore and report children with suspected non-accidental trauma. *Pediatr Radiol* 2010;40:932–938.
2. Al-Holou WN, O'Hara EA, Cohen-Gadol AA, et al. Nonaccidental head injury in children. Historical vignette. *J Neurosurg Pediatr* 2009;3:474–483.
3. American Academy of Pediatrics Committee on Child Abuse and Neglect. Shaken baby syndrome: rotational cranial injuries—technical report. *Pediatrics* 2001;108:206–210.
4. Bandak FA. Shaken baby syndrome: a biomechanics analysis of injury mechanisms. *Forensic Sci Int* 2005;151:71–79.
5. Barlow KM, Minns RA. Annual incidence of shaken impact syndrome in young children. *Lancet* 2000;356:1571–1772.
6. Caffey J. The whiplash shaken infant syndrome: manual shaking by the extremities with whiplash-induced intracranial and intraocular bleedings, linked with residual permanent brain damage and mental retardation. *Pediatrics* 1974;54:396–403.
7. Case ME, Graham MA, Handy TC, et al. Position paper on fatal abusive head injuries in infants and young children. *Am J Forensic Med Pathol* 2001;22:112–122.
8. David TJ. Shaken baby (shaken impact) syndrome: nonaccidental head injury in infancy. *J R Soc Med* 1999;92:556–561.
9. Duhaime AC, Christian CW, Rorke LB, et al. Nonaccidental head injury in infant; the "shaken-baby syndrome." *N Engl J Med* 1998;338:1822–1829.

10. Feldman KW, Bethel R, Shugerman RP. The cause of infant and toddler subdural hemorrhage: a prospective study. *Pediatrics* 2001; 108:636–646.
11. Furness P. Shaken baby syndrome: report of pathologist meeting. *BMJ* 2010;340:c2397.
12. Geddes JF, Hackshaw AK, Vowles GH, et al. Neuropathology of inflicted head injury in children. I. Patterns of brain damage. *Brain* 2001;124:1290–1298.
13. Geddes JF, Vowles GH, Hackshaw AK, et al. Neuropathology of inflicted head injury in children. II. Microscopic brain injury in infants. *Brain* 2001;124:1299–1306.
14. Gerber P, Coffman K. Nonaccidental head trauma in infants. *Childs Nerv Syst* 2007;23:499–507.
15. Morad Y, Kim YM, Mian M, et al. Nonophthalmologist accuracy in diagnosing retinal hemorrhages in the shaken baby syndrome. *J Pediatr* 2003;142:431–434.
16. Morad Y, Wygnanski-Jaffe T, Levin AV. Retinal hemorrhage in abusive head trauma. *Clin Experiment Ophtalmol* 2010;38:514–520.
17. Mraz MA. The physical manifestations of shaken baby syndrome. *J Forensic Nurs* 2009;5:26–30.
18. Newton AW, Vandeven AM. Update on child maltreatment. *Curr Opin Pediatr* 2008;20:205–212.
19. Petitti N, Williams DW III. CT and MR imaging of nonaccidental pediatric head trauma. *Acad Radiol* 1998; 5:215–223.
20. Roche AJ, Fortin G, Labbe J, et al. The work of Ambroise Tardieu: the first definitive description of child abuse. *Child Abuse Negl* 2005;29:325–334.
21. Spevak MR, Kleinman PK, Belanger PL, et al. Cardiopulmonary resuscitation and rib fractures in infants: a postmortem radiologic–pathologic study. *JAMA* 1994;272: 617–618.
22. Uscinski R. Shaken baby syndrome: fundamental questions. *Br J Neurosurg* 2002;16: 217–219.
23. Vicenzini E, Pulitano P, Cicchetti R, et al. Transcranial Doppler for brain death in infants: the role of the fontanelles. *Eur Neurol* 2010;63:164–169.
24. Vinchon M, de Foort-Dhellemmes S, Desurmont M, et al. Confessed abuse versus witnessed accident in infants: comparison of clinical, radiological, and ophthalmological data in corroborated cases. *Child Nerv Syst* 2010;26:637–645.
25. Wells RG, Vetter C, Laud P. Intracranial hemorrhage in children younger than 3 years: prediction of intent. *Arch Pediatr Adolesc Med* 2002;156:252–227.

Clinical Problem 18

Maternal Brain Death

■ THE COMMON CLINICAL QUESTIONS

In order to salvage the fetus, is prolonged support possible in brain dead mothers? What is the outcome of a fetus after maintenance of a brain-dead mother?

■ THE FACTS

Obstetric admission to the ICU often involves hypertensive emergencies, but maternal death is uncommon.[19] Brain death during pregnancy, particularly in the last trimester, is equally rare. In one series, postdelivery catastrophic neurologic illness resulting in brain death was found in 11 of 252 patients (4%).[13] In our experience with over 300 brain death determinations, only 1 patient was in the early stages of pregnancy.

A major ethical quandary presents when a patient is diagnosed with brain death and carries a potentially viable fetus. Support of the brain dead mother would be provided until the baby could be delivered. Typically, a fetus of 16 weeks or older could prompt such support. Because the survival rate of the neonate is approximately 80% and neurologic morbidity is less than 10%, somatic support could be provided until the gestational age of 28 weeks, but earlier delivery of an immature—and more medically and neurologically complicated—infant has been described.

The cost of ICU care is very high, and is followed in successful cases by the high costs of postneonatal care of the immature infant. Nonetheless, in the reported cases of premature birth, the babies had normal developmental milestones despite having low Apgar scores. Follow-up into adolescence is, however, not available.

Long-term support of a brain-dead pregnant patient is complicated, and it is most likely that unsuccessful cases have not been reported in the literature. The medical literature suggests that there are approximately 30 reported cases of prolonged support of a brain-dead mother since 1982. (A selection of cases with reasonable documentation is shown in Table 6-13.)[1,2,4,6,8,12,14,15,21] There has not been a successful neonatal outcome reported in the US or Europe in the last decade.

It is also possible that some patients were not officially declared brain dead. In several instances, the apnea test may not have been performed for fear of causing

TABLE 6-13   *Cases of Prolonged Support of the Fetus after Diagnosis of Maternal Brain Death*

Case Reports	Details of Brain Death Examination N/NN	Ancillary Test	Gestation at Diagnosis	Gestation at Delivery	Fetal Outcome	Support for Complications
Dillon et al.[3]	N	EEG	23 weeks	24 weeks	Normal at 3 months	BP fluctuations and shock prompted cesarean section
Heikkinen et al.[7]	N†	EEG	21 weeks	31 weeks	Normal at 8 months	DI developed 3rd week and hypotension 2nd week
Field et al.[15]	NN	EEG	22 weeks	31 weeks	Normal at 18 months	Sepsis, DI
Bernstein et al.[2]	NN	EEG	15 weeks	32 weeks	Normal at 11 months	VAP, DI, bradycardia
Wuermeling[20]	NN	EEG/Doppler	13 weeks	19 weeks	Died	Sepsis
Nettina et al.[14]	NN	—	27 weeks	33 weeks	No follow-up	Pulmonary edema, DI
Vives et al.[19]	NN	EEG	27 weeks	27 weeks	Within 2 days delivery, no follow up	
Lewis and Vidovich[11]	NN	—	25 weeks	32 weeks	Live birth; good outcome at 1 year	DI, sepsis
Spike[16]	NN	EEG/nuclear scan	17 weeks	31 weeks	Apgar score 8; no follow-up	DI
Lane et al.[10]	N*	—	13 weeks	19 weeks	Fetus died	DI, VAP
Hussein et al.[9]	NN	—	26 weeks	28 weeks	Live birth; good outcome at 2 years	
Souza et al.[15]	NN	TCD	25 weeks	28 weeks	Apgar 10, normal at 3 months	DI, VAP
Mejia, et al.[13]	NN	EEG	17 weeks	25 weeks	Live birth, no outcome	Cardiac arrest, DI
Yeung, et al.[21]	NN	EP	15 weeks	27 weeks	Apgar 8, died of necrotizing enterocolitis	DI

*Serial exams mentioned but no details. †Apnea test not performed.

Abbreviations: DI, diabetes insipidus; N, neurologist involved; NN, no neurologic details or neurologist involved; TCD, transcranial Doppler; VAP, ventilator-associated pneumonia.

hypoxemic injury to the fetus. Obviously, the vast majority of the brain-dead mothers were not considered organ donors, and thus a full neurologic evaluation was likely not completed. Details on brain death testing in the published reports are absent, and in most reports there was no documented neurology or neurosurgery involvement. It is therefore far more likely that these patients may still have had some retained medulla oblongata function that would make long-term hemodynamic support much more feasible. Moreover, sudden marked difficulties with treatment of hemodynamic support—using progressively more combinations and higher doses of intravenous fluids and inotropic medications—have been described after several weeks of support, suggesting that the catastrophically injured mothers became brain dead later.

Most of the problems associated with prolonged support are potential injuries to the fetus. Hyperglycemia in the mother may occur, temperature regulation may be difficult, and infectious complications may lead to premature spontaneous abortion. Prolongation of the pregnancy sometimes is achieved with magnesium sulfate infusion. In general, long-term support includes adequate hemodynamic support with vasopressors, control of poikilothermia using either cooling or warming, and use of parenteral alimentation guided by serial measurements of 24-hour urea nitrogen excretion and serum prealbumin levels. Suggestions on supportive care have been published, but there is virtually no experience in how to adequately support these brain-dead mothers.[4]

Generally, documentation of gestation time by ultrasound of more than 16 weeks may result in the decision to support a comatose patient with a major catastrophic neurologic injury. A fetus less than 16 weeks of age warrants extraordinarily long ICU support, almost certainly with an unsuccessful outcome.

If there is no realistic possibility of delivery of a live neonate, withdrawal of care in the ICU is likely to proceed. Support of the family—who likely has seen the moving fetus during ultrasound—requires extra attention. Legal advice should be sought, and decisions may be more complicated because some countries recognize a legal standing of the fetus. Organ donation in a brain-dead mother with a live fetus is also ethically charged, and some organ procurement agencies have not wanted to proceed because the inevitable death of the fetus may then be linked to organ donation (clamping of the aorta will lead to immediate death of the fetus).

■ REFERENCES

1. Anstotz C. Should a brain-dead pregnant woman carry her child to full term? The case of the "Erlanger Baby." *Bioethics* 1993;7:340–350.
2. Bernstein IM, Watson M, Simmons GM, et al. Maternal brain death and prolonged fetal survival. *Obstet Gynecol* 1989;74:434–437.
3. Dillon WP, Lee RV, Tronolone MJ, et al. Life support and maternal death during pregnancy. *JAMA* 1982;248:1089–1091.
4. Esmaeilzadeh M, Dictus C, Kayvanpour et al. One life begins, another ends. Management of a brain dead pregnant mother–a systematic review. *BMC Medicine* 2010;8:74.
5. Field DR, Gates EA, Creasy RK, et al. Maternal brain death during pregnancy. Medical and ethical issues. *JAMA* 1988;260:816–822.

6. Hauksson A, Akerlund M, Melin P. Uterine blood flow and myometrial activity at menstruation, and action of vasopressin and a synthetic antagonist. *Ann NY Acad Sci* 1994;734:47–56.
7. Heikkinen JE, Rinne RI, Alahuhta SM, et al. Life support for 10 weeks with successful fetal outcome after fatal maternal brain damage. *Br Med J* 1985;290:1237–1238.
8. Hurtado GF, Juarez MZ, Sandoval Munro RL, et al. Apoyo nutricio en una mujer embarazada y con muerte cerebral. Informe de un caso y revision de la literatura. *Nutr Hosp* 2007;22:503–506.
9. Hussein IY, Govenden V, Grant JM, et al. Prolongation of pregnancy in a woman who sustained brain death at 26 weeks of gestation. *BJOG* 2006;113:120–122.
10. Lane A, Westbrook A, Grady D, et al. Maternal brain death: medical, ethical, and legal issues. *Intensive Care Med* 2004;30:1484–1486.
11. Lewis DD, Vidovich RR. Organ recovery following childbirth by a brain-dead mother. A case report. *J Transpl Coord* 1997;7:103–105.
12. Mallampalli A, Guy E. Cardiac arrest in pregnancy and somatic support after brain death. *Crit Care Med* 2005;33:S325–S331.
13. Mejia R, Badariotti G, De Diego B, et al. Brain death in a pregnant woman and fetus survival. *Medicina (Buenos Aires)* 2008;68:447–452.
14. Nettina M, Santos E, Ascioti KJ, et al. Sheila's death created many rings of life. *Nursing* 1995;23:44–48.
15. Souza JP, Oliveira-Neto A, Surita FG, et al. The prolongation of somatic support in a pregnant woman with brain-death: a case report. *Reprod Health* 2006;3:3.
16. Spike J. Brain death, pregnancy, and posthumous motherhood. *J Clin Ethics* 1999;10:57–65.
17. Suddaby EC, Schaeffer MJ, Brigham LE, et al. Analysis of organ donors in the peripartum period. *J Transplant Coord* 1998;8:35–39.
18. Togal T, Yucel N, Gedik E, et al. Obstetric admissions to the intensive care unit in a tertiary referral hospital. *J Crit Care* 2010;25:628–633.
19. Vives A, Carmona F, Zabala E, et al. Maternal brain death during pregnancy. *Int J Gynaecol Obstet* 1996;52:67–69.
20. Wuermeling HB. Brain-death and pregnancy. *Forensic Sci Int* 1994;69:243–245.
21. Yeung P, McManus C, Tchabo JG. Extended somatic support for a pregnant woman with brain death from metastatic malignant melanoma: a case report. *J Matern Fetal Neonatal Med* 2008;21:509–511.

Legal Challenges in Brain Death

■ THE COMMON CLINICAL QUESTIONS

What are the most common legal challenges that may come to the courtroom? How have the court rulings been? How do physicians handle criminal cases resulting in brain death?

■ THE FACTS

In the early days of transplantation, liability and fear of unjust litigation by those involved in organ procurement may have been common.[1] It prompted the development of the Uniform Determination of Death Act.[4,5] Concerns have also been raised about whether court action could arise from declaring patients dead by neurologic criteria involving murder cases. Defendants of first-degree murder would charge that physicians caused the death of the patient and that removal of life support measures from a brain-dead victim was the proximate cause of death.[2] The courts have been clear and firm in their rejection of these claims.

In all court cases recently reviewed, only 5% actually addressed disputes on the diagnosis of brain death.[3] From this review it appears that nothing in the court cases has the potential to change the current medical standard of brain death determination and—as usual—the law is not a guide for medical practice. Adherence to accepted guidelines, such as these issued by the American Academy of Neurology (Chapter 2), remains the norm. The court judgments listed in Table 6-14 best summarize the current law.

The legal challenges have involved documentation. Accurate diagnosis of brain death has a profound influence on the availability and monetary amount of personal claims for damages or reimbursement that may arise from the eventual death of the patient. Legal precedent suggests that practitioners may also best ensure their protection from claims brought against them by family members or other patient representatives by timely documentation of brain death. Physicians and hospitals must also be aware that courts have established that medical liability for malpractice, and for pain and suffering claims, continues until the time of formal brain death diagnosis.

The documentation of brain death has a profound influence on the property interests of the heirs of the deceased. Courts have accepted documentation of brain death noted in a physician's note predating a death certificate as a "stop" to changes

TABLE 6-14 *Areas of Emphasis in Court Cases Involving the Diagnosis of Brain Death*

	I. Importance of Documentation Involving Timing of Death	
Case Citation	Court Decision	Physician Consequence
Cavagnaro v. Hanover Ins. Co.	Following injuries suffered in automobile accident, hospital expenses in maintaining and continuing intensive care support systems after confirmation of irreversible brain death are not reimbursable through "no fault" insurance payouts because they are not incurred to "preserve life and relieve the patient as much as possible from pain and disability".	Proper and timely determination of brain death by physician may impact availability of insurance proceeds to reimburse hospital expenses for care provided to an accident victim.
Ajnoha v. J.C. Penny Life Ins. Co.	Jury should be allowed to hear conflicting physician expert opinions as to both diagnosis and timing of brain death when making judgments on availability of insurance proceeds payable to decedent's beneficiaries.	Physicians charged with diagnosing brain death may have profound influence on the availability of time-sensitive insurance proceeds offered to decedent's beneficiaries. Disputes between physician experts as to time or diagnosis of brain death will be left to jury to decide.
Bassie v. Obstetrics & Gynecology Assoc. of Northwest Alabama	Once person is diagnosed as brain dead, the person is both medically and legally dead and heirs may not subsequently file personal injury claim on the decedent's behalf; remedy is limited to wrongful death.	Viability of legal claims brought on behalf of patient may be dependent on time of brain death diagnosis, both accurate and time-sensitive documentation by diagnosing physician is imperative.
Mineroff v. Silber	Claims allowed for medical malpractice and pain and suffering between the time of initial diagnosis of brain death and final declaration of brain death after discontinuation of intensive care support.	As legal awards for malpractice and pain and suffering up to the declaration of brain death are allowable, timely documentation of brain death can limit ongoing damages claims.
Estate of Sewart v. Taff	Time listed in death certificate establishes time of death when determining sequence of death for transfer of money to a will beneficiary. Without expert testimony to contrary, individual cannot be diagnosed as legally brain dead at a point prior to the documented date and time supplied on death certificate.	Because property and money exchanges between beneficiaries of a decedent's will often hinge on time of brain death diagnosis, it is important for physician to accurately document time of brain death.

(Continues)

TABLE 6-14 *Areas of Emphasis in Court Cases Involving the Diagnosis of Brain Death* (Continued)

	I. Importance of Documentation Involving Timing of Death	
Case Citation	Court Decision	Physician Consequence
Crobons v. Wisconsin National Life Ins. Co.	Physician documentation of a diagnosis of brain death within the medical record that predates the formal timing of the death certificate determines legal time of death for purposes of life insurance payout.	As beneficiaries to life insurance policies may be changed up until the death of a patient, the time of brain death diagnosis is highly determinative of life insurance payouts. If the patient record documents a diagnosis of brain death that predates the formal certification of death by "death certificate," the documentation in the patient record supersedes and determines the time of death.
Farlow v. Roddy	Decedent's heirs may collect damages for pain and suffering that occur prior to the final declaration of brain death even if the brain death occurred within minutes of the insult to life.	As legal claims for pain and suffering may occur until brain death is declared, both accurate and time-sensitive physician diagnosis and documentation of brain death are important.

	II. Family Interference or Involvement With Brain Death Diagnosis	
Case Citation	*Court Decision*	*Physician Consequence*
Virk v. Detroit Receiving Hosp. and Univ. Health Ctr.	Physician may discontinue intensive care support measures once diagnosis of brain death is established, even when against family wishes and what might be construed as murder within the Islamic faith.	Formal diagnosis of brain death enables physician to remove intensive care support measures despite family members' objection.
Matter of Long Island Jewish Med. Ctr.	Hospital may terminate intensive care support measures from brain-dead patient against family wishes as long as facility has met standards set forth by state law ensuring that reasonable accommodation for religious or moral objection be addressed.	Once brain death is confirmed and any requirements under state law for religious or moral objections to be heard have been met, hospitals may terminate intensive care support measures against family wishes.
In the Matter of Alvarado v. New York City Health & Hosp. Corp.	Hospital may remove supportive care from newborn against family wishes when following determination of death in state Department of Health regulation that is both consistent with current medical knowledge and law.	Hospitals may terminate intensive care support measures against family wishes at diagnosis of patient's brain death.
Strachan v. John F. Kennedy Memorial Hosp.	Hospital may be found negligent for failing to turn over a dead body to family when hospital continued intensive care support measures after formal diagnosis of brain death and despite family's refusal to further consider organ donation options.	Hospital may not continue intensive care support measures (pending possible organ donation or otherwise) against family's wishes once patient has been formally diagnosed as brain dead.

Gallups v. Cotter	Physicians who, upon a formal diagnosis of brain death, terminated intensive care support measures against family wishes found not guilty of intentional or reckless tort of outrage.	Physician who terminates intensive care support measures upon a proper diagnosis of brain death, yet against family wishes, is not liable for emotional distress caused to family members of deceased.
Jacobsen v. Marin Gen. Hosp.	Coroner or medical examiner is authorized to dispose of unclaimed body for the purpose of organ transplantation after certain period of time following diagnosis of brain death. Once a diagnosis of brain death is confirmed and a proper search for next of kin has occurred for preset period of time, unclaimed body may be released for organ procurement without risk of liability if relatives to deceased are later found.	Physician documentation of brain death plays important role in establishing time required before organ procurement from unclaimed body can take place.
Smith v. Methodist Hosp. of Indiana	Hospital has no legal duty to disclose the incompetent (brain dead) patient's condition to the patient's family because information is not related to course of medical treatment.	Physician or other hospital representative has no legal duty to report the status of a brain-dead patient to decedent's relations, as this information has no ongoing medical relevance to the care of a patient in such condition.

Source: Adapted from Burkle CM, Schipper AM, Wijdicks EFM. Brain death and the Courts.[3] Used with permission from *Neurology.*

made by insurance beneficiaries (*Crobons v. Wisconsin National Life Insurance Company*). When only death certificate documentation exists, courts have refused to allow into evidence conflicting arguments as to the time of death that may be made by persons outside the medical field (*Estate of Sewart v. Taff*). Physicians must therefore be cognizant that the accuracy and timeliness of brain death formulation may have a bearing on inheritance of a deceased person's property.

Another theme in courts involves the emotionally laden area of dispute between family members and the medical profession with regard to withdrawal of support. Courts have routinely held that physicians may terminate care of a brain-dead patient even when this conflicts with the wishes of the family (*Virk v. Detroit Receiving Hospital and University Health center, Matter of Long Island Jewish Medical Center, In the Matter of Alvaradov. New York City Hospitals Corp.*). Furthermore, a 1988 Alabama Supreme Court decision assured physician immunity for such decisions on termination against families' wishes when it held that a practitioner is not liable for the emotional stress caused to family members stemming from the conflict (*Gallups v. Cotter*).

When evaluating whether a medical malpractice is the proximate cause of death, the courts look at the *relatedness* of the medical or surgical procedure to the injury the patient may have suffered outside of the clinical setting. The courts again suggested the importance of *relatedness* when it established that life support cessation and subsequent organ donation would not have resulted had the victim not suffered from (being *related* to) the initial out-of-hospital injury.[3]

Brain death in homicidal conduct poses significant challenges. When the case comes to trial, clinicians who have determined brain death may be deposed. Investigations may involve scrutiny of specific errors that can be technical—for example, failure to completely document a neurologic examination or to perform an apnea test inappropriately, which results in marked hypoxemia and cardiac arrest, or failure to measure a $PaCO_2$ level, which is considered a generally accepted standard. When the homicidal conduct involves drugs, brain death examination should not be completed; such an examination constitutes lack of adherence to professional standards. The nature and location of the injuries needs to be documented for medicolegal purposes. For example, if a patient is shot in the heart and dies from anoxic encephalopathy, then surgeons would probably restrict organ donation to locations outside the chest area, but the other tissue could still be used after external photographic documentation.

After death is declared, the coroner or medical examiner should be contacted. This person takes jurisdiction of the body until an autopsy and other evidence gathering is complete.

■ REFERENCES

1. Beresford HR. Legal aspects of termination of treatment decisions. *Neurol Clin* 1989;7:775–787.
2. Beresford HR. Brain death.*Neurol Clin* 1999;17:295.
3. Burkle CM, Schipper AM, Wijdicks EFM. Brain Death and the Courts . *Neurology* 2011 76:837–841.
4. Morenski JD, Oro JJ, Tobias JD, et al. Determination of death by neurological criteria. *J Intensive Care Med* 2003;18:211–221.
5. Uniform Determination of Death Act, 12 uniform laws annotated 589 (West 1993 and West supp (1997)).

Clinical Problem 20

Family Opposition to Accepting Brain Death

■ THE COMMON CLINICAL QUESTIONS

What should be done if the family refuses withdrawal of support? What should be done if religious reasons are mentioned?

■ THE FACTS

Family opposition to brain death may occur, and is most often as a result of a specific cultural view. Brain death has been accepted by all major religions (Chapter 3). However, in New York and New Jersey, devout Orthodox Jews can demand that the attending physician continues support and respects their religious belief that cardiac arrest is the only sign of death.[3] In 1991, New York and New Jersey enacted such a law providing this exception.

If families fail to accept brain death as death, there are two options. First, the physician should consider to maintain full support for 2 to 3 days and ask for assistance from a hospital ethics committee to explain to the family that brain death is death of the person. Spiritual counsel may be sought. Physicians should appreciate sensitivities of the family members in question and try to achieve closure. In our limited experience, this approach has worked best. Continuing support should be full support. It is questionable practice to maintain mechanical ventilation and stop administering vasopressors causing hypotension (such an action is reminiscent of the so-called slow code).

Second, if the family refuses to agree and remains intransigent, legal advice should be obtained. A local judge will then decide and can be expected to declare the patient dead, which would then allow withdrawal of support.

On rare occasions, families may request certain rituals after the diagnosis of brain death has been made.[1] A comprehensive discussion has been recently published describing a request for the administration of an unknown herbal supplement that the family believed could have a potential impact. Other requests may involve certain washings or administration of certain substances (often Chinese medicine). Some request can generally be honored. It has been called "compassionate futility," but such an approach will not be acceptable to most physicians.[1,2] Physicians are in no way obliged to administer such medicine, particularly if this would lead to a delay in the diagnosis of brain death or potentially jeopardize organ donation. One request may be followed by other requests, which could lead to prolonged continued care of a patient who has been declared dead. Honoring the request may also imply that physicians are now considering the possibility that this intervention might have an effect. Others have rightfully argued that to support such beliefs would "violate the intellectual integrity of medicine as a profession."[2] Brain death is death of the person. If there is no organ donation, withdrawal of support is the appropriate course of action.[2] No intensive care physician has the obligation to care for a legally deceased person and hold a bed (causing potential of refusal of other sick patients).

■ REFERENCES

1. Appelbaum AI, Tilburt JC, Collins MT, et al. A family's request for complementary medicine after patient brain death. *JAMA* 2008;299:2188–2193.
2. McCullough LB. Request for complementary medicine after brain death. *JAMA* 2008;300:1517.
3. Olick RS. Brain death, religious freedom, and public policy: New Jersey's landmark legislative initiative. *Kennedy Inst Ethics J* 1991;1:275–292.

Sperm and Oocyte Retrieval in Brain Death

■ THE COMMON CLINICAL QUESTIONS

What are the ethical concerns related to sperm and oocyte retrieval in brain death? Given a strong desire of the family to proceed, what are some of the positions? What is the necessary documentation that would allow retrieval?

■ THE FACTS

Occasionally, a request for sperm retrieval and storage is proposed by the wife of a patient declared brain dead.[15-18] And, a husband may request oocyte retrieval for future insemination on the assumption that this was the patient's wish. Postmortem oocyte retrieval has not been reported in the literature, and the practice is unknown.[5,6] There are a number of ethical questions to be asked. They include the ownership rights (spouse versus parents), the expense of retrieval and storage, and the future well-being of a single-parent child. The intent of the deceased, particularly if the person has expressed a desire for conception, should also be considered. Sperm or oocyte retrieval is different ethically than organ donation. The former is intended for the patient's husband or wife and is simply a matter of gratification; the latter involves saving the lives of others.

The technique of sperm retrieval can be multifold. It may include vibratory stimulation, transrectal electroejaculation, or, most commonly, orchiectomy of one or both testicles. This provides immature sperm, but this can be used for in vitro fertilization. These procedures can be interpreted as invasion of the body's integrity, particularly if there is no consent. Posthumous semen procurement requires approval and is often refused by the courts.[1-3,7,14] Hospital policies may exist and often specifically require an advance directive, written or verbal, with evidence of implied consent from the patient. This is often lacking, but the request should still be carefully vetted.

A recent review pointed out possible ICU medications that could result in sperm dysfunction. These include epinephrine and norepinephrine; the latter alters testosterone, and it may cause ischemia to the seminiferous organs. Calcium channel blockers also inhibit sperm activity and spermatogenesis.[2] There is no systematic study of the success of the retrieval procedures, particularly in patients

TABLE 6-15 *Issues to Discuss with the Family Prior to*
Oocyte or Sperm Retrieval

- *Documentation*: Virtually every hospital policy demands some form of documentation.
- *Success rate*: Unpredictable and less than 30% in artificial stimulation (may be less than 15% in women at ages 40–42). There is the possibility of decreased sperm quality from critically ill patients.
- *Timing of posthumous reproduction*: Unknown, but a 1-year waiting period has been suggested.
- *Expenses*: Very high costs involved in the fertility procedures needed to have the child and raise the child. Probably not covered by insurance plans.
- *Ethics*: Stigma of raising a child or children without the biological parent.
- *Inheritance*: The child could be considered the rightful heir to the parents' estate, directly affecting other family members.

who are brain dead.[3,12,13] The results in patients in a persistent vegetative state cannot be extrapolated to brain death.[4,9]

Again, the physician should inquire about an expressed desire to have children. Documentation of pregnancy wishes is needed, but is rarely available. Strong indications include recent discontinuation of oral contraceptives, attending a fertility clinic, or prior discussion with family members. It will be difficult to find convincing evidence in most instances. Another complicating matter is that a gestational carrier may be uncertain, and often some commitment from a family member is needed or at least suggested. Finally, oocyte retrieval follows ovarian hyperstimulation for 7 to 10 days, and in unstable organ donors this may be a medical challenge.[6] The effect of vasopressors on oocytes is not known. After being harvested, the oocytes would be fertilized and cryopreserved or preserved unfertilized.[11] Embryo cryopreservation introduces a new set of legal and ethical problems involving the discarding of embryos.

The American Society for Reproductive Medicine's Ethics Committee has stated that "a spouse's request that sperm or ova be obtained terminally or soon after death without the prior consent or known wishes of the deceased spouse need not be honored."[6] In both instances, the ethical issues extend to the life of a potential motherless or fatherless child, social stigmatization, and possible other disadvantages, such as financial difficulties without a father. Some have termed such a child a *commemorative child*, but the long-term consequences are not known. Furthermore, the success rate of the entire procedure is less than 30%.[8]

A summary of all of the major issues is found in Table 6-15, and most physicians involved in these requests will be uncomfortable in handling these issues. The legal standing involves only the husband or wife, not the future grandparents. Generally, hospitals may require to have, in writing, clear evidence of a prior desire for posthumous donation by the deceased patient. Advice from an ethics committee and the hospital's legal department is also required.[10,11]

■ REFERENCES

1. Assisted reproductive technology success rates: national summary and fertility clinic reports. Atlanta: Centers for Disease Control and Preservation, 2006. Available at http://www.cdc.gov/art/ART(2006)/PDF/(2006)ART.pdf.
2. Bahadur G. Death and conception. *Hum Reprod* 2002;17:2769–2775.
3. Batzer FR, Hurwitz JM, Caplan A. Postmortem parenthood and the need for a protocol with posthumous sperm procurement. *Fertil Steril* 2003;79:1263–1269.
4. Brown CVR, Foulkrod KH, Dworaczyk S, et al. Barriers to obtaining family consent for potential organ donors. *J Trauma* 2010;68:447–451.
5. Christmas AB, Burris GW, Bogart TA, et al. Organ donation: family members not honoring patient wishes. *J Trauma* 2008;65:1095–1097.
6. Ethics Committee of the American Society for Reproductive Medicine. Posthumuous reproduction. *Fertil Steril* 2004;82:S260–S262.
7. Finnerty JJ, Thomas TS, Boyhle RJ, et al. Gamete retrieval in terminal conditions. *Am J Obstet Gynecol* 2001;185:300–307.
8. Fishbach RL, Loike JD. Postmortem fatherhood: life after life. *Lancet* 2008;371: 2166–2167.
9. Kramer AC. Sperm retrieval from terminally ill or recently decreased patients: a review. *Can J Urol* 2009;16:4627–4631.
10. McLean SA. Post-mortem human reproduction. Legal and other regulatory issues. *J Law Med* 2002;9:429–437.
11. Mutter GL, Hornstein MD. Factors associated with disposition of cryopreserved reproductive tissue. *Fertil Steril* 2003;80:584–589.
12. Powner DJ, Rumohr JA, Lipshultz LI. Sperm retrieval during critical illness. *Neurocrit Care* 2010;12:445–449.
13. Pozda R, Miedema F, Matthews M. Sperm collection in the brain dead patient. *Dimens Crit Care Nurs* 1996;15:98–104.
14. Soules MR. Commentary: posthumous harvesting of gametes—a physician's perspective. *J Law Med Ethics* 1999;27:362–365.
15. Strong C, Gingrich JR, Kutteh WH. Ethics of postmortem sperm retrieval: ethics of sperm retrieval after death or persistent vegetative state. *Hum Reprod* 2000;15: 739–745.
16. Tash JA Applegarth LD, Kerr SM, et al. Postmortem sperm retrieval: the effects of instituting guidelines. *J Urol* 2003;170:1922–1925.
17. Townsend MF III, Richard JR, Witt MA. Artificially stimulated ejaculation in the brain dead patient: a case report. *Urology* 1996;47:760–762.
18. Webb SM. Raising sperm from the dead. *J Androl* 1996;17:325–326.

Organic Donation and the Hemodynamically Unstable Donor

Organ Donation and the Hemodynamically Unstable Donor

■ **THE COMMON CLINICAL QUESTIONS**

How should patients with unstable blood pressure be managed? How should patients with recurrent cardiac arrhythmias be managed?

■ **THE FACTS**

After consent—in the United States and many other countries—the management of the organ donor is directed by an organ procurement organization. This allows the agency to shepherd the organ donor to the operating room and provides an opportunity for the agency to develop extensive experience. Following the determination of brain death, a comprehensive proactive management protocol is initiated.[2,4,14,16,18] Attending physicians are often involved in the management of the patient before consent for organ donation has been obtained. Before the organ donor is transferred to their care, blood pressure can be significantly unstable and poorly responsive to vasopressors.

Hemodynamically unstable donors have been noted in 70% to 90% of series of potential organ donors.[7,9,17] In these patients, fluid resuscitation and a combination of vasopressors is not sufficient to maintain arterial blood pressure adequately. Most organ donors—even in the short time between brain death declaration and transfer to the operating room—have an incremental need for multiple vasopressors and vasopressin to maintain adequate blood pressure. The role of the anterior pituitary in hemodynamic instability is not completely clear.[6,10] Cortisol secretion after corticotropin (ACTH) stimulation is reduced. Moreover, abnormal triiodothyronine (T3) levels are found in up to 80% of donors, with barely detectable levels in more than 10% of tested organ donors.[9] Loss of sympathetic tone and vasodilation contribute to blood pressure instability. Hemodynamic instability, therefore, is more likely a result of reduced afterload than poor cardiac contractility.[3] Nonetheless, coronary perfusion after brain death is poorly autoregulated, partly due to endothelial dysfunction that impairs endothelial-dependent vasodilatory mechanisms.[20,21] Cardiac arrest during organ procurement has been reported in several series and varies from 7% to 15%.[1,11,19]

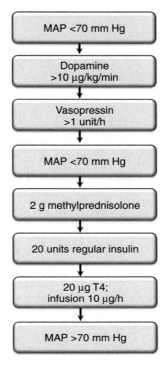

Figure 6-9 Treatment options for hypotension in an unstable organ donor. MAP, Mean Arterial Pressure.

An example of a management protocol in these more complex organ donors is shown in Figure 6-9. The approach includes fluid resuscitation, administration of packed red cells if the hemoglobin level is less than 9 g/dL and the hematocrit is less than 30%, correction of any hypothermia, and use of vasopressors. Pulmonary artery catheters are rarely used. Intravenous infusion of vasopressin may also reduce the dose of inotropes or vasopressors.[12,15] High-dose corticosteroids are not only used to reduce the systemic inflammatory response (Chapter 5), but their administration has also specifically resulted in improved lung function and better blood pressure management. In several studies of hemodynamically unstable donors, pharmacologic support was reduced with T4 administration.[8,13,22] Moreover, addition of a thyroxine (T4) protocol has increased the number of organs per donor used.[17]

Cardiac arrhythmias are more common, and in our series we have seen mostly ventricular dysrhythmias (in 14% of donors).[5] Others have reported nonspecific tachycardia or bradycardia, atrial tachycardia, and ventricular fibrillation.[1] Cardiac arrhythmias are common during organ procurement. In many patients, ventricular arrhythmias occur, often in the form of nonsustained ventricular tachycardia. Intravenous loading with amiodarone may prevent recurrence (a single dose of

TABLE 6-16 *Common Cardiac Arrhythmias*

Arrhythmia	Therapy
Sinus tachycardia	Fluids, vasopressin, esmolol (0.5 mg/kg bolus)
Sinus bradycardia	Atropine (0.5–1 mg bolus)*; temporary cardiac pacing
Atrial fibrillation with rapid ventricular response	Diltiazem (0.25 mg/kg bolus; infusion 5–15 mg/h)
Ventricular tachycardia	Amiodarone (150 mg IV) or cardioversion
Torsade de pointes	Substitute potassium and provide magnesium sulfate (1–4 g/h infusion)

* ineffective after brain death.

adenosine 6 mg IV may be needed first to differentiate ventricular tachycardia from supraventricular tachycardia). Preexisting atrial fibrillation and an increased ventricular response may be observed and is best controlled with a diltiazem infusion. Sinus tachycardia is due to multiple causes, including fluid deficit or fever. Sinus bradycardia is commonly a result of sudden catastrophic injury, usually without hypotension. Treatment of cardiac arrhythmias is summarized in Table 6-16.

■ REFERENCES

1. Delaunay L, Denis V, Darmon PL, et al. Initial cardiac arrest is a risk factor for failure of organ procurement in brain-dead patients. *Transplant Proc* 1996;28:2894.
2. Dictus C, Vienenkoetter B, Esmaeilzadeh M, et al. Critical care management of potential organ donors: our current standard. *Clin Transplant* 2009;23:2–9.
3. Dimopoulou I, Tsagarakis S, Anthi A, et al. High prevalence of decreased cortisol reserve in brain-dead potential organ donors. *Crit Care Med* 2003;31:1113–1117.
4. DuBose J, Salim A. Aggressive organ donor management protocol. *J Int Care Med* 2008;23:367–375.
5. Dujardin KS, McCully RB, Wijdicks EFM, et al. Myocardial dysfunction associated with brain death: clinical, echocardiographic, and pathologic features. *J Heart Lung Transplant* 2001;20:350–357.
6. Gramm HJ, Meinhold H, Bickel U, et al. Acute endocrine failure after brain death? *Transplantation* 1992;54:851–857.
7. Jenkins DH, Reilly PM, Schwab CW. Improving the approach to organ donation: a review. *World J Surg* 1999;23:644–649.
8. Masson F, Thiociope M, Latapie JM, et al. Thyroid function in brain-dead donors. *Transplant Int* 1990;3:226–233.
9. Najafizadeh K, Radipei B, Ghorbani F, et al. Organ experience with organ procurement from hemodynamically unstable brain dead patients. *Ann Transplant* 2009;14:20–23.
10. Novitzky D, Cooper DK, Rosendale JD, et al. Hormonal therapy of the brain-dead organ donor: experimental and clinical studies. *Transplantation* 2006;82:1396–1401.
11. Nygaard CE, Townsend RN, Diamond DL. Organ donor management and organ outcome: a 6-year review from a level I trauma center. *J Trauma* 1990;6:728–732.
12. Pennefather SH, Bullock RE, Mantle D, et al. Use of low dose arginine vasopressin to support brain-dead organ donors. *Transplantation* 1995;59:58–62.
13. Rosendale JD, Chabalewski FL, McBride MA, et al. Increased transplanted organs from the use of a standardized donor management protocol. *Am J Transplant* 2002;2: 761–768.
14. Rosendale JD, Kauffman HM, McBride MA, et al. Aggressive pharmacologic donor management results in more transplanted organs. *Transplantation* 2003;75:482–487.

15. Rostron AJ, Avlonitis VS, Cork DMW, et al. Hemodynamic resuscitation with arginine vasopressin reduces lung injury following brain death in the transplant donor. *Transplantation* 2008;85:597–606.
16. Salim A, Martin M, Brown C, et al. Complications of brain death: frequency and impact on organ retrieval. *Am Surg* 2006;72:377–381.
17. Salim A, Martin M, Brown C, et al. Using thyroid hormone in brain-dead donors to maximize the number of organs available for transplantation. *Clin Transplant* 2007;21:405–409.
18. Shah VR. Aggressive management of multiorgan donor. *Transplant Proc* 2008;40: 1087–1090.
19. Solomon NA, McGiven JR, Alison PM, et al. Changing donor and recipient demographics in a heart transplantation program: influence on early outcome. *Ann Thorac Surg* 2004;77:2096–2102.
20. Szabó G, Buhmann V, Bahrle S, et al. Brain death impairs coronary endothelial function. *Transplantation* 2002;73:1846–1848.
21. Szabó G, Buhmann V, Vahl CF, et al. Endothelial function after brain death. *J Heart Lung Transplant* 2001;20:153.
22. Zuppa AF, Nadkarni V, Davis L, et al. The effect of thyroid hormone infusion on vasopressor support in critically ill children with cessation of neurologic function. *Crit Care Med* 2004;32:2318–2322.

Clinical Problem 23

Organe Donation in Prisoners

■ THE COMMON CLINICAL QUESTIONS

Is organ donation after execution allowed? How is organ donation after a major central nervous system (CNS) catastrophe in a prisoner handled?

■ THE FACTS

This major ethical problem is twofold. Most commonly, a prisoner is admitted to an intensive care unit after a catastrophic neurologic illness, and organ donation is considered as in any other situation. Transmission of disease has traditionally been an exclusion factor, with a significantly higher incidence of human immunodeficiency virus (HIV), hepatitis C virus (HCV), hepatitis B virus (HBV), and tuberculosis (TB) among prisoners than in the general population. However, if transmittable disease can be excluded, convicted criminals would be able to donate organs after consent has been obtained.

A much more controversial issue is whether prisoners on death row may become organ donors. In the United States, this practice has been opposed for a number of reasons.[1] Strictly speaking, it would place the organ transplant team in the execution room, and removing organs could equate the transplant team with the role of the executioner. In addition, the recipient should be informed that the donation came from an executed prisoner, which could result in refusal or at least an uncomfortable situation. The public trust in organ donation would be severely undermined, and protection from coercion and exploitation can hardly be guaranteed.[3,5,6] Medical organizations have therefore forcefully declined any participation of physicians with the death penalty. Similar arguments apply to prisoners offering kidney donation as a form of penitence or to commute a prior sentence.

Others differ and have pointed out that the 2.2 million prisoners in the United States could provide 22,000 kidney donations (assuming 1% participation).[2] In the literature, only a single case has been published of organ donation in a prisoner.[4] The United Network of Organ Sharing (UNOS) has rejected any such involvement and has argued strongly that "any notion that particular groups of people were receiving an increased number of death sentences to provide organs for the rest of society would really make it difficult to attempt to obtain consent for altruistic donation from these groups" (www.unos.org).

■ REFERENCES

1. An organ donation offer on death row is refused. *New York Times* 1998;9:A23.
2. de Castro LD. Human organs from prisoners: kidneys for life. *J Med Ethics* 2003;29: 171–175.
3. Hinkle W. Giving until it hurts: prisoners are not the answer to the national organ shortage. *Indiana Law Rev* 2002;35:593–619.
4. Magee E, Levy MH. Organ donation from prison. *MJA* 2007;186:156.
5. Mills MA, Simmerling M. Prisoners as organ donors: is it worth the effort? Is it ethical? *Transplant Proc* 2009;41:23–24.
6. Moser DJ, Arndt S, Kanz JE, et al. Coercion and informed consent in research involving prisoners. *Compr Psychiatry* 2004;45:1–9.

Clinical Problem 24

Organ Donation, Consent, and Costs

■ THE COMMON CLINICAL QUESTIONS

Who approaches the family for consent to donate organs? Who bears the costs of organ donation?

■ THE FACTS

The process of asking for consent to donate organs varies throughout the world. In the United States, it is preferable that neither medical nor nursing staff mentions the topic of donation to families. Consent is best obtained by a person not involved with care. Consent should be requested after the diagnosis of brain death has been made.

All organ procurement organizations (OPOs) train individuals to broach the topic of donation. In addition, some hospitals have specially trained and certified requesters. After the patient meets the criteria for brain death, the organ transplant coordinator normally asks the ICU staff or physician to let family know that they are present. This allows organ transplant coordinators to use an approach that is both respectful and positive. If a family raises the issue of donation first and tells the staff that they are not interested in donation, the nursing staff will still ask families if they would like to speak with a coordinator and have any questions answered. The organ transplant coordinator likes to offer the opportunity to everyone and explain the entire process. If families decline, the organ transplant coordinator will respectfully accept their decision.

One concern that has been identified is when the physician decides to perform a brain death examination only if the family agrees to donation. This would limit a detailed discussion with the family about the procedure and its benefits. Families may initially—in their grief—resent the suggestion of donation but, after some time has passed, may have a better understanding of its benefits for others. In all instances brain death should be determined first; and consent for organ donation is totally different process that comes later. (For legal concerns with delaying brain death determination, see Clinical Problem 19.)

The consent process should be informed and voluntary.[3-7] Organ procurement professionals serve as dual advocates, understanding the needs of those who wish to receive organs and those who would like to donate. Most organ procurement coordinators have a presumptive model for consent. That is, families will have to state a reason why they do not want to proceed.

Many reasons may explain refusal to obtain consent. Ethnicity may impact on consent; a recent study from Los Angeles county and University of Southern California Medical Center shows marked variability (declining organ donation: Causasian 21%, Hispanic 77%, African Americans 11%, Asians 26%). Some of the reasons for these major differences have been outlined in Chapter 3. In the US, these differences have remained constant over the years and it is unlikely they will change without a major effort to promote organ donation.[1]

There may be simple remedies. For example, we recently found that delay with brain death examination reduced the number of decisions to donate and resulted in a rate 10% to 20% lower than the usual 60% to 70% acceptance rate.[2] The time to decide to donate organs decreases as the time to declare brain death increases. Families at the bedside of a dying patient in the ICU are under tremendous stress. There may be some confusion as to why brain death examination takes so long. Often the family spends another night in the ICU. Frequently, they question why further testing is required and, even more, why a second examination is needed if their loved one is in fact dead. Therefore, prompt diagnosis of brain death after a comprehensive evaluation is key.

There are often questions about the costs of organ procurement. When families agree on organ donation, the cost is transferred. The family should be assured that the entire cost of the organ donation process is paid for by the OPO. Generally, this includes all costs from the time of the brain death declaration and consent until the donor's care is transferred after organ recovery to the medical examiner or funeral home. Paying the donor as a compensation for organ or tissue donation, however, is a much more complex ethical problem. Paying the family of the organ donor can be intimidating, particularly if the amount is extraordinarily high, and many of us would consider this inappropriate. Others have suggested that donations should be paid but then should be directed to a worthy cause.

■ REFERENCES

1. Branco BC, Inaba K, Lam L. Donor conversion and procurement failure: the fate of our potential organ donors. *World J Surg* 2011;35:440–445.
2. Lustbader D, O'Hara D, Wijdicks EFM, et al. Second brain death examination may negatively affect organ donation. Neurology 2011;76:119–124.
3. Salim A, Brown C, Inaba K, et al. Improving consent rates for organ donation: the effect of an in-house coordinator program. *J Trauma* 2007;62:1411–1414.
4. Siminoff LA, Gordon N, Hewlett J, et al. Factors influencing families' consent for donation of solid organs for transplantation. *JAMA* 2001;286:71–77.
5. Siminoff LA, Lawrence RH. Knowing patients' preferences about organ donation: does it make a difference? *J Trauma* 2002;53:754–760.
6. Siminoff L, Mercer MB, Graham G, et al. The reasons families donate organs for transplantation: implications for policy and practice. *J Trauma* 2007;62:969–978.
7. Siminoff LA, Traino HM, Gordon N. Determinants of family consent to tissue donation. *J Trauma* 2010;69:956–963.

Clinical Problem 25

Organ Donation and Directing the Gift

■ THE COMMON CLINICAL QUESTIONS

Can organs be directed to friends or family members? What are the restrictions if such a donation is considered?

■ THE FACTS

In the US it is legally allowed for families who consent to organ donation to request that the organs be directed to family members or friends. Any person who needs an organ transplant can receive it as a gift from a family member. Most commonly, this practice involves donation by living donors, but it can also apply to brain death donors. It is again important for physicians to ensure that the determination of brain death has been fully separated from any discussion of organ donation to eliminate any possible conflict of interest. Donating a gift to family members in DCD protocols might be more problematic because withdrawal of care could be seen as a way to facilitate organ donation. If family members can agree, the organ procurement agency would have to contact them. Family members, however, are unable to put certain restrictions on organ donation (e.g., refuse to donate an organ to a patient who might receive a liver transplant after alcohol and drug abuse). Another concern is that some family members do not wish to donate to another race. The UNOS has carefully worded their guidelines in this situation (Table 6-17). Directing a gift, however, is only the first decision in the entire process of matching the donor with the recipient, and an incompatibility may emerge.

TABLE 6-17 *UNOS Board of Directors Recommendations*

The following persons may become donees of anatomical gifts for the purposes stated:
Any hospital, physician, or surgeon, or procurement organization for transplantation therapy,
   medical or dental education, research, or advancement of medical or dental science.
Any accredited medical or dental school, college or university for education, research, advancement
   of medical or dental science, or therapy.
   (a) Designated individual for transplantation or therapy needed by that individual

(Continues)

TABLE 6-17 (Continued)

(b) The gift may be made to a designated donee or without designating a donee. If the donee is not designated or if the donee is not available or rejects the anatomical gift, the anatomical gift may be accepted by any hospital.

(c) If the donee knows of the decedent's refusal or contrary indications to make an anatomical gift or that an anatomical gift by a member of a class having priority to act is opposed by a member of the same class or a prior class under Section 3 (a), the donee may not accept the anatomical gift.

(d) Donation of organs may not be made in a manner which discriminates against a person or class of persons on the basis of race, national origin, religion, gender or similar characteristic.

Source: UNOS Website: www.unos.org/resources/bioethics.

■ INDEX

Page numbers followed by "*f*" and "*t*" indicate figures and tables, respectively

AAN. *See* American Academy of
    Neurology
AAP. *See* American Academy of Pediatrics
ABC of Brain Stem Death, 15, 15*f*
acetaminophen
    acid-base abnormalities induced by, 159*t*
    serum toxicology assays available for, 163*t*
acid-base disturbances, 158–59, 159*t*
acidosis, 158–59, 159*t*
adult brain death
    ancillary tests for, 46–53, 47*t*, 48*t*,
        49*f*, 50*f*
    neurologic examination of, 32–41, 33*t*,
        35*f*, 36*t*, 38*f*, 41*f*, 44*f*, 45*f*, 46*f*
Africa, neurologic criteria for
    death in, 21–22
African-American, cultural views on brain
    death in, 72–73
Ajnoha v. J.C. Penny Life Ins. Co., 205*t*
Alaska, brain death examiners in, 58*t*
alcohol
    acute intoxication with, 162
    methyl, 163*t*
alkalosis, 37, 158
Alvarado v. New York City Health &
    Hosp. Corp., 206*t*
American Academy of Neurology (AAN)
    brain death determination 1995
        guideline by, 19–20, 19*f*
    brain death determination 2010
        guideline by, 150
American Academy of Pediatrics
    (AAP), 53–56, 54*f*, 54*t*
    death determination guidelines
        of, 151
amitriptyline, half-life of, 36*t*
amphetamines, urine toxicology assays
    available for, 164*t*
ancillary tests, 46–53
    BAEP, 47*t*, 52–53
    bispectral index scale monitor, 48
    cerebral angiogram, 48–49, 169*t*
    confounders, 168–70, 169*t*
    CT angiogram, 47*t*, 51, 169*t*

EEG, 46–48, 47*t*, 49*f*, 50*f*, 169*t*
    false negative with, 166*t*
    false positive with, 166*t*
    MRI, 47*t*, 53
    nuclear brain scan, 169*t*
    pitfalls of, 169*t*
    reliability, 165–67, 166*t*
    SSEP, 47*t*, 52–53, 169*t*
    transcranial Doppler, 47–48, 47*t*,
        51–52, 169*t*
anencephaly, 193–95, 194*f*
    characteristics of, 193
    diagnosis of, 193
    International Federation of
        Gynecology and Obstetrics
        on, 195
    intubation for, 193
    organ donation with, 194–95
anesthetics, acid-base abnormalities
    induced by, 159*t*
antibiotics, undetectable by toxicity
    screen, 163
apnea, neurologic criteria with, 4
apnea test, 33*t*, 41–45
    acceptable conditions for, 43
    breathing during, 184–86, 185*f*
    catheter for, 43
    CO_2 retention with, 179–80, 180*f*
    ECMO with, 190–91, 191*t*
    no breathing with, 43–45
    terminating, 181–83
Argentina, organ procurement
    organization for, 100*t*
Aristotle, 3
arterial tone, brain death
    with, 119–20, 121*f*
Asia, neurologic criteria for
    death in, 20, 21*f*, 22–24
asymmetric opisthotonic posturing of
    trunk, 175*t*
atonic syndrome, 84*t*
atracurium, half-life of, 36*t*
atrial fibrillation with rapid ventricular
    response, 216*f*

Australia
neurologic criteria for death in, 23
organ procurement organization for,
100t
Austria, organ procurement organization
for, 100t
autoresuscitation, 83

baclofen overdose, brain death mimicked
by, 155–56
BAEP. See brainstem auditory evoked
potentials
Bangladesh, organ procurement
organization for, 100t
Baptists, beliefs about brain death
for, 70, 70f
barbiturates
acid-base abnormalities induced by, 159t
brain death mimicked by overdose of,
155–56
urine toxicology assays available for, 164t
Bassie v. Obstetrics & Gynecology Assoc.
of Northwest Alabama, 205t
battered baby. See shaken baby syndrome
Beecher, Henry, 8–10, 9f, 10f
Belgium, organ procurement organization
for, 100t
bispectral index scale monitor, 48
Bolivia, organ procurement organization
for, 100t
brain arrest, 84t
brain death
adult neurologic examination of, 32–41,
33t, 35f, 36t, 38f, 41f, 44f, 45f, 46f
absence of electrolyte, endocrine
abnormality in, 33t, 36–37
absence of residual paralytics
in, 33t, 36
coma in, 33–34, 33t
corneal reflex absent in, 33t, 39
cough reflex absent in, 33t, 40, 46f
eyes immobile in, 33t, 39
gag reflex absent in, 33t, 40, 46f
motor response to noxious stimuli
absent in, 33t, 40–41
no facial movement to noxious
stimuli in, 33t, 40, 45f
normal temperature in, 33t, 37
no spontaneous respirations in, 33t, 37
oculocephalic reflex absent in, 33t, 39

oculovestibular reflex absent in, 33t,
39–40, 41f, 44f
pupils non-reactive to bright light in,
33t, 38–39, 38f
sedative drug effect absent in, 33t,
34–36, 36t
systolic blood pressure in, 33t, 37
alternative terms for, 84t
ancillary tests for, 46–53
BAEP, 47t, 52–53
bispectral index scale monitor, 48
cerebral angiogram, 48–49, 169t
confounders of, 168–70, 169t
CT angiogram, 47t, 51, 169t
EEG, 46–48, 47t, 49f, 50f, 169t
false negative with, 166t
false positive with, 166t
MRI, 47t, 53
nuclear brain scan, 169t
pitfalls of, 169t
reliability, 165–67, 166t
SSEP, 47t, 52–53, 169t
transcranial Doppler, 47–48, 47t,
51–52, 169t
anencephaly and, 193–95, 194f
apnea test for, 33t, 41–45
acceptable conditions for, 43
catheter for, 43
no breathing with, 43–45
beliefs about, 69–77
clinical determination in children
of, 53–56, 54f, 54t
clinical problems in, 149–223
controversy with, 84–90, 84t, 86t, 89f
brainstem formulation of death, 85
critical vital systems, 85
dissatisfaction with term "brain
death," 84–85, 84t
EEG activity remaining, 86
somatic integration argument in, 89
transplantation, 86
criticism with, 81–93
critique of, 90–92
cultural views on, 72–75, 74f
African-American, 72–73
Chinese, 73
gypsies, 73
Japanese, 73–75, 74f
Native American, 73
Roma, 73

documentation for, 56
errors in determination of, 56–57, 56t
family opposition to accepting, 209–10
history of, 3–26
hospital guidelines for determination
 of, 151f
legal challenges in, 204–8, 205t–207t
legal definitions of, 57–59, 57t, 58t
maternal, 200–202, 201f
mimics of, 155–56, 155t
obligations with, 57t, 58t
pathology of, 28–42, 28f, 30f–31f, 33t, 35f,
 36t, 38f, 41f, 44f, 45f, 46f, 112–20
 arterial tone in, 119–20, 121f
 circulation in, 119–20, 121f
 coagulopathy in, 111, 112f, 119
 diabetes insipidus, 111, 112f, 114
 hypothalamic-pituitary function in,
  113–16, 114f
 kidney function in, 119
 liver function in, 119
 myocardial function in, 116–17
 pulmonary function in, 118
 systemic inflammatory response
  in, 113
procurement after, 97–145
 avoidance of injury to organs in, 122t
 cardiovascular management for,
  121–23
 coagulation management for, 124
 complications impacting donation
  with, 111–12, 112f
 contraindications to, 108t
 donation protocols for, 109–11, 110t
 donation requests for, 102–6, 103t,
  104t, 106f–107f
 donor management orders for, 125–27
 electrolyte management for, 123–24
 evaluation/management forms
  for, 128–45
 glucose management for, 123–24
 imminent neurologic death in, 97
 medical management of donor
  for, 111–20, 112f, 114f, 121f
 medical supportive care
  for, 120–21, 122t
 medication used for, 122t
 organizations for, 99–102,
  100t–101t, 102f
 organ suitability in, 106–9, 108t, 109t

respiratory management for, 123
 transition to organ donation,
  97–98, 98f
 recoveries from, 56–57, 56t
 religious beliefs about, 69–72, 70f
  Buddhism, 71–72, 76f
  Catholic Church, 70, 70f
  Christianity, 69–70, 70f, 76f
  Confucian, 73, 76f
  Hindu, 76f
  Islam, 70–71, 76f
  Jehovah's Witnesses, 72
  Judaism, 71, 76f
  resolution of conflict from, 75–77, 76f
  Roman Catholic Church, 70, 70f
  Shinto, 74, 76f
 sperm/oocyte retrieval in, 211–12, 212t
 uncertainty with, 81–84, 82f
brain death syndrome, 84t
brainstem auditory evoked potentials
 (BAEP), 47t, 52–53
brainstem death, 85
brainstem lesion, primary, 171–73, 172f
brain tumor and organ donation, 107
Brazil, organ procurement organization
 for, 100t
Buddhism, beliefs about brain death
 in, 72, 76f
Bulgaria, organ procurement
 organization for, 100t

Canada
 neurologic criteria for death in, 20
 organ procurement organization
  for, 100t
carbamazepine, serum toxicology assays
 available for, 163t
carboxyhemoglobin, serum toxicology
 assays available for, 163t
cardiac arrhythmias
 atrial fibrillation with rapid ventricular
  response, 216f
 complications of brain death
  with, 111, 112f
 hemodynamically unstable donor with,
  215–16, 216f
 sinus bradycardia, 216f
 sinus tachycardia, 216f
 torsade de pointes, 216f
 ventricular tachycardia, 216f

cardiac data, evaluation/management
    forms, 136
cardiocirculatory death, 83
cardiopulmonary resuscitation (CPR),
    187–89, 188t
  brain death following, 187
  hypothermia induced for comatose
    patients following, 187–89, 188t
Catholic Church, beliefs about brain
    death in, 70, 70f
Cavagnaro v. Hanover Ins. Co., 205t
central nervous system (CNS), sedative
    drug effect absent in, 33t,
    34–36, 36t
cerebral angiogram, 48–49
  pitfalls with, 169t
children
  anencephaly with, 193–95, 194f
  determination of brain death
    in, 53–56, 54f, 54t
  ECMO for, 190
  shaken baby syndrome, 196–98, 197f
Chile, organ procurement organization
    for, 100t
China
  cultural views on brain death in, 73
  neurologic criteria for death in, 20,
    21f, 22
Christianity, beliefs about brain death
    in, 69–70, 70f, 76f
circulation, brain death with, 119–20, 121f
clergy
  meaning of brain death clarified by, 75
  mediation between family and
    physician, 75
  role in intensive care unit, 69
  views on organ donation, 72, 102
clinical mimics, 155–56
  baclofen overdose, 155–56
  barbiturate overdose, 155–56
  delayed vecuronium clearance, 155–56
  Guillain-Barré syndrome, 155–56
  hypothermia, 155–56
  warning signs for, 155t
clinical problems in brain
    death, 149–223
  acid-base disturbances, 158–59, 159t
  ancillary tests
    confounders, 168–70, 169t
    reliability, 165–67, 166t

anencephaly and brain death, 193–95,
    194f
apnea test
  breathing during, 184–86, 185f
  CO_2 retention and, 179–80, 180f
  terminating, 181–83
cardiopulmonary resuscitation, 187–89,
    188t
clinical mimics, 155–56, 155t
ECMO, 190–91, 191t
electrolyte abnormalities, 160–61, 161t
family opposition to accepting brain
    death, 209–10
intoxications, acute, 162–64, 163t, 164t
legal challenges in brain death, 204–8,
    205t–207t
maternal brain death, 200–202, 201f
organ donation
  consent/costs with, 220–21
  directing organs given, 222, 222t–223t
  hemodynamically unstable donor
    with, 214–16, 215f, 216f
  prisoners, 218–19
primary brainstem lesion, 171–73, 172f
qualification of examiner, 150–54,
    151f, 153f
shaken baby syndrome, 196–98, 197f
sperm/oocyte retrieval in brain death,
    211–12, 212t
spinal reflex interpreting, 174–76, 175t
ventilator autocycling, 177–78, 178t
clonazepam, half-life of, 36t
CNS. See central nervous system
CO_2 retention, apnea test with,
    179–80, 180f
coagulation, organ donation management
    with, 124
coagulopathy, complications of brain death
    with, 111, 112f, 119
cocaine
  acid-base abnormalities induced
    by, 159t
  urine toxicology assays available
    for, 164t
codeine, half-life of, 36t
Colombia, organ procurement
    organization for, 100t
coma
  irreversible apneic, 84, 84t
  neuroimaging explaining, 33t, 34, 35f

coma dépassé, 4–5, 5f
Confucian, beliefs about brain death in,
    73, 76f
corneal reflex absent, 33t, 39
cortisol, 115
cough reflex, 33t, 40, 46f
CPR. See cardiopulmonary resuscitation
Creutzfeldt-Jakob disease, organ donation
    contraindicated by, 108t
Croatia, organ procurement organization
    for, 100t
Crobons v. Wisconsin National Life Ins.
    Co., 206t
CT angiogram, 47t, 51
    pitfalls with, 169t
Cuba, organ procurement organization
    for, 100t
cultural views on brain death, 72–75, 74f
    African-American, 72–73
    Chinese, 73
    gypsies, 73
    Japanese, 73–75, 74f
    Native American, 73
    Roma, 73
cyanide
    acid-base abnormalities induced
        by, 159t
    undetectable by toxicity screen, 163
Cyprus, organ procurement organization
    for, 100t
cytomegalovirus viremia, organ donation
    contraindicated by, 108t
Czech Republic, organ procurement
    organization for, 100t

DBD. See donation after brain death
DCD. See donation after cardiac death
dead-donor rule, 84
Defining Death: A Report on the Medical,
    Legal and Ethical Issues in the
    Determination of Death, 16–18, 17f
delayed vecuronium clearance, brain
    death mimicked by, 155–56
Denmark, organ procurement organization
    for, 100t
diabetes insipidus
    complications of brain death with, 111,
        112f, 114
    polyuria in diagnosis of, 114
diazepam, half-life of, 36t

digoxin
    serum toxicology assays available
        for, 163t
    undetectable by toxicity screen, 163
Dominican Republic, organ procurement
    organization for, 100t
donation after brain death (DBD)
    DCD v., 110t
    protocols for, 109–11, 110t
donation after cardiac death (DCD),
        82–83, 97
    DBD v., 110t
    IMD for, 98f
    protocols for, 109–11, 110t
donor hospital personnel form, 142
donor management record, 128–30
    admission course/comments in, 130
    consent information in, 128
    donor information in, 128
    tissue information in, 129
    UNOS reference codes in, 129
dopamine, brain death procurement
    with, 122t

echocardiography, 117
ECMO. See extracorporeal membrane
    oxygenation
EEG. See electroencephalography
electroencephalography (EEG)
    brain death ancillary testing with,
        46–48, 47t, 49f, 50f, 169t
    brain death history with, 3–4
    criteria to determine brain death
        with, 47t
    flat or isoelectric, 7, 11t
    Harvard Criteria with, 11t
    neurologic criteria with flat, 7–8, 11t
    pitfalls with, 169t
electrolytes
    abnormalities with, 160–61, 161t
    complications of brain death with, 111
    organ donation management with,
        123–24
Epstein-Barr virus, organ donation
    contraindicated by, 108t
Estate of Sewart v. Taff, 205t
Estonia, organ procurement organization
    for, 100t
ethanol, acid-base abnormalities
    induced by, 159t

ethics
  neurologic criteria with, 4, 6–7
  President's Commission on, 16–18, 17*f*,
    88–89, 89*f*
ethylene glycol
  acid-base abnormalities induced by, 159*t*
  serum toxicology assays available
    for, 163*t*
Europe, neurologic criteria for death in,
  20–21
Eurotransplant, 100*t*
evaluation/management forms, 128–45
  cardiac data, 136
  donor hospital personnel, 142
  heart data, 140
  initial physical assessment, 131
  intestine data, 140
  intraoperative management, 138
  lab profile, 132
  liver data, 140
  lung data, 140
  medications, 134, 138
  organ/tissue screening worksheet, 142
  pancreas data, 140
  pre-donor management culture
    results, 133
  pulmonary data, 137
  renal data, 139
  serologies, 135
examiner qualification, 150–54, 151*f*, 153*f*
  AAN guidelines for, 150
  AAP guidelines for, 151
  hospital guidelines for, 151*f*
  SCCM guidelines for, 151
extracorporeal membrane oxygenation
  (ECMO), 83, 190–91, 191*t*
  apnea test in patient on, 190–91, 191*t*
  children with, 190
  extracirculatory support with, 190
  unstable patient with, 191

family opposition to accepting brain
  death, 209–10
Farlow v. Roddy, 206*t*
fentanyl
  half-life of, 36*t*
  hypothermia and clearance change
    with, 188*t*
  undetectable by toxicity
    screen, 163

finger flexion, 175*t*
finger jerks, 175*t*
finger pinch, 175*t*
Finland, organ procurement organization
  for, 100*t*
flexion elevation of arm, 175*t*
flexion of trunk, 175*t*
flexion-withdrawal reflex, 175*t*
France, organ procurement organization
  for, 100*t*
fungal infection, organ donation
  contraindicated by, 108*t*

gag reflex, 33*t*, 40, 46*f*
Gallups v. Cotter, 207*t*
gangrenous bowel, organ donation
  contraindicated by, 108*t*
Georgia
  brain death examiners in, 58*t*
  organ procurement organization for,
    100*t*
Germany, organ procurement organization
  for, 100*t*
glucose, organ donation management with,
  123–24
glycosuria, 6
gonadal hormones, 115
graft rejection, 113
Greece, organ procurement organization
  for, 100*t*
growth hormone, 115
Guillain-Barré syndrome, brain death
  mimicked by, 155–56
gypsies, cultural views on brain
  death in, 73

Harvard Ad Hoc Committee to
  Examine the Definition of Brain
  Death, 8–10, 9*f*
Harvard Criteria, 4, 11–13, 11*f*, 11*t*, 12*f*
  controversy with, 84
  flat EEG in, 11*t*
  movement/breathing in, 11*t*
  reflexes in, 11*t*
  unresponsiveness in, 11*t*
head turning to side reflex, 175*t*
heart
  kanji, 74, 74*f*
  management form with data on, 140
  transplantation, 82

hemodynamically unstable donor, 214–16
  cardiac arrhythmias with, 215–16, 216f
  management protocol for, 215, 215f
  vasopressors for, 214
hepatitis B
  organ donation contraindicated by, 108t
  prisoner organ donors with, 218
herpes simplex, organ donation
      contraindicated by, 108t
higher brain death, 85
Hindu, beliefs about brain death in, 76f
HIV infection
  organ donation contraindicated by, 108t
  prisoner organ donors with, 218
Hodgkin's disease, organ donation
      contraindicated by, 108t
Hong Kong, organ procurement
      organization for, 100t
hormonal resuscitation therapy (HRT),
      brain death procurement with, 122t
HRT. See hormonal resuscitation therapy
Hungary, organ procurement organization
      for, 100t
hydrogen sulfide, undetectable by toxicity
      screen, 163
hypercalcemia, values requiring correction
      for, 161t
hyperglycemia, 6
  complications of brain death with, 112f
  pregnant brain dead patient with, 202
  values requiring correction for, 161t
hypernatremia, values requiring correction
      for, 161t
hypoglycemia, values requiring correction
      for, 161t
hyponatremia, values requiring correction
      for, 161t
hypotension
  complications of brain death with, 111, 112f
  neurologic criteria with, 4
hypothalamic-pituitary
      function, 113–16, 114f
  blood supply for, 114f
  cortisol with, 115
  diabetes insipidus diagnosed with, 114
  gonadal hormones with, 115
  growth hormone with, 115
  pancreatic dysfunction with, 116
  prolactin with, 115
  thyroid function with, 115

hypothermia
  brain death mimicked by, 155–56
  CPR and comatose patients with
      induced, 187–89, 188t
  neurologic criteria with, 4
hypoxia, complications of brain death
      with, 111

Iceland, organ procurement organization
      for, 100t
imminent brain death (IMD), 98, 98f
imminent neurologic death, 97
infection
  fungal, 108t
  HIV, 108t, 218
  parasitic, 108t
  retroviral, 108t
  West Nile virus, 108t
initial physical assessment form, 131
International Federation of Gynecology
      and Obstetrics, 195
intestine, management form with
      data on, 140
intoxications, acute, 162–64, 163t, 164t
  acetaminophen, 163t
  alcohol, 162
  amphetamines, 164t
  antibiotics, 163
  barbiturates, 164t
  carbamazepine, 163t
  carboxyhemoglobin, 163t
  cocaine, 164t
  cyanide, 163
  digoxin, 163, 163t
  ergot alkaloids, 163
  ethylene glycol, 163t
  fentanyl, 163
  halogenated hydrocarbon solvents, 163
  hydrogen sulfide, 163
  iron, 163t
  isoniazid, 163
  lithium, 163, 163t
  LSD, 163
  methemoglobin, 163t
  methyl alcohol, 163t
  nitrogen dioxide, 163
  opiates, 164t
  PCP, 164t
  phenobarbital, 163t
  propoxyphene, 164t

intoxications, acute (*continued*)
  salicylate, 163*t*
  theophylline, 163*t*
  toxins, 163
  transferrin, 163*t*
  valproic acid, 163*t*
intra-abdominal sepsis, organ donation
  contraindicated by, 108*t*
intraoperative management, 138
Iran, organ procurement organization
  for, 100*t*
Ireland, organ procurement organization
  for, 100*t*
iron, serum toxicology assays available
  for, 163*t*
Islam, beliefs about brain death
  in, 70–71, 76*f*
isoniazid, undetectable by toxicity
  screen, 163
Israel, organ procurement organization
  for, 100*t*
Italy, organ procurement organization
  for, 100*t*

Jacobsen v. Marin Gen. Hosp., 207*t*
Japan
  cultural views on brain death
    in, 73–75, 74*f*
  neurologic criteria for death in, 22–23
  organ procurement organization
    for, 100*t*
Japan Organ Transplantation systems
  (JOTs), 75
Jehovah's Witnesses, beliefs about brain
  death in, 72
Jews
  conservative, 71
  orthodox, 71
  reform, 71
JOTs. *See* Japan Organ Transplantation
  systems
Judaism, beliefs about brain death
  in, 71, 76*f*

kanji, 74, 74*f*
Kentucky, brain death examiners
  in, 58*t*
ketamine, half-life of, 36*t*
kidney, brain death with function
  of, 119

labetalol, brain death procurement
  with, 122*t*
lab profile, evaluation/management forms
  with, 132
Latin America, neurologic criteria for
  death in, 20
Latvia, organ procurement organization
  for, 100*t*
Lazarus phenomenon, 83, 175
legal challenges in brain death, 204–8,
  205*t*–207*t*
  Ajnoha v. J.C. Penny Life Ins. Co., 205*t*
  Alvarado v. New York City Health &
    Hosp. Corp., 206*t*
  Bassie v. Obstetrics & Gynecology
    Assoc. of Northwest Alabama, 205*t*
  Cavagnaro v. Hanover Ins. Co., 205*t*
  Crobons v. Wisconsin National Life Ins.
    Co., 206*t*
  directing organs donated, 222, 222*t*–223*t*
  documentation of time of
    death in, 205*t*–206*t*
  Estate of Sewart v. Taff, 205*t*
  family interference/involvement with
    death diagnosis in, 206*t*–207*t*
  Farlow v. Roddy, 206*t*
  Gallups v. Cotter, 207*t*
  Jacobsen v. Marin Gen. Hosp., 207*t*
  Long Island Jewish Med. Ctr., 206*t*
  Mineroff v. Silber, 205*t*
  Smith v. Methodist Hosp.
    of Indiana, 207*t*
  Strachan v. John F. Kennedy Memorial
    Hosp., 206*t*
  Virk v. Detroit Receiving Hosp. and
    Univ. Health Ctr., 206*t*
leukemia, organ donation contraindicated
  by, 108*t*
Libya, organ procurement organization
  for, 100*t*
LifeSource
  evaluation/management forms
    for, 128–45
    cardiac data, 136
    donor hospital personnel, 142
    heart data, 140
    initial physical assessment, 131
    intestine data, 140
    intraoperative management, 138
    lab profile, 132

liver data, 140
lung data, 140
medications, 134, 138
organ/tissue screening worksheet, 142
pancreas data, 140
pre-donor management culture
   results, 133
pulmonary data, 137
renal data, 139
serologies, 135
follow-up letter to organ donor family,
   106f–107f
organ donor management
   orders for, 125–27
lithium
serum toxicology assays available
   for, 163t
undetectable by toxicity screen, 163
Lithuania, organ procurement organization
   for, 100t
liver
brain death with function of, 119
management form with data on, 140
Long Island Jewish Med. Ctr., 206t
lorazepam, half-life of, 36t
LSD, undetectable by toxicity screen, 163
lungs
brain death with function of, 118
management form with data on, 140
Luxembourg, organ procurement
   organization for, 100t
lymphoma, organ donation
   contraindicated by, 108t

magnetic resonance imaging (MRI), 47t, 53
Malaysia, organ procurement organization
   for, 100t
malignant neoplasms, organ donation
   contraindicated by, 108t
Malta, organ procurement organization
   for, 100t
maternal brain death, 200–202
cases of prolonged support with, 201t
complications with, 200
hyperglycemia with, 202
magnesium sulfate infusion for
   support of, 202
mechanical asystole, 83
mechanical ventilation, neurologic
   criteria with, 6

medications, evaluation/management
   forms with, 134, 138
melanoma, organ donation contraindicated
   by, 108t
meningitis, organ donation contraindicated
   by, 108t
methanol, acid-base abnormalities induced
   by, 159t
methemoglobin, serum toxicology assays
   available for, 163t
Methodists, beliefs about brain death for,
   70, 70f
methyl alcohol, serum toxicology assays
   available for, 163t
Mexico, organ procurement organization
   for, 100t
Michigan, brain death examiners in, 58t
midazolam
half-life of, 36t
hypothermia and clearance
   change with, 188t
Mineroff v. Silber, 205t
mode of death, 88
Mollaret, P., neurologic criteria in
   paper by, 6–7, 6f
morphine, half-life of, 36t
MRI. See magnetic resonance imaging
multiple myeloma, organ donation
   contraindicated by, 108t
multisystem organ failure (MSOF),
   organ donation contraindicated
   by, 108t
myocardial function
brain death with, 116–17
echocardiography for screening of, 117
intracranial hemorrhage with
   dysfunction of, 117
plasma catecholamines with, 116

National Institutes of Health (NIH),
   neurologic criteria for, 15–17
Native American, cultural views on brain
   death in, 73
neck-abdominal muscle
   contraction, 175t
neck-arm flexion, 175t
neck-hip flexion, 175t
neck-shoulder protrusion, 175t
Netherlands, organ procurement
   organization for, 100t

neurologic criteria for death
AAN on, 19–20, 19f
Africa on, 21
Asia on, 20, 21f, 22–24
Australia on, 23
bilateral mydriasis with, 7
Boston Children's Hospital on, 20
Canada on, 20
cardiac arrest with, 6
China on, 20, 21f, 22
EEG in, 7–8, 11t
ethics with, 4, 6–7
Europe on, 20–21
France, 4–5, 5f
international guidelines on, 20–24, 21f
Japan on, 22–23
Latin America on, 20
mechanical ventilation with, 6
New Zealand on, 23
NIH, 15–17
President's Commission on, 16–19, 17f, 18t
reflexes, absent with pain, 4, 7
respiration, absent, 7
Royal Colleges of Physicians, 13–15,
14f, 14t
United Kingdom, 13–15, 14f, 14t, 15f
United States, 4, 6–8, 15–20
neurologist, critiques against brain death
by, 86t
neurology
ancillary tests for, 46–53, 47t, 49f, 50f
BAEP, 47t, 52–53
bispectral index scale monitor, 48
cerebral angiogram, 48–49, 169t
confounders of, 168–70, 169t
CT angiogram, 47t, 51, 169t
EEG, 46–48, 47t, 49f, 50f, 169t
false negative with, 166t
false positive with, 166t
MRI, 47t, 53
nuclear brain scan, 169t
pitfalls of, 169t
reliability, 165–67, 166t
SSEP, 47t, 52–53, 169t
transcranial Doppler, 47–48, 47t,
51–52, 169t
apnea test in, 33t, 41–45
acceptable conditions for, 43
catheter for, 43
no breathing with, 43–45

brain death diagnosis with, 27–58
children's brain death determination
with, 53–56, 54f, 54t
clinical examination of, 32–41, 33t, 35f,
36t, 38f, 41f, 44f, 45f, 46f
absence of electrolyte, endocrine
abnormality in, 33t, 36–37
absence of residual paralytics
in, 33t, 36
coma in, 33–34, 33t
corneal reflex absent in, 33t, 39
cough reflex absent in, 33t, 40, 46f
eyes immobile in, 33t, 39
gag reflex absent in, 33t, 40, 46f
motor response to noxious stimuli
absent in, 33t, 40–41
no facial movement to noxious stimuli
in, 33t, 40, 45f
normal temperature in, 33t, 37
no spontaneous respirations
in, 33t, 37
oculocephalic reflex absent in, 33t, 39
oculovestibular reflex absent in, 33t,
39–40, 41f, 44f
pupils non-reactive to bright light in,
33t, 38–39, 38f
sedative drug effect absent in, 33t,
34–36, 36t
systolic blood pressure in, 33t, 37
documentation for brain death
determination with, 56
errors with brain death in, 56–57, 56t
legal definitions with brain death in,
57–59, 57t, 58t
pathology of brain death in, 28–42, 28f,
30f–31f, 33t, 35f, 36t, 38f, 41f, 44f,
45f, 46f
recoveries from brain death
in, 56–57, 56t
New Jersey, brain death examiners
in, 58t
New York, brain death examiners in, 58t
New Zealand
neurologic criteria for death in, 23
organ procurement organization
for, 100t
NIH. See National Institutes of Health
nonaccidental head injury. See shaken baby
syndrome
normothermia, 37, 43, 87

Norway, organ procurement organization for, 100t
nuclear brain scan, pitfalls with, 169t

oculocephalic reflex, 33t, 39
oculovestibular reflex, 33t, 39–40, 41f, 44f
oocyte retrieval, 211–12, 212t
opiates
   acid-base abnormalities induced by, 159t
   urine toxicology assays available for, 164t
OPO. See organ procurement organizations
organ donation
   anencephaly with, 194–95
   avoidance of injury to organs in, 122t
   brain tumor and, 107
   cardiac arrhythmias with, 215–16, 216f
   cardiovascular management for, 121–23
   coagulation management for, 124
   complications of brain death impacting, 111–12, 112f
   consent/costs with, 220–21
   contraindications to, 108t
   directing organs given, 222, 222t–223t
   donor management orders for, 125–27
   electrolyte management for, 123–24
   evaluation/management forms for, 128–45
   glucose management for, 123–24
   hemodynamically unstable donor with, 214–16, 215f, 216f
   imminent neurologic death for, 97
   medical management of donor for, 111–20, 112f, 114f, 121f
   medical supportive care for, 120–21, 122t
   organizations for, 99–102, 100t–101t, 102f
   organ suitability in, 106–9, 108t, 109t
   prisoners, 218–19
   protocols for, 109–11, 110t
   reasons/factors for declining, 104–5, 104t
   religious beliefs about, 72
   requests for, 102–6, 103t, 104t, 106f–107f
   respiratory management for, 123
   transition from brain death to, 97–98, 98f
organ procurement organizations (OPO), 58, 99–102, 100t–101t, 102f
   list of world, 100t–101t
organ/tissue screening worksheet, 142
orthodox Jews, 71

Pakistan, organ procurement organization for, 100t
pancreas, management form with data on, 140
pancuronium, half-life of, 36t
papaverine, acid-base abnormalities induced by, 159t
PCP, urine toxicology assays available for, 164t
pediatrics
   anencephaly with, 193–95, 194f
   brain death determination for, 53–56, 54f, 54t
   ECMO for, 190
   shaken baby syndrome, 196–98, 197f
persistent vegetative state, irreversible coma v., 84
phenobarbital
   half-life of, 36t
   serum toxicology assays available for, 163t
phenylephrine, brain death procurement with, 122t
plantar flexion of toes, 175t
pneumonia, organ donation contraindicated by, 108t
poisoning. See also intoxications, acute
   alkalosis with, 37, 158
   pupil response to light with, 162
   self, 28
Poland, organ procurement organization for, 100t
Polyuria, neurologic criteria with, 4
Portugal, organ procurement organization for, 100t
pre-donor management culture results, 133
pregnant brain dead patient, 200–202
   cases of prolonged support for, 201t
   complications with, 200
   hyperglycemia with, 202
   magnesium sulfate infusion for, 202
President's Commission for the Study of Ethical Problems in Medicine and Biomedical and Behavioral Research
   controversy with, 85
   ethics, 16–18, 17f, 88–89, 89f
   neurologic criteria in report by, 16–19, 17f, 18t
primidone, half-life of, 36t

prisoner as organ donors, 218–19
procurement, 97–145
    avoidance of injury to organs in, 122t
    cardiovascular management for, 121–23
    coagulation management for, 124
    complications impacting donation with,
        111–12, 112f
    contraindications to, 108t
    donation protocols for, 109–11, 110t
    donation requests for, 102–6, 103t, 104t,
        106f–107f
    donor management orders for, 125–27
    electrolyte management for, 123–24
    evaluation/management forms for,
        128–45
    glucose management for, 123–24
    imminent neurologic death in, 97
    medical management of donor for,
        111–20, 112f, 114f, 121f
    medical supportive care for, 120–21, 122t
    organizations for, 99–102, 100t–101t, 102f
    organ suitability in, 106–9, 108t, 109t
    respiratory management for, 123
    transition to organ donation, 97–98, 98f
prolactin, 115
propofol, hypothermia and clearance
        change with, 188t
propoxyphene, urine toxicology assays
        available for, 164t
Puerto Rico, organ procurement
        organization for, 100t
pulmonary function, brain death with, 118
pulmonary system, management form with
        data on, 137
pupils
    non-reactive to bright light in, 33t,
        38–39, 38f
    response to light in intoxications, 162

Qatar, organ procurement organization
        for, 100t

rabies, organ donation contraindicated
        by, 108t
reflexes
    abdominal, 175t
    absent, 4, 7, 11t
    asymmetric opisthotonic posturing of
        trunk, 175t
    corneal, 33t, 39

cough, 33t, 40, 46f
finger flexion, 175t
finger jerks, 175t
finger pinch, 175t
flexion elevation of arm, 175t
flexion of trunk, 175t
flexion-withdrawal reflex, 175t
gag, 33t, 40, 46f
head turning to side, 175t
neck-abdominal muscle contraction,
    175t
neck-arm flexion, 175t
neck-hip flexion, 175t
neck-shoulder protrusion, 175t
neurologic criteria with, 4, 7
oculocephalic, 33t, 39
oculovestibular, 33t, 39–40, 41f, 44f
plantar flexion of toes, 175t
spinal, 174–76, 175t
tonic neck, 175t
unilateral extension-pronation, 175t
reform Jews, 71
religious beliefs, 69–72, 70f
    Buddhism, 72, 76f
    Catholic Church, 70, 70f
    Christianity, 69–70, 70f, 76f
    Confucian, 73, 76f
    Hindu, 76f
    Islam, 70–71, 76f
    Jehovah's Witnesses, 72
    Judaism, 71, 76f
    resolution of conflict from, 75–77, 76f
    Roman Catholic Church, 70, 70f
    Shinto, 74, 76f
remifentanil, hypothermia and clearance
        change with, 188t
renal system, management form with data
        on, 139
respiration
    absent, 7
    no spontaneous, 33t, 37
    organ donation management
        with, 123
retroviral infections, organ donation
        contraindicated by, 108t
rocuronium, half-life of, 36t
Roma, cultural views on brain
        death in, 73
Roman Catholic Church, beliefs about
        brain death in, 70, 70f

Romania, organ procurement organization
for, 100*t*
Royal Colleges of Physicians, neurologic
criteria in, 13–15, 14*f*, 14*t*
Russia, organ procurement organization
for, 100*t*

salicylates
acid-base abnormalities induced by, 159*t*
serum toxicology assays available for,
163*t*
Saudi Arabia, organ procurement
organization for, 101*t*
Scandiatransplant, 100*t*
SCCM. *See* Society of Critical Care
Medicine
SCCM/AAP guidelines, 53–56, 54*f*, 54*t*
serologies, evaluation/management
forms with, 135
severe acute respiratory syndrome,
organ donation contraindicated
by, 108*t*
shaken baby syndrome, 196–98
epidemiologic study on, 196
pathologic examination for, 198
subarachnoid hemorrhage with, 197*f*
subdural hematomas with, 197*f*
Shinto, beliefs about brain death in, 74, 76*f*
sinus bradycardia, 216*f*
sinus tachycardia, 216*f*
Slovak, organ procurement organization
for, 101*t*
Slovenia, organ procurement organization
for, 101*t*
Smith v. Methodist Hosp.
of Indiana, 207*t*
Society of Critical Care Medicine (SCCM),
53–56, 54*f*, 54*t*
death determination guidelines of, 151
somatic integration argument, 89
somatosensory evoked potentials (SSEP),
47*t*, 52–53
pitfalls with, 169*t*
Spain, organ procurement organization for,
99, 101*t*
sperm retrieval, 211–12, 212*t*
spinal reflex interpreting, 174–76, 175*t*
SSEP. *See* somatosensory evoked potentials
Strachan v. John F. Kennedy Memorial
Hosp., 206*t*

strychnine, acid-base abnormalities
induced by, 159*t*
Sweden, organ procurement organization
for, 101*t*
Switzerland, organ procurement
organization for, 101*t*
systemic inflammatory response, 113

Taiwan, organ procurement
organization for, 101*t*
TCD. *See* transcranial Doppler
theophylline, serum toxicology assays
available for, 163*t*
thiopental, half-life of, 36*t*
thyroid function, 115
toluene, acid-base abnormalities induced
by, 159*t*
tonic neck reflexes, 175*t*
torsade de pointes, 216*f*
total brain failure, 84, 84*t*
total brain infarction, 84*t*
transcranial Doppler (TCD), 47–48, 47*t*,
51–52
pitfalls with, 169*t*
transferrin, serum toxicology assays
available for, 163*t*
transplantation
controversy with brain death and, 86
early, 81–82
Eurotransplant, 100*t*
graft rejection with, 113
heart, 82
Japan system for, 75
Scandiatransplant, 100*t*
Trinidad and Tobago, organ procurement
organization for, 101*t*
tuberculosis
organ donation contraindicated
by, 108*t*
prisoner organ donors with, 218
Turkey, organ procurement organization
for, 101*t*

UAGA. *See* Uniform Anatomical Gift Act
UDDA. *See* Uniform Determination of
Death Act
Ukraine, organ procurement organization
for, 101*t*
Uniform Anatomical Gift Act (UAGA),
58–59

Uniform Determination of Death Act
(UDDA), 57–58, 57*t*, 150
death defined for, 83
unilateral extension-pronation reflex, 175*t*
United Kingdom
neurologic criteria in, 13–15, 14*f*, 14*t*, 15*f*
organ procurement organization for, 101*t*
United Kingdom criteria, 14–15, 14*t*
United Network of Organ Sharing
(UNOS), 72, 97
codes for donor management record, 129
imminent neurologic death for, 97
United States
neurologic criteria in, 4, 6–8, 15–20
organ procurement organization for,
101, 101*t*
UNOS. *See* United Network of Organ
Sharing
Uruguay, organ procurement organization
for, 101*t*

valproic acid, serum toxicology assays
available for, 163*t*
varicella zoster, organ donation
contraindicated by, 108*t*
vasopressin, brain death procurement
with, 122*t*
vecuronium
half-life of, 36*t*
hypothermia and clearance change
with, 188*t*
Venezuela, organ procurement
organization for, 101*t*
ventilator autocycling, 177–78, 178*t*
ventricular tachycardia, 216*f*
viral encephalitis, organ donation
contraindicated by, 108*t*
Virginia, brain death examiners
in, 58*t*
Virk v. Detroit Receiving Hosp. and Univ.
Health Ctr., 206*t*